to George and Dolly Mangun
with love and best wishes
Joanne Dobbs

10/13/13

"Written by his wife, Joanne, with skill, sensitivity, and honesty, *The Life of Charles W. Denko* takes you on an inspiring lifelong journey of learning that reflects Chuck's humility, his intellect, and his compassion, and demonstrates how he turned every difficulty into opportunity. It was a joy to watch a man of great intelligence who was also truly humble and concerned about those around him. Chuck Denko was a valued friend, and Geneva College is honored to have his name on its Science Center."

— Charles N. O'Data, Vice President Emeritus, Geneva College, Beaver Falls, Pennsylvania

Earlier Books

The Psychiatric Aspects of Idiopathic Hypoparathyroidism: Case Report and Survey of the World Literature (under Joanne D. Denko, M.D. and Rudolf Kaelbling, M.D.)

Through the Keyhole at Gifted Men and Women: A Study of 159 Members of the Mensa Society (under Joanne D. Denko, M.D.)

A Handful of Ashes: One Mother's Tragedy (under Victoria C. G. Greenleaf, M. D.)

Fighting the Good Fight: One Family's Struggle Against Adolescent Alcoholism (under Victoria C.G. Greenleaf, M. D.)

Into a Mirror and Through a Lens: Forty Poems on the Mother/ Child Relationship from Conception to Marriage (under Victoria C.G. Greenleaf, M. D.)

Interlink: and Other Nature/Humankind Poems (under Victoria C.G. Greenleaf, M. D.)

Envy: A Survey of Its Psychology and History (under Victoria C.G. Greenleaf, M. D.)

The Life of
Charles W. Denko, Ph.D., M.D.

Joanne D. Denko, M.D., M.S.

Cypress House

The Life of Charles W. Denko, Ph.D., M.D.

Cypress House
155 Cypress Street
Fort Bragg, CA 95437
(800) 773-7782

www.cypresshouse.com

Cover and book design by Mike Brechner/Cypress House
Cover Photograph by Bachrach Photographers, Holliston, Mass.

Publisher's Cataloging-in-Publication data

Denko, Joanne Decker, 1927-
The Life of Charles W. Denko, Ph.D., M.D. / Joanne D. Denko, M.D., M.S.
p. cm.
Includes bibliographical references.
ISBN 978-1-879384-91-0

1. Denko, Charles W., 1916 - 2005. 2. Denko, Charles W., 1916 - 2005 --Family. 3. Poliomyelitis --Patients --United States --Biography. 4. Physicians -- United States --Biography. 5. Rheumatologists --United States --Biography. 6. Russian Americans --Biography. I. Title.
R154 .D46 2012
610/.92 --dc23 2012931901

First edition

Printed in the USA

2 4 6 8 9 7 5 3 1

Dedication

To the memory of Chuck's parents, Wasil and Evdokiya,
and teachers, particularly A. K. Anderson, Ph.D.,
Chuck's mentor and friend, who encouraged his education,
and to Charles J. Malemud, Ph.D., his colleague and friend,
who supported him in his life work,
This book is lovingly dedicated.

Joanne D. Denko
2012

CONTENTS

Foreword

Back in the 1970s and '80s, Chuck and Joanne Denko would sometimes generously invite me to a concert or an astronomy event. I appreciated these invitations more than I can say. They warmed. They illuminated. And sometimes on these outings, it was my role to offer an arm to Chuck to steady him where the way was dark, steep, or uncertain.

One such night was the occasion of Johann Sebastian Bach's 300th birthday — a showcase of the birthday boy's greatest hits to be rendered with almost rabid enthusiasm on a cathedral organ.

The steps up to the main doors of the ersatz Gothic structure did *not* spill leisurely onto the sidewalk, but had been short-spaced by some penny-pinching committee of long ago. Thus the risers were higher than the steps. *Nasty.*

Nevertheless, Chuck and I assaulted the steps like mountaineers, neither of us wanting to grunt and strain — nor, Lord forbid, gasp. I could sense the heaviness and effort of Chuck's disadvantaged side, the leg fashioned by his childhood polio. *Yet his other side was a revelation!* Light! Light as a Bachian fugue! Obviously, Chuck could have been a dancer. Indeed *was* one — as far as that could be accomplished.

Some months later it was my pleasure, once again, to offer an arm. It was a cold winter's night, and what lay before us was a challenging field of corn stubble that reared upward in the darkness to the brow of a ridge. Silhouetted against the sky was a line of large telescopes and enormous binoculars mounted on tripods. Vague figures dodged between and around the instruments. Magic was in the air — *tonight a comet was visible!*

Chuck and I entered the cornfield, then hesitated. Clumpy furrows with tough stalks formed a nightmare staircase that became a tangle of spikes at the top. In the darkness, it was going to be a struggle. We plunged forward. Up we went. Up. Stepping over. Stepping around. Pausing. Waggling. Tipping. Stepping back. Stumbling to avoid a hole. Teetering again. It was a tough puzzle.

After several minutes, our eyes adjusted, and we were climbing with confidence, even a hint of ease. Chuck was so focused on reaching the top of the ridge, I swear nothing short of a landslide could have stopped him.

Now, years later, it strikes me that the treacherous cornfield furrows, each more tricky and ankle-turning than the one below, paralleled the challenges of Chuck's life — a metaphor, if you will, of all that could have stood in his way but had not. *Tonight a comet was visible!* The moment was now. The adventure was on. Soon another gem would have been lived — the numbing cold and aching legs forgotten.

As so now I wonder... who *really* offered an arm?

— *Charmaine Severson*

Preface

On Valentine's Day, 2000, my late husband Chuck and I welcomed Kristina Joanna Thomas, our first of six grandchildren. Already in my early seventies and he in his early eighties, we realized that we were unlikely to see them into adulthood or even their teen years. Nevertheless I wanted to make them familiar with their lineage, or at least leave for them the possibility of this knowledge when they would be of an age to delve into it. This would need to be accomplished before the passing of my entire generation, with the loss of such memories with us and our children. I pondered how to implement this project.

I conceived of a collection of vignettes written by all living ancestors (and some in collateral lines) about their lives and times. I had a number of ideas for this kind of vignette about my own life and those of my parents (I had no siblings), cousins, aunts and uncles, and grandparents. I even remembered one uncle, Orson Fall, who had fought in the renowned trenches of World War I, and I had a story about one grandfather coming to Ellis Island. Over the many years of our marriage, I had heard reminiscences from my husband about his life before we met in medical school, and I visualized his anecdotes in similar format. I imagined the same kinds of stories from my grandchildren's mothers and maternal relatives (our three children being boys), but I knew only superficially the families of my daughters-in-law, living states away, unlike in former times when most people married within their own community, and therefore I did not know what they might contribute. I could conceptualize all these vignettes brought together in a book like a mosaic, which would be available for all the grandchildren and their cousins in later years. Unless I preserved those stories in hard copy, they would all be lost shortly after our children no longer remembered them. I could picture a book in hardcover, being kept and opened by at least some of the six. It would be like a Denko time capsule.

Clearly, time was not on my side. I would have to begin immediately harvesting such memories from everyone able and willing to make the effort necessary to crystallize them into written words.

I began by explaining my project to my husband Charles (Chuck), to our sons and their wives, to my brother- and sisters-in-law, and to my remaining cousins, and by requesting their help.

"Oh, you mean genealogy," was the usual response.

Correcting that idea, I would explain, "No, not the diagrammatic branching family trees with nothing but marriages and children, although the family tree will be the framework on which these memories are hung. Ours will go back only as far as living memory. What I am looking for are interesting and/or typical or atypical facets or events or work of each person's life and times. I recall, for example, my mother's stories about her nurse's training in Bronson Methodist Hospital in Kalamazoo, Michigan, and my father's World War I experience, being 4F because of severe myopia, and hence not army material. Therefore he got a job in the Quartermaster General's office in Washington, and lived with his cousin in a tent overlooking the Potomac. He must have been good at quartermastering because he always got the rock-bottom price for everything."

Sometimes I would have heard of a suitable topic from someone's life or ancestor's and suggest it for a vignette. I had heard a story about an ancestor on a collateral line of Kathy Venditto, Timothey's mother-in-law. In a time of terrible famine, her great-uncle at some remove, a wholesaler in Sicily, threw open the doors of his warehouse full of olives, olive oil, and cheeses to the starving populace. In recognition the king knighted him and gave him a coat of arms. For several years I have been asking for a vignette of that story, from Patricia's mother or someone else closer to the source, without results.

Often, even with my own cousins, I had no way to know the more telling features from their past. I never knew, for example, how much my cousin Leroy's summer vacations with me in Higman Park had meant to him until I received his contribution.

As their reports funneled in, I received stories about such things as how Annette Hudson, my son Nicholas's mother-in-law, treasured her Polish Christmas traditions, what life was like for students in my husband Chuck's high school during the Depression, what my son Nicholas and his wife Karen had to go through to adopt little Louis Alexandar and Jackson Gilberto in Ukraine and Guatemala respectively, what my cousin Eunice was doing the day Japan bombed Pearl Harbor and got us into World War II, and what it was like during the mid-twentieth century for Kristina Thomas's great-uncle to serve as a Catholic parish priest in towns in the South.

Still, I did not anticipate the reluctance of many relatives to put pencil to paper, and I was not prepared for the dearth of contributions I would receive from those one or more generations above our granchildren. With the exception of the Hudsons (Nicholas's wife's family), the great preponderance of my collection is about — and has been written by — those with the surname "Denko", including my late husband, our three sons, and myself. The vignettes I have are valuable but skew my results. My hope and plan were for a balanced collection, but you work with what you have.

At the end of the twentieth century, already in his eighties,

Chuck was diagnosed with Parkinson's disease. As it worked its inexorable course, he nevertheless struggled to finish his own life work (with the help of his colleague, former student, and friend, Charles Malemud, who generously contributed time and effort to get Chuck's data into publishable form and published), and to continue his marriage-long pattern of helping me with my projects, specifically in this case by working on vignettes.

As his cruel disease progressed, I was able to keep Chuck at home, with the help of a series of "home health aides", although the last, Valerij Onipko, a physician trained in Ukraine, was much more than that, more like a nephew.

As Chuck's condition deteriorated, one of the Parkinsonian symptoms he suffered was difficulty writing, and with it deterioration of his formerly excellent penmanship. Hence I needed to decipher some of his script from my knowledge of his life. Also, for him the act of writing itself became more laborious; he would need to put down ideas as they came to him, and I would have to rearrange them into chronological and logical sequence by transposing sentences. Nevertheless the memories and wording are his. When I had heard additional explanatory material, I have inserted it in parentheses over my initials, or in endnotes.

The vignettes Chuck wrote for this project have included recollections, both those that he has shared with me during our long married life together and others that occurred to him as germane to my project. As a result of his input, my complete collection has become even more unbalanced, this time in the Charles W. Denko direction.

As I worked with my material, I came to realize that Chuck's contribution overshadows the rest and warrants its own hardcover. Unlike other academics and scientists, whose lives are interesting to live but less so to read about, Chuck did many fascinating things outside the lab, including his assignments when he was sent by the army to work in the Occupation. It is of value to examine what he has done by seizing a variety of seemingly disconnected opportunities and ideas and bringing them together. Therefore I began separating out his portion, along with his ancestral material, and leaving my history, the Hudson material, and the rest for a second book, companion to the first. Thus all the family history I have collected will be available for the grandchildren, as originally planned, but in two books, the biography of their grandfather and the companion book of the other ancestors. As I worked with Chuck's material, I realized that perhaps his story might have a wider appeal, as inspiration to the young and others who have never met him, possibly for use in schools. It is also of interest because of his travel, not only work-related but travel related to the manmade and natural wonders of the world.

In the late nineteenth century, Horatio Alger wrote "rags-to-riches" stories, narrating how a pencil sharpener could rise to industrial giant through frugality and hard work. Similarly, Chuck's biography is the story of a man born in poverty, unable to speak English, and with a severe handicap, who became a medical research scientist respected in his specialty throughout the Western world. His was a "scientific Horatio Alger" story and has lessons for us all.

My reaction, and that of most people assessing his life, is to find it a constructive and balanced life, contributing a rich legacy. He followed his own advice: "Work at something you enjoy, and love it."

Joanne D. Denko
2011

Acknowledgments

To Tom Pasko I am indebted for suggestions regarding the organization of this atypical biography.

I am grateful to Mary Anne Kehr for her painstaking proofreading and collection of repetitions that needed to be addressed.

I appreciate Kelly Patterson's secretarial skills and her help with my intractable computer.

Finally, as always, I acknowledge the help and advice of Joe Shaw, copyeditor and advisor for this and former books.

JDD

Charles Denko's Lineage

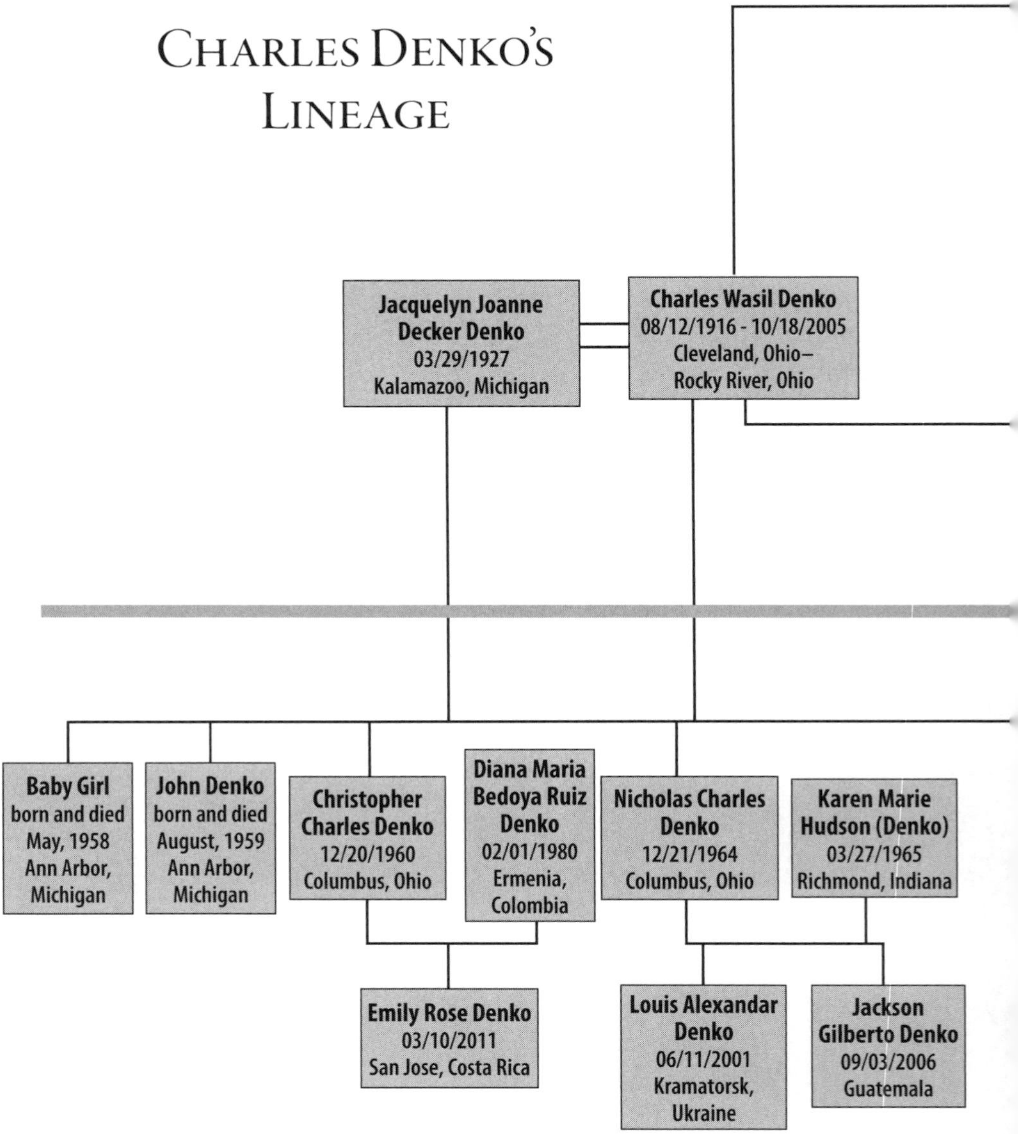

Jacquelyn Joanne Decker Denko
03/29/1927
Kalamazoo, Michigan
Charles Wasil Denko
08/12/1916 - 10/18/2005
Cleveland, Ohio–Rocky River, Ohio
Baby Girl
born and died May, 1958
Ann Arbor, Michigan
John Denko
born and died August, 1959
Ann Arbor, Michigan
Christopher Charles Denko
12/20/1960
Columbus, Ohio
Diana Maria Bedoya Ruiz Denko
02/01/1980
Ermenia, Colombia
Nicholas Charles Denko
12/21/1964
Columbus, Ohio
Karen Marie Hudson (Denko)
03/27/1965
Richmond, Indiana
Emily Rose Denko
03/10/2011
San Jose, Costa Rica
Louis Alexandar Denko
06/11/2001
Kramatorsk, Ukraine
Jackson Gilberto Denko
09/03/2006
Guatemala

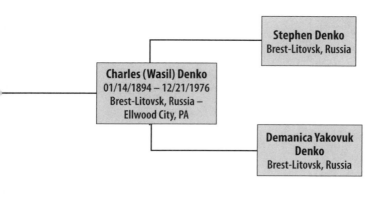

Stephen Denko
Brest-Litovsk, Russia

Charles (Wasil) Denko
01/14/1894 – 12/21/1976
Brest-Litovsk, Russia –
Ellwood City, PA

Demanica Yakovuk Denko
Brest-Litovsk, Russia

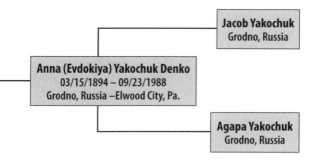

Jacob Yakochuk
Grodno, Russia

Anna (Evdokiya) Yakochuk Denko
03/15/1894 – 09/23/1988
Grodno, Russia –Elwood City, Pa.

Agapa Yakochuk
Grodno, Russia

Lisa Claire Thomas
03/24/1965
Scranton, Pennsylvania

Timothey Charles Denko
07/28/1966
Columbus, Ohio

Patricia Arlene Venditto Denko
08/12/1962
New Castle, Pennsylvania

Kristine Joanna Thomas
02/14/2000
Scranton, Pennsylvania

Madeleine Grace Denko
05/09/2001
Pittsburgh, Pennsylvania

Charles Michael Denko
11/26/2003
Pittsburgh, Pennsylvania

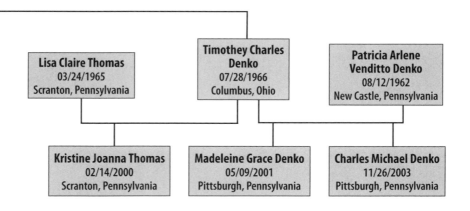

Timeline

1916
Born August 12 in Cleveland, Ohio, to Evdokiya Yakochuk Denko and Charles Wasil Denko.

1917
Suffered polio, producing shortening of left leg.
Family moved to Ellwood City, Pennsylvania.

1922
Walked with extreme difficulty; spoke only "peasant" Russian.
Entered first grade and teacher brought him up to speed in "perfect" English.

1922–1934
Educated in public schools of Ellwood City, Pennsylvania.
Teachers, townspeople, and priest reached out to educate and acculturate.

1924 or 1925
Shriners extended care (surgery and physical therapy) to greatly improve his gait and make normal life possible.

1934
Graduated from Ellwood City High School; valedictorian.
Won countywide competitive examination for Pennsylvania scholarship.

1934–1938
Studied at Geneva College, working for room and board.
Earned his B.S with highest honors.

1938–1943
Attended Pennsylvania State University, earning an M.S. in organic chemistry and a Ph.D. in physiologic chemistry.

1943
Taught in summer school at West Virginia University, Morgantown.

1944–1945
Worked as research chemist (SMA Research Laboratories), Wyeth Institute of Applied Biochemistry, Chagrin Falls, Ohio.

1945–1947
U.S. Army (Captain) Nutrition Officer, Biochemist, Microbiologist, Sanitary Corps, U.S. and E.T.O.

1947–1951
Johns Hopkins University School of Medicine, M.D.

1950
Married Jacquelyn Joanne Decker of Benton Harbor, Michigan.

1951–1952
Research and Education Hospitals, University of Illinois, in Chicago, Rotating Intern.

1952–1956
University of Chicago, Senior Assistant Resident, Postdoctoral Fellow; Research Associate (Instructor) Argonne Cancer Research Hospital.

1956–1959
University of Michigan; Instructor, Assistant Professor of Internal Medicine.

1959–1968
Ohio State University; Assistant Professor of Medicine.

1960
Birth of Christopher Charles Denko.

1964
Birth of Nicholas Charles Denko.

1966
Birth of Timothey Charles Denko.

1968–1987
Scott Research Laboratory, Fairview General Hospital, Cleveland; Director.

1968–2005
Case Western Reserve University, Cleveland, Ohio; Associate Professor of Medicine.

1974–1975
Australian National University, Canberra, A.C.T., Sabbatical.

1990
Second place for his life's work in rheumatology in the Carol Nachman Prize in Rheumatology.

1993
Member of American Chemical Society for fifty years.

2004
Longest of the over-fifty-year Ph.D.s at Pennsylvania State, recognition.

2005
Died at home. Buried in Locust Grove Cemetery, Ellwood City, Pennsylvania.

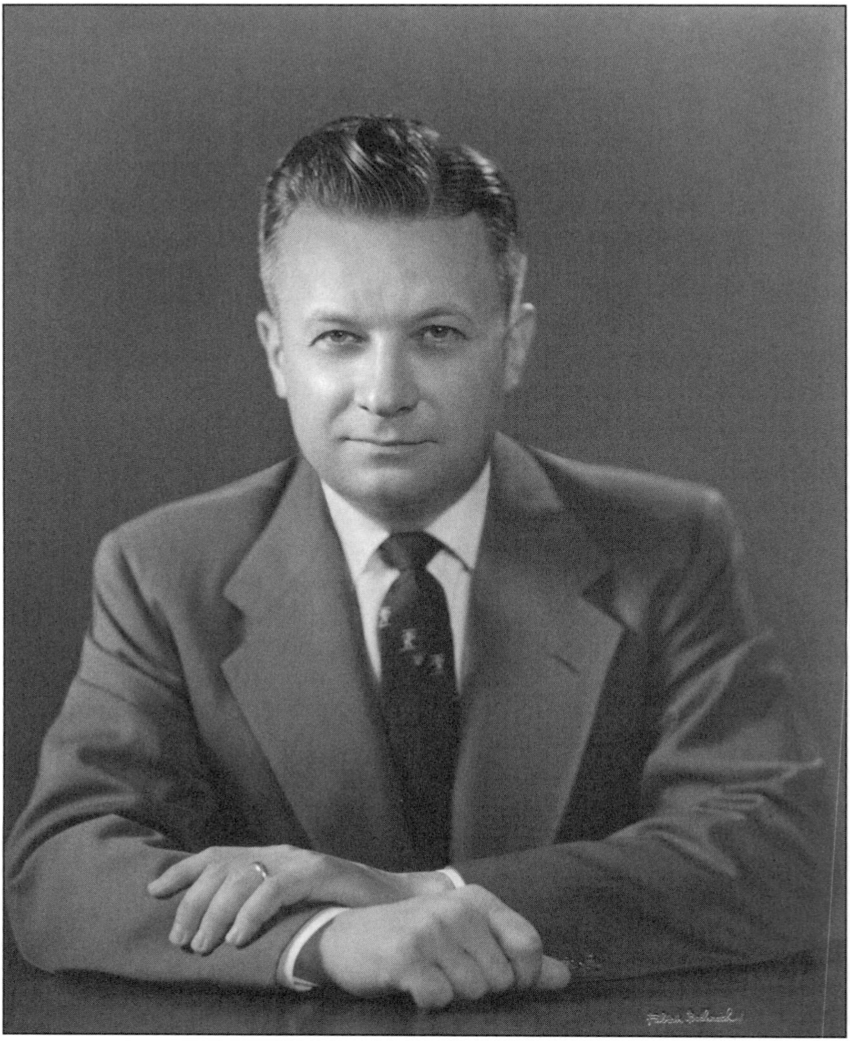

The Life of Charles W. Denko

Chemist and Physician

Scientist and Researcher

Teacher and Lecturer

Son and Brother

Husband and Father

Grandfather

Antecedents

Chapter I

Antecedents

By the strange workings of fate, Charles W. Denko began (8/12/1916) and ended (10/18/2005) his life in Cleveland, Ohio, with several other addresses, schools, laboratories, practices, professorships, lectureships, and a sabbatical in between.

As a birthplace, Cleveland was determined by the trajectory of two young immigrants from Byelorussia (now Belarus), Wasil and Evdokiya, who came, like millions of others seeking a better life, specifically to a city needing laborers in the steel mills and already an enclave of Eastern European immigrants. From the same village back "home", they met and married (see their wedding picture) in their new home, and Charles was their first child, baptized in St. Theodosius Cathedral, with its magnificent chandelier, a gift from the czar. Soon Wasil, a steel worker with brawn and a highly intelligent problem solver, investigated other steel towns, looking for the smallest because Evdokiya did not like loud, bustling, dirty Cleveland. Hence Charles grew up in Ellwood City, Pensylvania.

We turn now to his accounts.

JDD

Family History of the Denko (Denyko) Family

At the western end of the map of the former Soviet Union, almost at the border of Poland, in the smallest type and near the large city of Brest,[1] is the town of Kobrin. The former USSR, then the largest country in the world by area, is now divided into fifteen countries, including Belarus. In those days Byelorussia, meaning "White Russia", was a province of Russia.

Two explanations are given for this designation. One is that it is derived from the people, who carried an admixture of Swedish blood from the blond Swedes, who invaded down the Bug River (pronounced "Boog"), the border with Poland, said to be a mile wide and a foot deep, a source of fish to augment the food supply. An alternative theory holds that "White Russia" comes from the traditional dress, consisting of a white shirt or tunic with red trim.

In the 15th or 16th century, envoys came from the court of Moscow to invite the region of White Russia to become part of Greater Russia. Inhabitants in white tunics greeted them, and, as was the custom, scattered salt and bread as symbols of welcome. They subsequently accepted the offer.

Early in the 20th century, from the town of Kobrin came emigrants looking for opportunity in the New World.

A young man of nineteen, Vassily (Wasil) Denyko arrived in New York in April 1912. Vassily had watched nautical history in the making when the *Carpathia,* the ship on which he traveled in steerage, went to the aid of survivors of the *Titanic,* hauling them from the icy waters onto the deck of the *Carpathia,* making the European emigrants give up their beds to the survivors in shock, and sleep on the deck for the remainder of the voyage.

After landing in New York, where the immigration officer

highhandedly changed the name Vassily to Charles and shortened Denyko to Denko, Vassily gradually worked his way to Cleveland via short farm jobs in New York State. With his powerful muscles, he found work in the booming steel industry that soon supplied the raw material for ordnance for World War I.

In 1914 a teenaged orphan girl, Evdokiya Yakochuk, unable to speak or read English, traveled alone across the Atlantic and by train directly to Cleveland, with a job waiting as a domestic.

The two met, married, and started a family. Their eldest, Charles Wasil Denko, at age one, suffered a bout of polio, which left him with a shortened left leg and a very difficult walk. Vassily's hopes to attend night school came to nothing because of his added responsibilities with his growing family.

CWD

Note

All notes are by Joanne D. Denko. Contributions by others are over their initials or signatures.

1. Formerly Brest-Litovsk.

My Two Grandfathers

My grandfathers lived in neighboring villages of Kobrin and environs in Byelorussia. I have forgotten which grandfather went with which offspring, but no matter since they both had similar lives except that my maternal grandfather was really my mother's uncle since she was sent to live and work with him when she was orphaned at about ten.

My father's father had three sons and several daughters. The girls were expected to marry, but the farm would not support three sons. Therefore it was decided that the eldest would remain on the land. Of the other two, one joined the army and was killed in service. My father had the best deal, in that the family scraped together money to send him to the Land of Opportunity in 1912.[1]

The grandfathers' winter occupations set them somewhat apart.[2] One man carved wooden spoons and related kitchen items. The other grandfather repaired shoes and boots during the long cold winters. Once, when I complained about a fall snow in my hometown in Western Pennsylvania, my father pointed out that I should consider myself lucky. "When I was your age, I had to chase the cows in my bare feet," he pointed out.[3]

Neither grandfather survived World War I. Since the relatives lived near the German border, occasional mail would get through. A letter arrived for my father years ago. It was from Canada, not from a relative, but from an acquaintance who emigrated from Byelorussia. In Canada, he had learned the trade of electrician and found work in construction. His family was well. My father invited him to visit, even offering to pay expenses, but he did not wish to travel as far as Pennsylvania. Our parents had no car and no desire to leave on a long trip to Alberta.[4]

Thus we lost track of this tie to the "old country".[5]

CWD

Notes

1. See my poem "One Family's Homecoming" in *Into a Mirror and Through a Lens.*

2. CWD thought it too obvious to mention that in summer they both worked on farms to grow food for people and animals for the long winter.

3. He was referring to the fact that the only way they had to warm the animals in winter was to run them. This was not limited to Russia. I recall reading in one of Laura Ingalls Wilder's books,

Farmer Boy, about her husband's childhood in upstate New York, that they ran the animals the same way in winter. That family grew or made everything they needed, including straw hats, except the new stove.

4. One long trip across the Atlantic was enough to last a lifetime.
5. Years later, when Chuck and I drove across Canada, we visited a provincial park in which was preserved a small house that had been the home of immigrants from the former Soviet Union. Hooks on the walls were for hanging up clothes. The house even featured the kind of stove on the flat top of which family members could sleep for warmth. The western plains of Canada attracted those immigrants, being similar to the steppes of Russia, with fertile soil for farming.

Denko Relatives in Russia

After World War II my father received a letter from a relative back in Byelorussia. She related that when the Germans came, they herded the villagers into a barn and then set it afire. She escaped only because she had been visiting that day in a neighboring village.[1]

CWD

Note

1. Years later, at the Cleveland Cinemateque, Chuck and I saw a Russian film under the translated title *Come and See,* directed by Elen Klimov. This film dealt with the same phenomenon Chuck's relatives had experienced, and the historic note at the end related that more than 600 villages had suffered this fate at the hands of the invading Germans. Since the inhabitants

were obviously noncombatants, the strategy was evidently to get agricultural workers out of production to create food shortages. We found it remarkable that although the Jewish Holocaust receives (deserved) attention for the six million Jews who perished, neither the Russian war casualties, including civilian deaths in large cities like Leningrad and in villages like Chuck's relatives', nor the Stalin-inflicted deaths, such as starvation in the Ukraine in the 1930s, and deportation to the Gulag of political prisoners, are publicized, at least not to the extent that the Jewish Holocaust is legitimately kept fresh in our minds.

My Father's Last Letter From Home

Shortly after the end of World War II, my father received a letter from his sister who was living in a village back home. The letter was posted from Dobrenichin, Byelorussia, near a collective farm about fifty miles east of Brest. With the letter was a snapshot showing several women, two elderly, three or four younger, and one young male, probably a teenager. In her letter the sister explained that this was a family portrait including all of the remaining Denyko/Denko family. No one else was left. She further imputed the fact that there were no other males in the Denyko/Denko line due to the devastation of the war. Only two women survived at collective farms. The writer was satisfied with food and housing. She felt well cared for. She was content.[1]

CWD

Note

1. Did she have to fear censorship? Is being "satisfied with food and housing... well cared for... content" what they really

want from government? A nanny state? When Chuck and I traveled in Russia we observed, on the streets, many women in pairs and groups and only an occasional man, often an elderly veteran with war decorations on his civilian clothes. The war produced an entire generation of women with little opportunity for marriage.

Recollections of My Father

He was known as "Big Charlie" and I as "Little Charlie" on those relatively rare occasions when we were working together. My father was a great hulk of a man weighing about 200 pounds, while I was a high school student, eager to work but without the avoirdupois of a career manual laborer. He considered my amateurish efforts worthwhile but hardly on his level. With my bad leg, I would not, of course, work where he earned his living, in the steel mill, although it had been my mother's ambition and dream to pack two "buckets", one for my father and one for me to take to work in the factory together. Sometimes we would go together to help with farm work on the farm of a friend of "Big Charlie's" from the Old Country. My father believed in honest work.

Wasil, as he was called in the family, with the equivalent of a third grade education in Russia, was a highly intelligent man and a talented problem solver. When my mother was unhappy living in big, bustling, noisy Cleveland, having come from a small village, my father inquired where he could find the smallest town with a steel mill (where he knew he would be a welcome worker with his brawn), and that was how the family grew up in Ellwood City, Pennsylvania.[1] We were close enough to the woods that he could take us kids out mushroom hunting, as they had done in Russia and do to this day. Nearby woods furnished a bit of nut harvest.

My father served in many ways like a social worker, helping newcomers without knowledge of the language or culture find work and get established without allowing the locals to take advantage of the "greenhorns". He would let such men sleep on an old couch in the basement and shovel coal into the furnace to keep the house warm overnight, or help in the garden where he raised much of our food, or do odd jobs painting around the house, which he had the foresight to build on an alley to try to avoid the dust of the unpaved but much busier street — an alley just five minutes' walk from his job at the mill.[2] Wasil was pleased to be able to get to work on time if he left home at the first whistle.[3]

He was the Ann Landers of the newly arrived immigrants. One friend wanted to get married, so he asked my father for advice on judging a young lady who had caught his eye. "Take her out for dinner and see how much she eats" was Wasil's sage advice.

To the young man's delight, "She just picked at her food," he reported.

"Then she should be an economical wife," Wasil reassured his friend.

But after the wedding he learned that she was on to that trick and had eaten before the date so as to give the impression of being a light eater.[4]

Many years later, when I had already completed my doctorate in chemistry and was partway through medical school, I came home on a school vacation. Wasil met me at the door waving an official-looking letter from the city. Glancing at it quickly, I saw that it pertained to property he had bought in the country and contained several legalistic phrases, which I did not want to try to interpret. I told him he should either go to the union office or ask my lawyer friend for the explanation.

"How many years have you been going to school?" he asked.

Not anticipating what was coming, I quickly added up twelve through high school, four more of college, and yet another four of graduate school. "Twenty," I told him.

"Twenty years?" he repeated. "In Russia if we sent a horse to school twenty years, he'd know an answer to that." My father could be sarcastic.[5]

We went through the Depression, and part of the time my father had only part-time work. He knew about economies — ends of lunchmeat at reduced price. I was in college before I knew that cookies came round and unbroken. He would take me shopping with my little wagon to bring home the food for our growing family.[6]

Knowing that he enjoyed an advantage with his muscle mass, he would help other workers at the steel mill lest they fall behind, explaining "That skinny Italian also has a family to feed."[7]

CWD

Notes

1. Noted for its "tube mill", where seamless tubes were made by piercing a solid cylinder of steel.

2. That house built on an alley was another thing that astonished me, both when I heard about it and when we pulled in on my first visit to meet the family.

3. Judging intelligence by these kinds of creative and novel ways to work toward goals, Wasil was clearly highly intelligent. Now we sometimes call this "thinking outside the box".

4. Wasil hadn't learned that handling food in the kitchen doesn't tell the whole tale about economy. After I had been taken to meet the family, he told Chuck that I should be an economical wife because I put away small helpings of leftovers into the fridge, amounts his sisters would have thrown away. It had taken him many years to realize that the reason his food came in little portions was that the women gave him the leftovers to finish them up. This he approved. True, I

was saving with food, but later, when we were planning to marry and he found out that I had in mind a trip to Europe, he advised against it: "Don't go. The roads are bad, and the plumbing is terrible." He didn't realize that we weren't going for roads or plumbing.

5. I must add that from the question and its timing, my innocent and unsuspecting husband-to-be should have expected something like this.

6. Unlike many men, Wasil delayed smoking until the children were self-sufficient. He was always happy when Chuck, having had lunch with his friend Tkach, White House physician, would bring him a cigar with the White House logo on it.

7. The story by Chuck's sisters was that this family fed the meat, which was in short supply in the Depression, to the father so he could keep up at the mill, even with Wasil's help. The children did well despite their lower protein diet. A brother who became a teacher wrote and published a family history praising the mother.

The Inspector General

George Muller, husband of Chuck's sister Helen, once told us about an experience he had with Wasil when the two were in what sounded like a crossroads general store.

Wasil, with his imposing height and his usual air of self-assurance, would stroll around, take an item off the shelf, inspect it, replace it, and repeat this behavior with other items. George said that the shopkeeper began to get nervous, and he, George, began to get embarrassed.

Hearing the story, I was reminded of a novella by Gogol, *The Inspector General,* about a government official expected in a provincial town. When a stranger arrives, he is assumed to be the inspector, and everyone attempts to hide everything corrupt that he has been up to, and also to wine, dine, and bribe the stranger. This has been made into the most hilarious movie I have ever seen, *The Inspector General,* starring Danny Kaye.

It sounds as though the shopkeeper was similarly afraid that Wasil was some kind of official who had come on government business and might find out his shady or illegal secrets.

My Mother's Story

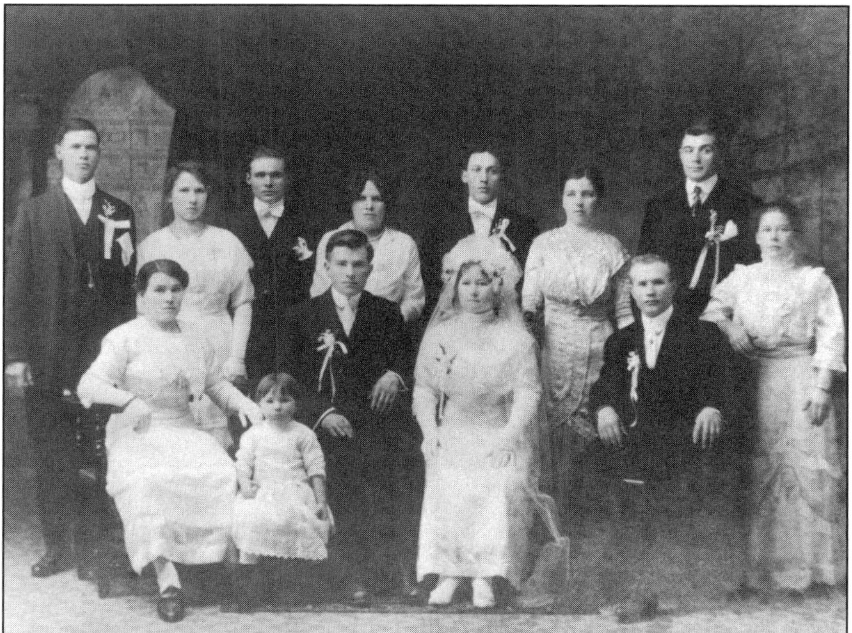

Wasil and Evdokiya's wedding picture.

My mother, Evdokiya, was an orphan girl in Byelorussia. After the death of her mother, she was sent to live with an uncle and worked in her late teens for a neighbor on a farm. The Orthodox priest helped guide her, and arranged for her to emigrate to the "Land of Opportunity", and the city of Cleveland, with a large Russian population. Evdokiya's farmer/employer was good to her, and sold a cow to raise money for the ocean passage to Baltimore and a railroad ticket to Cleveland. She was a passenger on the last ship to leave Liebau,[1] on the Baltic, in 1914 before World War I.

With contacts in Cleveland, the priest had found work for her as a maid and cook for a Jewish family with a bakery. There she learned Jewish cooking and baking.[2]

Wasil had already made his way to Cleveland, where they met and married on Hallowe'en, 1915.[3] Soon they moved to Ellwood City. Not only were the surroundings greener, but also the steel-mill pay was better.

Wasil also had a friend on a nearby farm, where they would visit, sometimes help with farm work, and have picnics.

Back to my mother: I came home one vacation from graduate school to a very quiet house.[4] After settling down, my mother said, "Chuck, I have a surprise for you. Munya, clear the table." A sheet of paper and a pen materialized. I was puzzled by this strange behavior and wondered what was happening. My mother carefully arranged the paper, took the pen, wrote something, and handed it to me. The words were "Evdokiya Denko". "Now," she said, "I can sign any papers you want, the way you told me." But she never progressed in literacy beyond these simple words.

She was always very proud of me. When I went off to graduate school, my mother, speaking in broken English with the adjective after the noun, as in several European languages, proudly told the milkman, "My boy's in the State Pen!" A few miles apart, but vastly different in significance, were Pennsylvania State University and the State Penitentiary.[5]

CWD

Notes

1. Now Liepaja, Latvia.

2. There are the usual types of stories about incoming immigrants learning the ways of this country. Soon after arrival, she ate a piece of pie (from the bakery?). When they asked how she liked it, she said she thought the crust was tough. It turned out that she had eaten the cardboard on which it came.

3. The wedding photo shows Evdokiya as a lovely young bride.

4. A sure tip-off that something was in the wind.

5. Her courage in conditions of deprivation (not reading, never fluent in English) is shown in the story of her trip (with three small children in tow according to Helen) from Western Pennsylvania to the Shriners Hospital in St. Louis. By Helen's account, when they had to change trains in Chicago, Evdokiya left Helen watching John while she went to inquire about the connection. When she returned, to her horror Helen had not been able to control John, who had wandered off. Evdokiya ran around frantically screaming, "My baby! My baby!" (probably in Russian) until he was found. At the hospital, not only did she check (were his fingernails clean?) but also learned to perform the physical therapy to help him recover and continue to improve his gait after his return home. (See the vignette about the Shriners Hospital.)

Unbreakable Dishes and Homemade Weapons

My late mother-in-law was an honest and truthful person, and it never occurred to her not to expect the same from others. Munya told me two anecdotes that illustrated this.

In the days when she was coping with a young family, peddlers were still a feature of American life. One day a peddler offered her "unbreakable dishes". In times when the children were always breaking something, this seemed like what we have come to call a "no-brainer". And so she invested.

When Munya got home, she proudly displayed her acquisition. "Look, Munya, they're unbreakable," she exclaimed as she dropped them to the floor!

She was like a mother tiger when it came to defending her children. A neighborhood girl teased and taunted Chuck over his crippled leg. First Evdokiya tried to work with the girl's mother, to no avail. Then, angry over the mother's failure to restrain the child, Evdokiya poured a panful of dirty dishwater from the second floor onto the head of the woman walking below. For this she was taken to court and had to pay a ten-dollar fine but concluded, "The satisfaction was worth ten dollars." And there were no more problems from the neighbor child.

She treated the children's minor abrasions and breaks in the skin with hydrogen peroxide, pointing to the bubbles as proof that the medication was working. Apparently she, like other contemporary mothers, prohibited scratching, lest infection set in. I surmised this when I asked Chuck to scratch between my shoulder blades where I couldn't reach, and he gently rubbed with his fingertips, tickling and making it itch all the more. I had to teach him how to scratch!

Siblings

Chapter II

Chuck's Siblings and Their Families

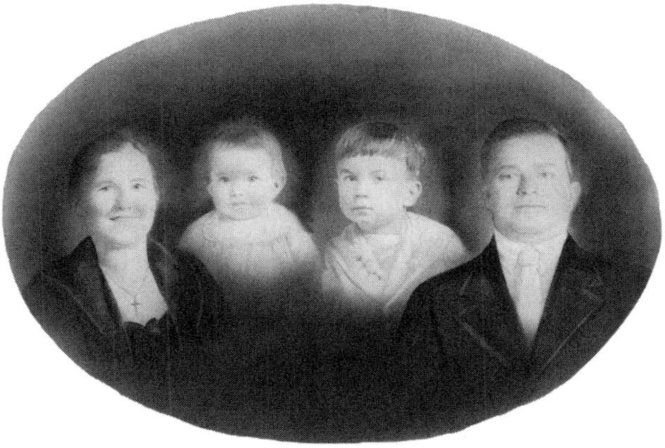

Charles's parents, Evdokiya and Wasil Denko, with Charles and baby sister Munya.

After Chuck's birth and the family's subsequent move to Ellwood City, Chuck was followed, at intervals of about two years, by Munya (Eastern European for Mary), Helen, Ivan (later Anglicized to John), and two later boys, Peter and Andrew. Andrew died in infancy. Peter was born with a congenital heart lesion at a time long before Blalock and Taussig at our institution, Johns Hopkins, developed surgical repair for many of these conditions. Peter never enjoyed a normal life, suffering frequent convulsions from diminished blood supply to the brain, causing intellectual loss and finally requiring care in an institution. Chuck and I visited him there, taking clothes, but he did not recognize his brother, and died in his early twenties.

Munya, two years younger than Chuck, married Paul Lyttle, and they had one child, Bobby. Paul was a few years older than Munya and died in his early fifties. At that time Munya came home to live at 11 Glen Avenue with her parents. (Even before her move home, just a block and a half, I noticed that rarely did a day pass without her touching base with her mother. I have never known anyone else with such a close bond to her mother.) Munya kept books for several small businessmen in the area. When I knew her, she had set up a "sandwich shop" at one entrance to the steel mill. She featured ethnic food (including borsch) and sandwiches, and the men knew which soup to expect on which day of the week. Wasil helped with heavy lifting, in bringing in supplies. Originally Helen was a partner, but sold out her interest at her husband's insistence so he could pursue his outdoor activities and buy a boat and have a cottage at Tionesta in the mountains of Western Pennsylvania. Munya carried on alone with the sandwich shop until the mill closing ended its usefulness. Munya was lucky in that her kidney cancer announced its presence by bleeding early enough that she was cured by nephrectomy. She died in her early eighties from another malignancy.

Their son, Bobby, went to Gannon College in Erie, Pennsylvania, became a specialist in clean water (clean water inspector), and supervised updating the water systems in Lima, Peru; Caracas, Venezuela; and several cities in California. He married Margaret DeFonde. She was never known by any name other than Togi, and even her mother could not cite the origin of the nickname. When the priest asked Margaret to "take this man", etc., people looked around to see whom Bobby was marrying. Nicholas and Timothey were in the wedding, as ring bearer and assistant, wearing black velvet Lord Fauntleroy suits with short pants, but they had mistakenly put on each other's jackets and we didn't notice until the photos showed Timothey's hands almost covered by sleeves, and Nicholas's sleeves a third of the way up to his elbows (see companion book's vignette on weddings and the photograph of Nicholas and Timothey in each other's jackets).

Togi worked for many years in the Sky Bank, later supervising all the tellers. Bobby and Togi also had just one child, Mary Anne. She married Timothy Anderson, and they also have one child, Dorian Kane. Timothy and his father alternate shifts running a large wholesale refrigerated-food warehouse in Ellwood City, and Mary Anne keeps their books.

Munya took over the household tasks as her mother aged. Helen also came from her home in Zelienople a day a week to help with heavy cleaning. Wasil, their father, never regained his health after being hit by a car and suffering leg injuries. Evdokiya, their mother, lived into her nineties.

One of Helen's recollections is that she had attacks of herpes simplex (cold sores) so severe that her whole lower face was swollen. She would stay home from school because of embarrassment. When she graduated from high school, everyone was pressured by the uncertainties of war. George, in boot camp in the South, asked her to visit him before he was shipped out, and, of course, persuaded her to marry him. One consideration was that as a married man his pay was increased, with the possibility of saving for the future.

Almost immediately he was sent to the "European" theatre for several years. Actually, he served in Africa against Rommel's forces and then proceeded up the spine of Italy. With his brawn he was assigned to the stevedore battalion and unloaded tons of war materiel for the men in combat. Like many returning veterans, he talked little about his war experiences, but he did tell Helen that the never-ceasing noises from the shelling were more than he could stand. The war changed his personality in the direction of increased irritability and less tolerance for stress. I believe that he probably suffered from what they then termed "combat fatigue" but that we now call "posttraumatic stress disorder"; he could have benefited from group therapy with other veterans.

He was a skilled mechanic and, home from the war, set up a car sales and service business with two friends. Whenever we went to Ellwood, we always had him do what I called a "history and physical" on our car, checking it out from nose to tail. We had always neglected it. His usual comment was something like "I don't know how that green Plymouth station wagon ever made it here." Muttering and shaking his head, he would add, "The points weren't even coming together." But he would fix it, and it took us across Canada from a meeting in Toronto to the Athabasca Glacier and back. When the frustrations of fine-tuning motors got to this perfectionistic mechanic, he developed an ulcer, eventually gave up the repair business, and went to work in a factory until heart trouble produced his disability. He had open-heart surgery in its infancy and survived three decades. He loved fishing, and once took his nephew (see Christopher's vignette "Uncle George" in companion book). Helen and George did not have any children. Just a few years older than I, as a young woman Helen had a similar "pear" body shape. When she began to put on weight, she gave me her dresses in the style that suited us both, shirtwaist, fitted blouse and full skirt, in bright printed materials.

Helen never had a full-time job. As mentioned, she worked for a time in the sandwich shop. She cared for several housebound invalids (living within walking distance). Sometimes when we traveled, she would come to care for our child or children, alternating with my mother. Although she had all the emergency phone numbers, she worried about not driving, especially when we lived in the country on Watt Road. I am surprised now that Chuck and I were not concerned about this lack of backup in case of emergency. Helen loved to tell the story about walking outdoors with little Nicholas and suggesting that he "smell the pretty flower". He stood up and backed away with a swollen nose, from a bee sting.

We shall look at Chuck's brother's life and family separately.

John V. Denko, M.D., and Family

Of the five physicians in our immediate Denko family (John, CWD, JDD, NCD, and TCD), Chuck's brother John was first.

When Chuck was courting me and telling me about his family, he kept referring to "Ivan", pronounced the same as "Yvonne", and I finally asked how *she* was a *man*. It turned out that about this time Ivan changed to the Anglicized equivalent, "John". Chuck attributed this idea to Gloria. Madeleine sent me copies of a collection of postcards and letters that Chuck had sent "Ivan" while in the service, but by the time I first met him he was going by "John". The youngest of the surviving children, John's life pattern resembled his brother's.

Like his older brother, John was soon recognized as gifted and given educational stimulation. He attended Antioch College in Yellow Springs, Ohio, one of the first colleges that offered a program of study and working alternate quarters. (Recently on the brink of closing, Antioch has now had a reprieve, at least temporary.) John's work was in the auto industry in Detroit, I believe at the Ford plant. He did further undergraduate work at Denison University in Newark, Ohio, and finally completed his B.S. at the University of Chicago, where he also earned his M.D., sent by the navy. While in Chicago, he married Gloria Sandalis, a contralto, who had taken second place in the All-Chicagoland Annual Talent Contest. Gloria had an upside-down smile. (Gloria's parents were delightful; see vignette "The Sandalises".)

After his graduation from medical school, John owed medical time, in payment of which he served in the U.S. Public Health Service. He was stationed in Seattle, where he was the public health officer for the state of Washington and the then territory of Alaska, where he handled an epidemic. As his discharge time approached, he wrote what then seemed to me an enormous number of letters (150) about where he should settle as a pathologist, and chose Amarillo, Texas, where his friend Ralph Zientek was already practicing and in need of another pathologist. Ralph died tragically at an early age, as did Del Bergenstal, another University of Chicago friend of John's, who was the same man who taught Chuck radioisotope techniques in medical research. John was active in the social life of Amarillo, and served on various boards, including the Symphony Board. He established a department for the training of pathology technicians at Canyon College. Also, he testified against a company in a successful court case concerning industrial pollution, which was held responsible for disease and death.

John and Gloria had three children. Kathy, the youngest, born in Amarillo, has spent her entire life there, active in social and cultural affairs such as ballet and a pageant about the history of the area. She married Michael Edmund McAfee, who began a career in the beef business. However, when concerns about eating too much fatty red meat affected that industry badly, he wisely took up nurse's training and became an emergency-room nurse. They had one child, Ryan Scott McAfee, who, after majoring in communications and trying several lines of work, is now studying alternative medicine.

John and Gloria's middle child, John Scott, who goes by Scott (his grandmother Fanchon Scott Sandalis's maiden name), studied both engineering and law and became a patent lawyer, finally running his own firm in Austin, Texas. He and his wife, Anne, have two sons, Alexander Landis and Jackson Landis (see John's letter of tribute to his Uncle Chuck).

John and Gloria's eldest child, Madeleine, went to Bryn Mawr and received an M.F.A. in dance at the Tisch School of the Arts at New York University. She spent several years in the publishing industry, but was always interested in dance, both ballet and modern, and now teaches dance and violin. She married late, Steve Carter, a reporter specializing in education news for

The Oregonian, Portland, Oregon's newspaper. By this marriage Madeleine acquired a stepson, Leland Nelson Carter. She is what I think of as "Denko glue", keeping in touch with the rest of us. Interested in her roots, she has traced her ancestry on her maternal grandfather Sam's side back to Greece and visited there twice, where all sixty-six of her Sandalis relatives met her at the airport. She is a freelance writer, and her account in *The Oregonian* of her and Steve's visit to Greece includes a photograph of one of the large feasts they gave to celebrate her visit. She has also been in contact by letter with the Denko survivors in Belarus, and we have discussed a trip there (Christopher also expressed interest), but even now travel in the erstwhile Soviet Union is fraught with problems and uncertainties and expectations of bribes.

After twenty-five years of marriage, John and Gloria were divorced, and Gloria continued work as entertainment editor for the two Amarillo newspapers, the *Amarillo Globe-Times* and the *Amarillo Sunday News-Globe.* Not long after remarrying, she developed a bile duct carcinoma, a rare malignancy, and died in her sixties.

A few years after the divorce, John married Susan Sheldon of the Weirton Steel family, who had three children by a former marriage to Denny Fraze, a mathematics professor. They were David (now a financial advisor), Michael (now deceased), and Wendy, married to Mauricio Aguilar (a restaurateur) with three children (Shelby Weir, Wesley, and Walker). Susan inherited money that, by the terms of the will, had to be spent for a house in California, which she built in a gated community in Rancho Santa Fe, where she and John retired. All of us have been entertained there.

I admired John for several things. I have observed that most people stop growing after they leave formal education. Not John. He pursued several interests, one of which was searching for fossil bones of camels and other prehistoric animals in the canyon north of Amarillo, where he took us on one of these explorations. He also was an inveterate photographer, and after the extended family had been together for a visit or wedding, he would send copies of many photos. With his second wife, Susan, John traveled to many parts of the world, and we would share experiences and ideas.

When Chuck had been diagnosed with Parkinson's disease, John and Susan invited him out to California, along with Timothey, Patricia, and baby Madeleine. They were good at caring for someone in decline and keeping him entertained. On another trip, when Chuck and I were both in California, John took us, among other places, to Torrey Pines State Park to see the tree for which it was named, endemic to their area. He also took us to see the century plant in bloom. He was an ideal host, knowledgeable about the interesting and unique features of his area and willing to share them.

Tragically, when John had a medical checkup, he was found to be in good health, but advised to get a colonoscopy, he did not heed this advice. A cancer of the ascending colon, diagnosable early only by colonoscopy, caused his death. I had been having sigmoidoscopies and colonoscopies, but this sad event sent the other relatives for their gastrointestinal studies.

The Sandalises

When, in the 1950s, we spent five years in Chicago for our training, the parents of Chuck's brother John's wife, Gloria, often invited us over for dinner on Sunday. (I would refer to the Sandalises as my "parents-in-law-in-law".) Gloria's mother, Fanchon, came from a farm family in Kansas, and her brother teased her that she must have been part Indian because she liked jewelry so much. She recalled how, without electricity, their "washing machine" was agitated by a handle that she and her brother pushed back and forth, standing on opposite sides. She married Sam (Seraphim) Sandalis, who had emigrated from Greece but remained in close contact with and supported his mother and four sisters, and returned whenever possible to the land of his birth to visit his many relatives. Sam and "the Missus", as he referred to his wife, for many years ran a small restaurant in downtown Chicago, literally a "Mom and Pop" restaurant, in which she was the marvelous cook. I smiled over Sam's way to evaluate a new city or town he might visit: he would look through the *Yellow Pages* to see how many Greek restaurants they had.

When they had us over on Sundays, I would bring our laundry to do in their washing machine. (Fanchon would usually do it while I fell asleep on the couch.) I can still taste her stewed chicken and gravy, over boiled potatoes, which she took out for me before mashing, to suit my preference. One Sunday Chuck and I arrived on the right day at the right hour, but the wrong week. Fanchon rose to the occasion and produced a dinner anyway, but I told Chuck to please keep out of the social arrangements, since he was the one who had messed up that time. The Sandalises had us over on the correct Sunday too, for some more delicious chicken and gravy. Once Sam told us that he sometimes became paralyzed, causing us to jerk to attention. Alarmed, we inquired further and learned that he meant that after a big meal he just couldn't keep his eyes open. Physicians need to evaluate how patients and others are using medical terms.

As happens far too often, Sam died shortly after retirement before an extended trip "home". "The Missus" survived Sam by many years, so long, in fact, that when Gloria developed a rare malignancy at a relatively early age in her sixties, Fanchon, in her nineties, was able to care for her. It is a terrible thing for an aging parent to lose an adult child to death — it turns nature on its head. But Fanchon believed that God kept her alive to be able to care for her child in her time of need.

Madeleine's Letter to Evdokiya

by Madeleine Denko-Carter

4221 SW Comus Street
Portland, Oregon 97219
May 31, 2000

Christ is risen! Christ is risen indeed! Easter 1973. It is nearly midnight outside the Russian Orthodox Cathedral in San Francisco, but inside, the church is lit by the candles held by each member of the congregation. "Christ is risen!" we exclaim again in Russian, and repeat over and over. As we breathe together the air redolent of incense and exhale as one, the candle flames flare, illuminating the darkness. I am in search of my beginnings. I want to understand my Russian soul.

Dear Grandma, the faces of the people in that church were radiant with hope as the priests, swinging incense, walked through the standing crowd, greeting all who came, making them feel welcome and at home. The smoke of the incense and the smoke from the candles rose through the church, the chants were repeated and repeated, and I felt a history I had never lived.

Evdokiya Yakochuk Denyko, in 1914 you came to the United States from Byelorussia as a teenaged girl. How brave you must have been, how bold to make your way. How kind and loving your relatives to raise your passage fare.

You left your village of Antapol, near the city of Brest, took the last ship leaving Tsarist Russia before World War I began, escaping the miseries and terror of the Russian Revolution. Uncle Charles tells me you arrived in Baltimore where they gave you the name of Anna. You forged on by train to Cleveland where a community of Russians awaited your arrival. In Cleveland, you worked in the home of a Jewish baker and his family. You were a good worker and there you acquired, says Uncle Charles, your taste for latkes and the like. And there you met Grandpa Wasil Denyko. He was from another village near Brest, I believe, a short distance from your native home.

I wish you could have told me these stories yourself, Grandma, but my Russian, learned in college, has never been fluent, and you, you lived here for seventy-three years and never really learned English.

I understand that yours was a Russian world. You and Grandpa married in Saint Theodosius Orthodox Cathedral, which was shown in the movie *The Deer Hunter,* and because you didn't like urban life, the two of you moved to Ellwood City, Pennsylvania. Even with its steel mill, it was a beautiful place. You loved the woods, the big rolling hills, and your friends.

And so there you raised your family. I always loved visiting your house, which Grandpa built in 1925 on an enormous lot. We could sit on the back porch swing and examine the mysterious jars of pickles and sauerkraut you made. "Oh, honey, so nice!" you would say to me, smiling and giving me a hug. I wanted so much to know who you were. Your eyes were so warm — and the food you prepared! This was how you took care of us all.

I understand why you wanted to live where other Russians lived. As you know, we moved to Amarillo from Seattle when I was five, and although my connection to the Texas Plains is deep, I never truly felt a part of it all when I was growing up. I never felt Anglo-Saxon enough. My name was unusual, and so my imaginary alias was Janie Anderson. My nose was too big, and so I longed for the smaller, upturned nose it seemed so many of the other girls had.

Someone once told me, "How exotic you look, how beautiful you are."

"When you smile you look like a blonde Chinese," another person said. Chinese? I thought. I wasn't Chinese.

One friend, who said she had never known anyone with my

kind of looks, saw the movie *What Soviet Children Think about the Bomb.* "They all looked like you!" she exclaimed. "It was incredible." I've not seen it yet. I'd love to see a movie filled with people who look like me.

Maybe it sounds like I'm complaining, Grandma, but I'm not. It's just that in a way I understand your staying close to those who were more like you, but I can't help wondering how you really felt about it all. Cooking, nurturing your five children, speaking with others who spoke Russian, unable to read most of what was printed in American newspapers or magazines. How did you see the world? What did you think about at night?

I tried to find my answers by being at your house and being in your presence. I visit a Russian church from time to time and ask, "Is this part of my life, and if so, in what way?" I am fascinated and somewhat intimidated by the ceremony and the ornate altar, curious about the chanting and the kissing of icons. What does it mean?" I ask. "And who am I now?"

When I read about or see the Russians on television these days, I am so disturbed. My people, I cry inside, my poor, long-suffering people.

And so I work to integrate the two, dear Grandma, the memory of the soul and a life not lived with the reality of my American days. I am an American, after all, and a blend of nationalities, yet something speaks to me from the Old Country. Remember, it says. Remember and you will know who you are.

This remembering speaks with no logic. It speaks with feeling. Its voice is connection. And so I speak to you, dear Evdokiya, my Grandma, and begin the conversation we never had. [1]

Love,
Madeleine

Note

1. This letter, written after Evdokiya's death, makes me wonder why Madeleine never asked any of those questions. She had an excellent interpreter. When Munya's husband, Paul, died, Munya returned to live with her parents. Therefore she was more fluent with the Byelorussian her parents spoke than Chuck, who, though able to carry on in Russian, did not have the advantage of using it daily.

The Garden Vegetables and Dad

A Story About John, Gloria, Madeleine, Scott, and Kathy Denko

Was it lunch? Was it dinner? It could have been either meal in summer, bright sun outside, the air conditioning keeping the house cool. "I'm going out to get the corn from the garden," said our father, who loved growing plants of all kinds: flowers, vegetables, trees, cacti, shrubs, we had them all. He rushed out the backdoor, and was gone for only a minute. He ran back into the house smiling, his hands filled with corn fresh from the stalks in our backyard. "Hurry!" he said. "The sooner we get them in the water, the sweeter they'll be."

Over at the sink he tore the husks away, rinsed them off, and dropped them, one, two, three, four, five fresh ears of yellow corn, into the giant pot of boiling water our mother Gloria had ready on the stove. "Fresh corn!" he said. "If you wait too long it gets starchy."

"If you wait too long it gets starchy," we kids repeated, hovering around the stove.

When it was done, our mother brought the steaming corn to the table on a platter and put one ear on each of our plates. I put butter on mine, and watched it melt over the kernels, smooth and yellow. "It's sweet," Dad said. "Mmmm, that's good!" He looked around the table to see if we were enjoying the corn as much as he was, which we were. We ate off the cobs, neatly in rows, or taking big, random bites. Sweet summer taste, from our garden!

Dad also grew tomatoes, red and fragrant with that strange green-and-red tomato smell, not really sour, but earthy and mysterious. We sat down another time to eat. "Color!" he said. "We need more color on the plate!" He disappeared into the yard again, returning with two fat tomatoes, one in each hand. He rinsed them at the sink, and rushed around the table as he sliced them onto our plates. Red circles of tomato slid onto our salads. "For you," he said to our mother, for she was first. "And you and you and you," he said to us kids. "That's good isn't it?" he said. He liked the color and fresh food, and combined his artist's eye with his doctor's knowledge of nutrition.

Madeline Denko-Carter
April 11, 2003

The Distaff Side of the Denko Family

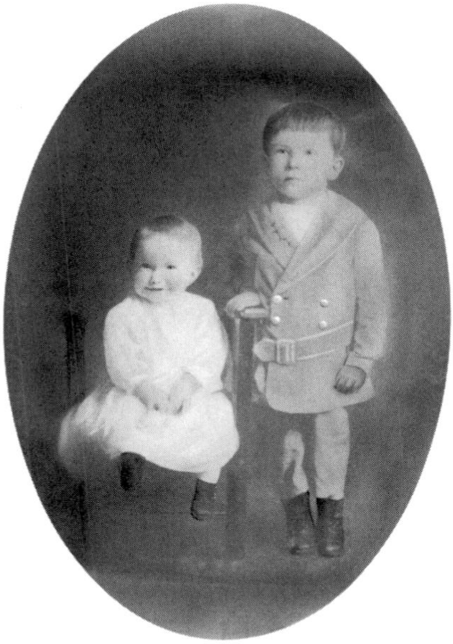

Charles at three, with baby sister Munya.

Denko women had different views on education as preparation for life from the men's. They were three: mother Evdokiya, elder daughter Munya (also known as Mary), and younger daughter Helen. They took the traditional view of their generation: that for women, finishing public high school was adequate education for life and work. Though both sisters were in the upper 10 percent of the class, they did not take up their father's offer to help them in college just as he had done for their elder brother Chuck and would do later for the younger, Ivan.[1] They assumed that with that high school standing they could get jobs in clerical work in retail establishments, light factory work, or office work.

Evdokiya was of course of the generation who worked very hard to raise a family, with several children and a husband. She also worked in the garden, although Wasil, the father, considered outside work the purlieu of the men and did most of the gardening on one half of a city plot. Besides vegetables, there were an apple tree, a pear tree, a sour cherry tree, and a peach tree.

The women specialized and were very competent cooks and house workers. Evdokiya told how, one day when she was about twelve, in Byelorussia where she grew up as an orphan, she was sitting on a porch swing, resting from her household duties on the farm when a Cossack asked why she wasn't working. She had a quick answer: "Why don't you make me go to school, not work?"[2] She was wanted for menial labor until her helpful relatives and the priest helped get her to America. Much later she went to night school and learned how to write her name.

CWD

Notes

1. Chuck's sisters did not value education for its own sake, like many today whose eyes glitter only at the thought of future earnings.
2. How many youths in a society with compulsory education appreciate being "made to go to school"?

Chocolate and Denko Siblings

In Western society, where virtually everyone favors chocolate almost above all other flavors, it is remarkable that neither Chuck nor Munya was partial to it. For many years Chuck never touched it, but in his last few years he would occasionally eat a little.

Munya's story about chocolate is that, as a child, she would always get chocolate ice-cream cones, because, not liking chocolate very much, she would lick them slowly and make them last a long time.

Movies in Mid-Century

Chuck's sister Helen's recollection of the World War II years, including when she had married George but of course was waiting for him at home, cited a movie price for everyone of just ten cents (I remember ten cents for children under twelve but twenty-five for those over). At eight to twelve dollars now, movie tickets must be among the greatest inflationary items.

Wasil Denko bought a piece of property out in the country — "down Burnstown", they always called it. The theater manager arranged with Wasil to erect a billboard there to advertise his films. Helen doesn't know what, if anything, Wasil was paid, but the family was given movie passes. Therefore each Saturday afternoon Evdokiya, Helen, and Bobby would go, regardless of what was showing.

The Story of the Munya Apple

The Munya apple story has its beginning in Tsarist Russia where Trofim, a friend of my father's, was born into a serf's family, and serfs worked the estates of the Russian upper classes. The serfs were taught agricultural art to produce necessities for the inhabitants of the estate. Trofim was born a serf and was to live and work as one.

Eventually the economic system of Russia was changed, permitting many serfs to migrate to the New World. Many became industrial workers, like our father and his friends in the mills. Wasil and Trofim and Rodion and their wives Evdokiya and Daria and Amana clustered around each other in areas of the U.S. where there were factory jobs, and steel paid well in those days. Women tilled the soil, usually of a city lot.

When Trofim had a break in his work,[1] he came to spend a few days or weeks with us. My father furnished a room near the furnace. In those days central heating meant shoveling coal around the clock.

One spring day I (CWD) noticed several small trees struggling for life. My mother said she had discarded cores from apples and put them in the ground to see what would come of it. The trees grew and in a few years came to the notice of Trofim. Our master gardener, alias Trofim, judged the apples No. 1 acceptable. Trofim took over and mated [cross-pollinated] several trees, and the matched trees' products were eaten, and those apples were also very good.[2]

One day on a trip to the nursery the owner [of the nursery] noticed one of the children [with an apple]. He took a bite and announced this to be a superior fruit — taste, appearance. We can start a new line.

I will name it the "Munya Apple" for how she took care of the trees. He made the decision that this was a superior product.

On my spring visit home I heard the bad news. All Munya apple trees were blown down.

He said he tried to save some of the Munya apples. Now we wait to see.

CWD (shortly before his death)

So I decided to trace, if possible, what, if anything happened to the "Munya apple". Munya's son, Robert Lyttle, told me that the Sturgis Orchard of the nearby village of Fombell had become involved. I called and left a message but received no return call. I wrote my question but received no response.

When I went to Ellwood City on other business, I decided to make one final effort. Although it was January and hardly an active season for an orchard, I drove out to Sturgis and found its roadside market closed, as expected. Still, I looked into the window, read a few notices, and planned to return in the spring.

At that point good luck favored me. A truck drove up, and a middle-aged man got out.

"Good afternoon, sir. Are you connected with Sturgis?"

"Yes, I am Aaron Sturgis."

And so I introduced myself as the widow of one of the Denko boys who had grown up in Ellwood City and explained my errand.

"Well, I'm the one who did it," said Aaron.

He went on to explain that he had gotten "budwood" from the graft in the backyard on Glen Avenue and had, in fact, planted twenty-five dwarf trees from that source. He found, however, that the apples they produced were what the original had been, the Cortland variety, a cross between Macintosh and Ben Davis. The latter had actually been brought from Eastern Europe, where it was called a Yupka. The Cortland was found to keep well through the winter because of a thick, waxy skin and was therefore very good for pies. Aaron told me that Munya said that when it was cut, the flesh did not turn brown from the iron in the knife. But it was not a new variety. Aaron said that he pursued this project as a favor to Munya, and they enjoyed it over the years. She had brought her sister out to the orchard once, and also her son.

You can just call me Sherlock.

Notes

1. The mill did not run full-time during the Depression.
2. Chuck has omitted something here about how Trofim had connections with a local nurseryman, and trees were transplanted to his nursery.

Recipes

Spaghetti Sauce

By John V. Denko, M.D.

Our father, John, always loved cooking and good food. Here is his basic recipe for spaghetti sauce. Some of the directions are a little general, so adjust according to your taste!

4 tablespoons olive oil (or safflower or canola oil), divided in half

1 onion, chopped

3–4 garlic cloves, chopped

1 pound mushrooms, sliced

1 pound ground meat, browned

Two or three ripe tomatoes, chopped, or canned tomatoes, cut up

1 green bell pepper, chopped

1 medium-size can tomato sauce

1 small can tomato paste

1 teaspoon basil

1 bay leaf

1 teaspoon tarragon (if you like it)

1–2 teaspoons oregano

1 teaspoon Italian seasoning (if you like)

Sauté the onion and garlic in half of the oil. In a separate pan, crumble and brown the ground meat, adding some oregano when it's almost cooked. Remove the onion and garlic from their pan, add the remaining oil, and lightly sauté the sliced mushrooms. Add the onion, garlic, and cooked meat back into the pan. Then add the other ingredients, stirring to combine. Simmer for about an hour, covered, then partially covered, stirring now and then. It is delicious.

Madeleine Denko-Carter

Stuffed Cabbage

From Munya Denko and Evdokiya Denko

Filling:

2 pounds ground beef (use ground chuck if you want)
4 onions, chopped
⅔ cup rice
2 teaspoons salt
½ tsp. pepper
2 tablespoons plain breadcrumbs
6 tablespoons Hunt's tomato sauce (from 8-oz. can)
2 heads cabbage
Optional: marrowbones for bottom of pan (ask your butcher to cut them into half-inch slices)

(Note from Madeleine Denko-Carter: This recipe is also very good without the bones.)

Sauté the onions in oil until soft. Add salt and pepper. Add the uncooked rice and sauté a little. Cool.

In a large bowl, add the cooled mixture to the meat with the breadcrumbs and tomato sauce. Mix to combine, and set aside.

To prepare cabbage

Cook the cabbage in a big pot of salted water so that you can carefully remove the leaves whole. Let the cabbage cool a bit—it will be very hot at first. Take off a few leaves at a time and put them on a large plate.

To make cabbage rolls

Place one cabbage leaf on a large plate. Put a couple of tablespoons of the meat mixture toward one end of the leaf. Roll it up halfway, then fold the sides in, and then finish rolling. Continue to make the rolls. You will have to transfer them to another dish for baking.

To prepare deep baking dish

Chop the cabbage that is left over, and put half of it in the bottom of the roasting pan or baking dish along with the rest of the tomato sauce. If you have any marrowbones, place them on the bottom of pan.

Put the cabbage rolls in the baking dish or roasting pan. Put the rest of the chopped cabbage on top, and cover with a 28-ounce can of whole tomatoes (about 3½ cups).

Bake, covered, for 2½–3 hours (350° F. for the first hour, then lower the heat to 325° and cook for 2 more hours).

Madeleine Denko-Carter

Munya Denko's Borsch

1 or 2 bunches of beets with stems and leaves (depending on how much soup you want to make)

(Optional): a pinch of salt

(Optional at end): a pinch of sugar

Wash the beets, stems, and leaves. Cut off the stems and leaves, and save them.

Peel and cut the root like French fries, then cut the stems, up to the leaves, into half-inch pieces.

Chop the leaves.

Cook the beet slices in enough water to cover them. The beets should float. Add a pinch of salt if you wish.

When the beets are tender, add the stems.

When the stems are tender, add the leaves and cook for 10 minutes.

Taste. If you like the taste, you're done. Or you can add a tiny pinch of sugar if you like. [1]

Serve with or without sour cream and dark bread. Can be served warm or cold.

CWD

Note

1. *I always add a teaspoon of vinegar to a soup bowl of borsch. On my Dutch side, vinegar is used for both flavor and preservative. It has surprised me that other northern cultures do not exploit this easy way to preserve food.*

Growing-Up Years

Chapter III

Chuck's Growing-up Years

What I know about Chuck's growing-up years I learned from him and his siblings. Thanks to his mother's push and his father's willingness to accommodate to her wishes, the children had the opportunity to grow up in a small Pennsylvania town in the foothills of the Appalachians, and on the Connoquenessing Creek, actually a non-navigable river with a relatively safe rock-protected inlet where they swam.

In a town where everyone knew each other, or at least the family, nobody could step far out of line without a report getting back to the parents.

Chuck had the advantage of being observed early as gifted, and various people made efforts to bring him into the Anglo-Saxon cultural mainstream.

He arrived in first grade severely crippled from an early bout with polio (see vignette "A Visit to the Shriners Sanitarium"), walking with great difficulty, and speaking only "peasant Russian". The teacher made sure that he entered second grade with good control of English.

She evidently got the word out. The Russian Orthodox priest heard of him and came over to get him to religion classes. The local Stevenson family, with the Presbyterian minister as father and three children older and younger than Chuck, included him in family events and outings (in their car!). Chuck remained friendly with all of them. After Art Stevenson and Chuck attended Geneva College, Art became a minister like his father, and he and his wife, Dottie, used money she inherited to buy a vacation house at Chautauqua. (Art was diagnosed with Parkinson's disease much younger than Chuck was diagnosed, and the advantage of Chautauqua was that all his ministerial friends came to Chautauqua in the summer and would visit him.) We also would visit them there, hear a lecture or two, and return to Rocky River the same night. (I still visit Dottie, now that we are both widows.) Chuck and I also kept in touch with Jane who, until her death, lived in Havre-de-Grace, Maryland, close to Johns Hopkins. We would sometimes see Bob, their brother, at Art's vacation home.

After his surgical repair by the Shriners, Chuck could, despite his limp, greatly expand his activities. He found a sport that did not depend on legs and was an archer in college. He announced sporting events on the town radio station, and he wrote news articles for the *Ellwood City Ledger.*

Chuck's sister, Helen, complained to me that after the family got the radio, when she had to scrub the kitchen floor on Saturday afternoons, Chuck wouldn't let her listen to popular music because he preempted the radio to hear the Metropolitan Opera.

My First Day of School

My early education was in the public schools of Ellwood City, Pennsylvania, beginning with my primary school three or four blocks from my home.

My mother came with me, bringing along one of our neighbors, a young lady fluent in Russian and English. She served as interpreter for the procedures of attending school, since my parents spoke only Russian. Thus I had had little exposure and that only to poor, ungrammatical English.[1]

This dedicated first grade teacher gave me special assignments to speed my learning English. I therefore spoke perfect English, without an accent, having learned it from textbooks and from my teacher.[2]

Years later when I traveled overseas the locals could not detect from my speech my origin.[3]

CWD

Notes

1. Recall that this six-year-old was still walking with great difficulty, from the worst effects of polio at age one.

2. In those days, teachers spoke close to perfect English, unlike now. My friend James Walker, himself a retired high school French teacher, explains this by the fact that back then teachers were usually single women from at least moderately well-to-do families, who devoted their entire lives to teaching.

3. Chuck did, however, pick up one western Pennsylvania speech idiosyncrasy, for a sensitive ear, i.e., "lenth" and "strenth" for "length" and "strength". Another was "crick" for "creek". We were told in my elementary school, Lafayette, north of Benton Harbor, Michigan, that of the then forty-eight states Michigan had the purest, least accented speech. When I began traveling around the country, I started to hear local usages that we did not have in Michigan.

A Visit to the Shriners Sanitarium (My Medical History)

We (several children) of our neighborhood were playing on the playground near the home of Metheny Buzard.[1]

Suddenly a car stopped, and the driver got out and motioned for us to come over to him. Even though this was not in those days a dangerous thing for children to do, Mrs. Buzard, the conscientious mother of an only child, came out and began to question the man in friendly conversation. She grasped the situation immediately and realized that the man, a member of the local Shriners chapter of businessmen, whose main project was to help needy children with orthopedic problems, had spotted an opportunity to help. Simply driving past, he had noticed that I was unable to participate in the children's play because of my polio-damaged leg.[2]

My case was presented to the Shriners' committee for consideration for medical attention — and approved. Since no specialized orthopedic physician was available locally, Mrs. Buzard conferred with my teachers and arranged with my parents for me to be evaluated by the orthopedic staff at the University of Pittsburgh. When my case was determined to be amenable to surgical treatment and physical therapy, I was sent to the Shriners Hospital in St. Louis. I was sent with another child, in the care of his college-aged sister.

They surgically removed a binding ligament, which produced foot-drop but greatly improved my walk. The other boy and I both underwent physical therapy for several months, and we both continued to improve.

My mother came out to St. Louis to check on me, despite having to bring along two younger siblings[3] because there was no one to care for them. (My next younger sister stayed home and cooked for my father.) In St. Louis they taught my mother how to continue my physical therapy at home, which she did, with an occasional visit to the local doctor, who supervised my care for several years until the therapy was tapered off.[4] The treatments were helpful to the point where I became able to walk well enough to find useful work as an adult.[5] Without the Shriners' help I would have become a dependent adult.[6]

CWD

Notes

1. Metheny later won the same countywide competitive examination for scholarship that CWD won in his graduation year—and became Ellwood City's postmaster. Chuck and I would visit him at the post office.

2. This is a marvelous example of the fact that in a given circumstance, what we observe is a function of what we take to the situation, based on our life experiences, as in the case of the Shriner. Louis Pasteur said it very well: "Chance favors the prepared mind", or, as he put it in French, "*Dans les champs de l'observation le hasard ne favorise que les esprits préparés.*" I favor the shortened translation because I believe that in *all* circumstances, not just "observation", the prepared mind has the advantage.

3. Helen remembers that Evdokiya had even the baby Peter along, making three children in tow.

4. We call this "maximal therapeutic advantage".

5. On vacations, Chuck even hiked long distances in the mountains. I observed that, like the tortoise in Aesop's fable, he had tremendous stamina, could continue long distances over a long period of time, while I found it hard to walk as slowly as he did, but would dart ahead, then rest while waiting for him to catch up.

6. Years later I wrote to the Shriners' headquarters about the productive life their charity had enabled, and received a reply to the effect that they can no longer dredge up such an old record, but they often receive letters like mine. Chuck's surgery was performed more than twenty years before I met him on his arrival in medical school at age thirty-one. Yet even as I write this, after his death, tears come to my eyes to think of the ripple effect of that stranger's intelligent kindness on Chuck's life, his army service, his subsequent research, practice, and career, my marriage, and our children's lives.

My Musical Career

My musical career had a hazy beginning. I remember being in the fifth grade in Ellwood City, a small town spread over the hills of western Pennsylvania. On the curriculum were classes in children's chorus, and every pupil was a member of the chorus. It was soon apparent that I had no singing talent. My teacher gave up on me but told me, in order not to ruin the effect, just to move my lips but emit no sound.

About a year later a musical contest to identify classical masterworks, naming the composers, was announced for sixth graders. Each sixth grade had been given a set of recordings to hear and practice identifying. The first prize was to be a silver dollar and a raincoat (offered by the local men's haberdashery), very useful in our rainy seasons. When the winner was announced, credit was given to the teacher. My sixth grade was the smallest in town, and my teacher was particularly proud that one of her students reflected positively on her. While I had no musical ability, I did have a good memory. When I was awarded the prize, not only did I get the silver dollar (which in those days paid for ten movie admissions, which I enjoyed very much) and the raincoat, but my teacher added her own accolade. She altered the school dismissal order, and I was given the position of leading the class out of sixth grade each day.

I remain a devotee of classical music to this day.[1]

CWD

Note

1. Chuck told me that he had taken piano lessons the summer before coming to Baltimore to enter medical school, but Poppy, his teacher, was never happy with his progress.

   Chuck drove several of us medical students to Philadelphia to attend an AMA convention, and we were singing songs in the car. When we asked why Chuck wasn't singing, he admitted that he couldn't. Yet, despite having little sense of rhythm, he loved to dance, and I would help by whispering the beat into his ear.

Chuck Denko, Boy Entrepreneur

In the early years of the 20th century, children went to their parents less often for money for goodies, and were turned down more often than now.

Chuck told me how when he wanted to go to a movie, he would need to buy a few newspapers at the print shop and sell them to workmen leaving the mill after their shift. A child's movie ticket was ten cents, and so he would buy five papers at three cents each, sell them for five, and have his admission price, but if he wanted a stick of licorice, that would require another nickel.

The special treat in Ellwood City and environs was a "Klondike", a chocolate-covered bar of ice cream costing five cents. In those days, an occasional one had strawberry ice cream instead of vanilla, and this entitled the lucky holder to another bar free.

Isaly's was the dairy store that featured these, and it has long since been bought out, but Klondikes live on in Ohio grocery stores, at six for $2.50 when they are on sale.

Our Gang

About the time we started high school we began an informal organization of teenaged boys. The usual size was six to ten youths usually in the same school year. No girls were permitted. The gang was only for socialization. One advantage over a tightly organized group was financial. No books were kept, as the Boy Scouts might want.

We members of these groups financed the buying of food. We usually earned small sums by doing small jobs for the store-owners where our parents shopped. We also sold junk to the junk dealers from New Castle. Occasionally we joined the girls in selling small packs of garden products such as leaf lettuce, green onions, and carrots. We took turns cooking until a member with special talent in cooking fish joined and was greatly welcomed by all.[1]

During summer months we gauged our activity to seasonal ones, such as camping. Swimming was a favorite activity.[2] For Hallowe'en we had a costumed group, and sometimes we won. We organized athletic teams to meet demands from playgroups, such as little leagues. We had volleyball teams, mushball, horseshoe teams, and swimming teams.

CWD

Notes

1. Fish from the Connoquenessing Creek, no doubt.
2. Chuck told me about swimming in the Connoquenessing Creek, a term in Pennsylvania for a much wider stream than what we called a creek in Michigan. Chuck once showed me a place where large rocks in the main stream had produced an eddy along the bank, with slow current, an ideal and safe pool for swimming.

Putting up the Aerial

At a time when radio was an important means of entertainment and education, even commercial information, my parents decided to buy one. Not just any radio, but a console. It was to be useful for a scholarly music lover (myself) and as a news source (for the whole family).

It was not a little radio to carry around but a monster that stood next to the phonograph and could play loud enough for all to hear. It was to have a large range. You could hear the station in Muscatine, Iowa.[1] Not that anyone knew anyone in Muscatine, but you could record in the log that you had heard Iowa, and not only Iowa, but you could explore around the country and the world, especially KDKA in Pittsburgh.

To maximize the benefits the radio was to have an aerial. The advantage to having the aerial was that you could listen to and explore everywhere. We were not satisfied to listen to KDKA and Muscatine. To remedy the range of the stations we needed an aerial, a wire stretching from our house to the neighbor's.

The news was out.

On the day in spring when we were to put up the aerial, neighbors gathered with their carpentry tools. My mother worked in the back of the house. The kitchen was the source of a light lunch.[2] The house electric wire thus furnished both the power source and the framework to support the aerial. It stretched from our porch to their porch. Since the wire crossed the alley on which we lived, the work had to be approved by the city engineer.

Now that I am an adult, I know my lessons in geography.[3]

CWD

Notes

1. Muscatine, a town of fewer than 50,000 in southeastern Iowa, apparently had a strong signal!
2. A "light" lunch in that household? Both qualitatively and quantitatively it must have been like the old days when all the harvesters were fed.
3. He is referring to the correlation between his grounding in geography in high school and at Geneva with the stations their radio brought in.

Science Teachers

The good they do keeps integrating the student into the adult world until student and teacher are satisfied with the product.[1]

Since I had become interested in technical aspects of modern civilization, Mr. Gills, my chemistry teacher, devised experiments that helped me learn in that direction. The physics course was of less interest to me.[2]

Biology proved as satisfactory as chemistry, under the teaching of Miss Helen Mathews. In her course we worked with plants, watering them, pulling weeds as needed, and with small animals such as frogs and tadpoles. In her course of general science we had to keep fish and plants balanced in a small aquarium, using only organisms available in the five-and-ten-cent store of those days. Thus we had them as pets but also learned to care for their needs.

Several other teachers also come to mind: Mr. Wilson in Latin, Miss Abraham in French, Mr. Caplan in Problems of Democracy, Mrs. Wilson in Geography. I had an excellent background in geography, a subject that, a few years later, was relegated to elementary school grades (or grade school or grammar school as it used to be called).[3]

A year or two ago I invited my remaining high school classmates to a reunion luncheon.[4] One told a moving story about Miss Abraham. He had dropped out to enlist in the army.[5] On his return, he showed up at school, expecting to graduate. His math teacher asked why he would try to finish high school and recommended that he just go to work. When he failed to appear in French class, Miss Abraham went to his home, talked to his father, and emphasized that he should complete his studies, including French. And so he made the effort and finally graduated with the later class.[6]

CWD

Notes

1. "The evil that men do lives after them; the good is oft interred with their bones." Chuck's experience from school is an excellent example of the reverse of Shakespeare's line from *Julius Caesar*. I am afraid Shakespeare came closer — Hitler, Stalin, Pol Pot, and modern dictators coming to mind.

2. With me, the opposite was true. I found physics fascinating because of new knowledge about radioactivity. I wrote a term paper on the subject in high school with equations, alpha particles, electrons, gamma radiation, etc. In college, at a

class reunion thirty years after graduating, a woman I did not remember came to thank me for getting her through physics. I might add that in those days there were no watered-down (household) chemistry courses. My mother's younger sister Edna had the opportunity to finish high school. I happened to see her grade card with an A in the only chemistry offered.

3. Chuck had further courses in geography at Geneva College, which stimulated his interest in the world and in travel.

4. Everyone a local classmate, Esther Gotjen, could find. (See Esther's letter to the *Ellwood City Ledger.)*

5. High school boys were told that their country would be better served if they graduated, but the war fervor was such that many signed up immediately.

6. I question whether a teacher would even be permitted to make such an outreach now, but at that time teachers had the freedom to be creative and to do what needed to be done.

High School During the Depression

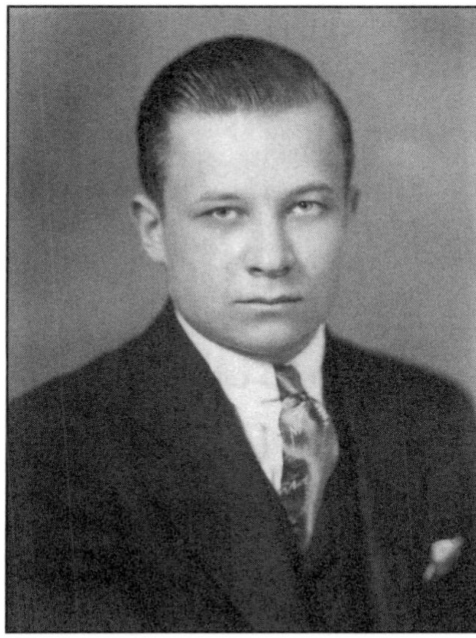

Charles's high school graduation photo at seventeen.

When I went to high school in the depression, few young people were pushed to "complete" their education in this way. In fact they had to be both ambitious and motivated, and many attended over the objections of their parents who, with many mouths to feed, needed supplemental income.

The same was true of black and white students, and we had no Asians in our community. I was friendly with students both inside and outside of my (Russian) ethnic group. This included a black boy I'll call Marvin, who somehow managed to get together enough money to buy a second-hand dump truck, with which he got odd jobs hauling and making deliveries. Sometimes he gave me a ride, and my father, well aware of the difficulties against which Marvin struggled, would give me a couple dollars and tell me to give them to Marvin for gas.[1] In later years Marvin went on to study law, thus making a living and helping his cohorts in need of legal assistance.

Rose (not her real name) was a black classmate of mine with whom I chatted about lessons. She was being raised by a mother who ran a boarding house. Often Rose would come without the assignment prepared. When I asked her why, she admitted that her mother had required her to service the boarders the previous night, leaving her no time or energy for lesson preparation. She attended high school when she could have made a living on her back with her mother pimping for her. I don't know what became of Rose, but I hope she somehow accomplished her goal of attending college to become a teacher.[2]

CWD

Note

1. About 20¢ a gallon.
2. In those days special colleges to prepare teachers were called "normal schools". Until recently I didn't know the meaning, but my editor has explained that the purpose of such schools was to establish teaching standards or *norms.*

Chuck's Lifelong Connection with Geneva College

When Chuck graduated from high school, Pennsylvania granted the winner of a competitive examination, held annually in each county, a four-year scholarship to any Pennsylvania school of the student's choice. Chuck won this, and knowing he needed guidance, went to his chemistry teacher for help in choosing. The teacher wisely advised that Chuck attend Geneva College in Beaver Falls, Pennsylvania, just ten miles from Ellwood City. This college was already known for its chemistry department and, a few years later, Geneva and a few other liberal arts colleges nationwide received special accreditation from the American Chemical Society for their excellent chemistry education.

An added advantage of Geneva was its proximity, with ease and cheapness of commuting. In those days, not only was hitch-hiking relatively safe, but some students drove and shared driving expenses. Room and board was not included by the state, but Chuck earned that by getting up at four to stoke furnaces at Geneva. His father, disappointed at being unable to attend night school in this country, was happy that the "Land of Opportunity" meant opportunity for subsequent generations. He helped Chuck with money for books and other expenses, and also helped John. My wise and generous father-in-law offered the same help to his two daughters, who declined. He also helped Chuck's brother's fiancée, Gloria Sandalis, with her tuition, and offered to help me when my father made threats of cutting me off, which fortunately came to nothing. Chuck's father understood that his sons needed intelligent and educated wives. The very year of our sabbatical was the only time that the exchange rate was in Australia's favor, and my father-in-law advanced us money from his pension fund, which we repaid with interest.

Chuck received an excellent education at Geneva. Besides chemistry and history, two of his main interests, Geneva offered geography courses, including not only physical but social and economic geography, from which he derived an exceptional knowledge of the world. His knowledge, particularly of Europe, was orders of magnitude greater than mine, which came along when geography was relegated to grade school and ended in seventh grade. Chuck joked that I should request refund of some of my college tuition money.

Over the years Chuck maintained close contact with Geneva, and it with him. In 1969 he was the Distinguished Alumnus of the Year. He returned to the college for meetings related to chemistry and sometimes gave talks. I also gave an occasional talk, e.g., to the premed students, and later became a visiting professor, conducting an occasional seminar on topics on which I had written.

My [Early] Career as a Chemist

In October 1943 I received my Ph.D. in biochemistry from Penn State, thus continuing my saga as a curious small-town boy facing an interesting future. I had already decided I wanted to use my talents working in the field of biochemistry solving the unknown problems facing us all, more specifically, those of my mentor, A. K. Anderson, professor of physiology, who was a victim of rheumatoid arthritis, of unknown cause but known destruction. He was already wheelchair-bound when I met him. I had a handicap myself due to polio, which did not interfere with any of my activities.[1] One of my jobs was to write Anderson's notes on the board before class.[2] Under his tutelage I was getting a good grounding in biochemistry.

One day in his office he looked at me over his glasses and said, "Denko, do you want a good problem for your thesis work?"

Now I had enough sophistication to know that you answer a question like that with "Yes, boss".[3]

His suggestion was, in fact, to find new treatments for rheumatoid arthritis. He went on, "I think you can do it with animal models." This quenched my objection.[4] Our first step was to find an animal model, and fortunately a paper by Albert Bruce Sabin contained the information I needed.[5] Anderson suggested that I should go to Cincinnati to work in Sabin's lab during summer vacation. From that experience I learned what I needed to carry on my project at Penn State. I planned various aspects of my study and began my work.

A year into it, my supervisory committee felt that my title did not fit, so I added a pharmacology section, adding useful information for the treatment of rheumatoid arthritis. But undesirable side effects surfaced. Gold was toxic, causing kidney failure in rats and sometimes in human patients. Eventually we found a way to reduce this toxicity by beginning with a small dose of the gold drug for the rats. By following certain kidney waste products, the physician could reduce kidney damage in humans.[6]

CWD

Notes

1. Is this really a "handicap", although admittedly a "disability", and one that may have spurred him to greater achievement.

2. What a great way to learn any subject!

3. Our sons and I always laughed when ideas of their father and "sophistication" were juxtaposed, since it was not sophistication in which he excelled, but intelligence, shown, for example, by his ability to see the connections between apparently unrelated situations. We must remember his background to see the distance he had come in areas of problem solving and

intelligent dealing with others of diverse backgrounds and orientations.

4. I.e., that they did not have patients.

5. This is the Sabin later famed for his oral polio vaccine. I ran two clinics that dispensed this vaccine when it first came out.

6. Chuck's synthesis of gold compounds, the only anti-arthritic known besides aspirin, became the bases for his dissertations for his M.S. and Ph.D. These were published as the second reference in his bibliography.

Shortly before Chuck left Penn State, *The New York Times* sent a reporter to interview Chuck and his research director. He never found out whether this information made its way into the newspaper, but, at my request, our daughter-in-law, Karen, Nicholas's wife, found it through a fifteen-minute search on the Internet. (See *New York Times* account in this volume.)

One bit of practical advice that Anderson gave Chuck was always to be on friendly terms with secretaries (now called assistants) because they know more than anyone else about what is really going on in the department.

In 2010, when I was starting stamp collections with my three older grandchildren, I taught each of them what their stamps commemorated in history or the natural world. For nine-year-old Louis, I had a fifty-five-cent stamp of Justin Morrill and explained that this man introduced in 1857 one of the two most important pieces of legislation ever to be passed by Congress: the Land Grant Act of 1862. This law set aside land for education in every state and territory applying for statehood. The new universities began with "Agriculture and Manual Arts", for which we needed educated men for improving those basic industries. As we moved westward, mining became important. I explained to little Louis that his grandfather Chuck had been educated as a chemist at Penn

State, Pennsylvania's Land Grant university. Several years later Louis's grandfather was educated as a physician at Johns Hopkins University, courtesy of the other of the most important laws, the GI Bill, which paid to educate veterans of World War II and the Korean Conflict.

War Years

Chapter IV

My War Years

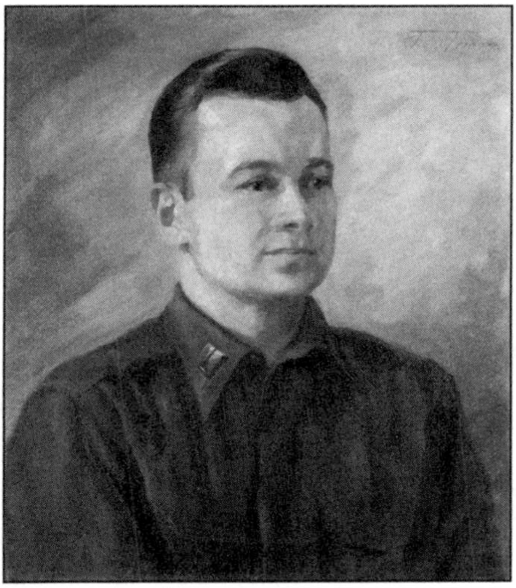

Captain Denko in 1945.

For the average male student at Penn State and other colleges and universities, the phrase "my war years" meant events beginning with a drawing of a number representing each possible birthday of the year, and ranging from having your birthday called first to the plain good luck of having such a high number as not to be called up, perhaps never. My roommate's number was called first, although he was exempt as will be explained.

To supply manpower for WW II, local boards had been designated to select the conscripts with the fairness of chance. On a beautiful summery day in State College, Pennsylvania, a large fishbowl was set up and filled with little slips of paper with numbers (corresponding to the days of the year) to identify by birthday conscripts to the army.[1] Each month another number was drawn.

In our apartment lived four graduate students (Iz, Murray, Cy, and myself), one of whom held number 156 (birthday in early June), making him eligible for the first call-up. However, students majoring in biochemistry had been declared essential for the war effort and could not be drafted. At a time when enlisting was not unheard of, our faculty advisors advised our group to finish our coursework. My case was different. I was deferred because a bout of polio had left me with a shortened left leg and therefore not draftable.

After completing my Ph.D., I started work at SMA (a research lab) in Chagrin Falls, Ohio.

In the summer of 1944 an army recruitment officer came to my work venue at SMA. After discussion, he agreed that, despite my shortened leg, I qualified for several military specialties. The officer offered me a commission as first lieutenant in the Sanitary Corps, which I joined in January 1945.[2] I was sent to a training camp at Carlisle Barracks in Carlisle, Pennsylvania, where I spent five weeks in the 80th Officers' Training Battalion (see vignette "War Games").

In the winter of 1944 I began my service time by organizing the Army Medical Lab in Chicago.[3]

In the fall of 1945 I was sent to the European Theatre as relief personnel for troops returning home. Based at the 98th General Hospital in Munich, I qualified for and was assigned to a variety of military duties: border station inspector for refugee health (as they were being brought from the Eastern Zone of occupation, they were dusted with sulfa to prevent typhus); repatriation of children to Eastern Zone (Jewish children looking "Aryan" had been removed by German troops from their homes in Poland, Czechoslovakia, and Byelorussia, to be raised as Aryan by German families); since I was somewhat familiar with the languages of the East Zone countries, I was assigned this duty;[4] smashing of empty penicillin vials, which were being scavenged to be used on the black market, filled with inert substances such as vegetable juice and sold as active medication, resulting in patients being treated with inert substances, thus causing more illness, even death;[5] sanitation and nutrition in a DP (displaced persons) camp. Inspecting the camp, I heard officials discussing a prisoner who was being held in camp, accused of spying and condemned to hang when the camp moved to Palestine. He had been accused by other Jews and believed he had not been given a fair trial. I intervened and alerted our criminal detective unit who investigated, found he had been tried properly and found innocent, and freed him. Several weeks later, I was walking down the street and he ran up, kissed my hand and arm, wept, and expressed his gratitude, as did his wife and daughter.

I mustered out with a captain's commission and was offered the rank of major if I had stayed.[6]

CWD

Notes

1. The navy, marines, and the then separate air force took volunteers.
2. Chuck was also offered a place on the Manhattan Project (on the atomic bomb), but declined because his chemistry was the wrong kind, M.S. in organic and Ph.D. in physiologic chemistry, oriented to human physiology and pathology.
3. There he did nutrition studies on COs (conscientious objectors) for the long-term effect of army rations on their bodies.

He had these subjects ingest for months the identical diet issued to service personnel on active duty, while he studied all their output of urine and feces. He found no deleterious effect on their nutritional status.

Items 3 through 8 in Chuck's bibliography are from work he did at the Nutrition Lab on the COs. The bibliography can be found at the end of this volume, and reprints of his papers are preserved in his archives at Geneva College in Beaver Falls, Pennsylvania.

4. See *Jewish News* article.

5. See vignette "An Empty Penicillin Vial Is Not Without Value"; also the film *The Third Man* (based on Graham Greene's novella) starring Orson Welles as Harry Lime, the black marketeer selling fake penicillin. The British version of the film shows a ward of patients given the fake penicillin and rendered vegetative.

6. Chuck continued in the reserves and spent one weekend a month on duty through a couple years of medical school.

Chuck told me that he had been assigned to investigate the allegations that wartime hardships had caused widespread malnutrition in German civilians. He tested their blood for vitamin levels and found them normal.

Chuck's experiences as a result of where he was at the time are included in vignettes. Another anecdote illustrates the fact that Captain Denko never really acquired what we might call "army-think". At the general's briefing sessions the general sat in front, with concentric semicircles of officers of ever-decreasing rank, with Chuck, as captain, in the outer ring. One day the general announced a policy, whereupon Chuck leaned forward to whisper to his friend in the next ring, "That's pretty arbitrary, don't you think?" With a completely straight face the friend replied, "No, not at all. That's just the way the general wants it."

When Chuck was in the army in the Occupation, in the Sanitary Corps, never anywhere near any combat zone, he went hiking in the Alps while on leave, fell, and suffered minimal damage with no impairment. By army rules he was given a purple heart.

A Visit with Russian Nobility — Émigrés from Tsarist Russia

At the mid-20th century, Russian immigrants included both the poor like my parents, former peasants who had come to the fabled land of opportunity, and the *nouveaux pauvre* (you've heard of the "nouveaux riche"), remnants of tsarist aristocracy and nobility who had escaped Communist bullets, and gotten out of the USSR ahead of the Bolsheviks, often with only the clothes on their backs, into which were sewn as many jewels as they could manage. Many of the latter were driving taxis in Paris, and if you asked to be taken to "the Cathedral", you were let out not at Notre Dame but at the Russian Orthodox Cathedral with its world-famous choir.[1] In our country these émigrés clustered in New York City and maintained a small subculture.

When I was in the army, I was stationed briefly in New Jersey and spent an occasional free weekend in the city with old friends, Walter and Nina Bouquet. They introduced me to Tanya, a graduate student in Russian, whose father was a professor of Russian at the University of Illinois at Urbana, and both elderly[2] parents were also employed as Russian translators at the United Nations. The father took me to a session of the Assembly where Nikita Kruschev[3] spoke. He used the Russian word *mir,* which has two meanings, "peace" and "world". On that occasion, the translator chose his unintended meaning. Kruschev banged his fist on the table and shouted, "We want peace", but was translated as saying,

"We want the world!" A near-riot broke out as the audience became unruly, jumping up and ignoring the Assembly police, protesting the second meaning, yelling, "They want the whole world!" while Kruschev himself was bellowing, "No! No! NO!" When the chairman could get order, the error was corrected.

On another visit to New York, when I called Tanya for our evening out, she informed me that we had an unusual invitation to a Christmas party put on by Tanya's parents and friends, this former Russian nobility. She explained this event as a gala evening hosted by Russian nobility. As a young Russian-speaking American officer, I was welcomed and taken on a tour and introduced to the various personalities around the ballroom, many wearing the jewels and tiaras from their former life that they had been able to get out of Russia and had not yet had to sell to live. The chambermaid who had made up my room at the Plaza Hotel was a former duchess, and a handsome white-haired man a count. Tanya explained that the partygoers did not want to exploit their former status. She introduced me to a tall elderly woman, Aleksandra Tolstoy, the youngest of eleven children of the novelist Leo Tolstoy, called by the Russian pet name Sasha.[4] Sasha prepared her father's novels on the wonderful new invention, the typewriter.[5] Sasha had managed to buy a vineyard along the Hudson, with a motel, so her friends could visit and talk as Russians are wont to do.[6] I was invited but unable to accept.[7]

After the war my father Wasil happened, in a group of Russians socializing in Pittsburgh at a picnic, to encounter the woman whose family had owned the estate in Byelorussia on which his family had worked as serfs and later as peasants.

This woman told my father proudly that her two sons had done well in business in this country. And so my father told her that he had two sons who were doctors.

"How can that be," she asked, astonished, "when you were once a peasant on our land?"

CWD

Notes

1. I learned that they sang a cappella because since ancient times musical instruments had been considered "idols". There also is said to be something remarkable about Russian voice boxes that permits the sopranos to sing very high and the basses very low.

2. He meant in their fifties.

3. The usual spelling is Khrushchev, but Chuck was always complaining that Russian words were transliterated through German. I left his transliteration, Kruschev. I always heard Kruschev with an "shch", not an "sch" in the middle. Also, Chuck always spelled Tchaikovsky, Chaikovsky.

   He was always interested in languages, and not just Eastern European languages. He would ask others, such as taxi drivers, how to say this or that in their language.

   When he had elderly patients who had come north from South Carolina, he would ask them about words in Gullah, a creole language based on an African language. They loved his expression of sincere interest.

   And he could learn by ear. I never could. I would have to see it written.

4. Sasha is used for both the feminine Aleksandra and the masculine Alexandar, my grandson's middle name. It has also become popular as its own name in our country.

5. In the terminology of the day, as the operator of the instrument, she was called Tolstoy's "typewriter".

6. Around the samovar?

7. He was shipped out to serve in the Occupation in Europe.

War Games

The army sent Chuck to Carlisle Barracks near Gettysburg, Pennsylvania, for five weeks, where he and the other officers-in-training were taught much that was useful throughout life, not just in service. Over our life together he would tell me about these experiences.

For example, in cooking class oriented to military life, they were told that so-called KP (kitchen patrol) as punishment resulted in a poor nutritional result, whereas assigning personnel to food service as a specialty gave it status, would keep the men well fed, and produced better morale. To assess results, the class members would stand at the end of the line where the men brought back trays and question them about the food that was being thrown out repeatedly. They found that one problem had resulted from the fact that, without instruction, the kitchen personnel had boiled large and small potatoes together, for the same length of time, turning out large hard rocks mixed with mush. A representative from Howard Johnson's Restaurant came to the Carlisle graduation and offered them all jobs as restaurant managers when their tour of duty was over.

In another course they were taught principles of packing and shipping. Parts for planes had been sent to the war theatre to be assembled there. One error was that all the propellers had been packed together, and the ship carrying them was sunk, so none of the planes could be completed until more propellers arrived.[1]

Finally, when they did field war games, with a mock battle, at Carlisle, they put Chuck in charge of casualties. On his clipboard he listed three levels of injury according to severity: (1) fatal cases — pain meds only in the field; (2) severe but salvageable — priority for triage to field hospital; (3) minor and less severely injured — later triage. His instructors were astonished by the intelligent design of his plan.

Note

1. Fifty years later, when Christopher and I went to Egypt for the typical Nile cruise, to see the ancient temples and pyramids, and a solar eclipse in the desert on the Sudan border, our route took us past El Alamein, site of a turning-point battle in the African campaign against Rommel and the German forces. We visited the British cemetery, where a single grave might contain body fragments of as many as five different unidentified soldiers (now they could be identified by DNA). Another older woman and I cried. The American indoor/outdoor museum exhibited planes used in combat, so small they looked as if two men could pick one up, with their propellers.

A Tale of Doctor Schilling — A Visit to Landshut

On a gloomy day in early spring I traveled from my base in Munich at the 98th General Hospital to an assignment that routed me near Landshut, the prison, built of massive dark blocks, where Adolf Hitler was incarcerated as a young man for his antigovernment political activity. I proceeded along walks with puddles of melting snow, following signs directing visitors to the office of the commandant, whose uniform showed him to hold the rank of captain.

"What can I do for you, Captain?" he asked.

"I'd like to visit Hitler's room."

"Fine. Follow me."

He led me down a long corridor and stopped before an iron door with iron bars. He opened the squeaking door, and we entered the small, sparsely furnished cell, with a large open volume. He led me to the window, waving his arms at various buildings. "Nothing to see here except prisoners," he said, but as we turned to go, he beckoned me and said, "I have someone for you to see especially because you're in the medical field. Tomorrow would be too late."

We passed down several long corridors, stopping at last at the door of a large cell in which sat a white-haired old man typing. "*Kommen Sie hier, bitte.*" But the old man kept typing.

I asked my guide who he was.

"He is a world-famous hematologist, here for medical war crimes.[1] Every time a patient needs a blood count, he does it for us."

"What do you do then?"

"What would *you* do?"

"I'd check it."

"Exactly what we do, too."

"What is he famous for?"

"The test devised by this old man for diphtheria helped millions, mostly children, in the past."[2]

I questioned my guide further. "What happens now?"

"Tomorrow he has an appointment with the gallows."

On my way out, I noticed that the gallows had been freshly painted.

CWD

Notes

1. Under Hitler, Schilling did worthless "scientific" tests on twins, infecting one with fatal disease organisms, keeping the twin for a "control", and sacrificing both.

2. Diphtheria had been a leading cause of death in small children. The Schilling test, later immunization (DPT), and finally antibiotics had virtually eliminated it in the industrial world. When we were in medical school, my mnemonic device for the Schilling test for diphtheria related to the Dick test for scarlet fever, i.e., the s's and d's crossed over.

A Page from the Book of Arch-Nazi Heinrich Himmler

In the American Army of Occupation in Europe after World War II, I served in the Sanitary Corps and was assigned to supervise public health measures in Southern Bavaria. One beautiful fall day in 1945 or 1946, I was driving along a winding highway and spotted an attractive stone house, the centerpiece of a well-kept estate. Since I had no need to hurry, I turned off the highway and stopped in front of the door. When I rang the bell, a neatly dressed middle-aged woman asked, "*Was wünschen Sie?*"

I answered in the army version of the local dialect, and we soon established that she was Czech, and I continued in my mixture of Russian and German (*Amerikanischer deutsch*), adequate with gestures and pointing.

She told me that this property had previously been a private home for a high-ranking Nazi leader, and Hitler had been a guest. Currently it was being used as a rest house for officers of the Occupation, and was used mainly on weekends and holidays. "I see by your uniform that you are an American officer, and so the club is for you." She offered to show me around, where the beautiful furnishings represented the life of the powerful. Then she produced tea and cookies.

I thought how I, son of American immigrants, was sitting in the chair of a Nazi leader. I began to leaf through various volumes in the library. She said, "I see that you are interested in books, and I suggest that you take a souvenir. Here is the book that Hitler used as an excuse to invade and conquer." She gave me the book *Baiern führen den Pflug nach Östen (Bavaria leads the Push toward the East*) by Heinz Hauzhofer and Johann V. Leers, © 1938, inscribed H. Himmler, April 1939.

The rest is history.

CWD

Two Is Better Than One

On a bright summer day in our little Town in the hills of western Pennsylvania, my mother, seated on the porch swing, said to my brother John and me, "I'm glad you could come home together this time." She was referring to the fact that it was only by chance that my brother and I, serving in different branches of the military (John in the navy, which put him through the University of Chicago Medical School, and he later repaid the time to the Public Health Service, and I in the army) arrived home together. Barring a family emergency or death, leaves to service personnel were not granted for family get-togethers.

My mother indicated that she wanted to go to Doude's, a small dry-goods store, to get emblems of our patriotism, i.e., two little flags, each with a blue star, which many families with military personnel would hang in the window. (A gold star represented a military death.)

Since we didn't have a family car, my brother and I spoke up quickly. "Mom, you don't need to walk downtown. We can get them and carry home any purchases."

Mother went on, "No, boys, thanks anyway, but I want to carry this one."

We persisted. Then she explained. "You know that Mrs. Jones behind the counter. She has been telling me about her son. He is a good officer. I want you to go with me. There is no other mother in town with two officer sons."

CWD

An Empty Vial Is Not Without Value

During my service in the US Army in World War II and the Occupation of Europe, I learned that some empty vials or bottles attained significant value as a result of their prior use and labeling for their contents. These bottles were small, able to hold one-half ounce of liquid, with a rubber stopper. They were very precious because they had contained the new miracle drug penicillin, in a very impure form, since the production process involved fermenting in huge vats to grow the mold *penicillium,* then separating the product from the culture medium. This penicillin was lifesaving in certain infections, and was used for some infections in servicemen. Our army shared the precious product when possible, but the supply was limited, and many civilians who might have been saved could not be, for lack of penicillin. By the law of supply and demand, this penicillin brought $50 a vial on the black market. This was bad enough in itself by subverting the precious supply, but worse, unscrupulous black marketeers would sell either penicillin diluted with tea, or a completely fake drug of the same amber shade as the impure product, in the recognizable vials.

The supply was under the control of the US Army, which shared with the civilian population, particularly for children with meningitis, as without it those children invariably died, and in children with other infections but little resistance resulting in part from poor diet in the war years.

Unscrupulous, criminal black marketeers would go through waste to find the bottles from used penicillin, into which to put their diluted (hence worthless) mixture so as to sell as many bottles as possible. Thus many died for lack of genuine treatment. Even worse was the fraudulently diluted penicillin because there might be enough potency to save the life of the child but leave him vegetative.

To combat this cruel and criminal activity, the army devised a method to stop this dangerous traffic by keeping the empty bottles out of the hands of black marketeers. I was given this detail and sent out under heavy guard to the outskirts of Vienna where the hospitals disposed of their used bottles, where I smashed them.

There is an old movie whose plot includes a black marketeer making a fortune on black-market penicillin. Orson Welles plays the part of Harry Lime in *The Third Man.* In the British version of the film, an army officer takes the American author to the ward of vegetative children to see what Lime's crimes have caused.

CWD

Visiting our Allies

Russian Zone, Berlin, 1945–46
Two Social Events Soviet Army Style[1]

On a bright spring day I decided to visit the territory controlled by our allies, the victorious Russian army. I made my way from my billet in West Berlin to a city park via public transport. Spring flowers and shrubbery, bright spots of yellow, red, white, and blue dotted a green background. In other areas a brown background was prominent where the public walked. I took my camera out of my pouch and turned around for a good picture.

At that moment a Russian major spoke to me in Russian. "There are better scenes ahead." I responded in Russian, and he tried to sell me his binoculars. As we chatted, I told him my parents were from Byelorussia, more specifically from the city of Brest, a border town of 30,000 inhabitants. He went on to say that that was his last campaign.[2] He added, "The fighting was fierce." When the battle was over, the town was back in the hands of the Russian army. But he described the destruction. "There was not a wall left standing that stood as high as I am." He was about six feet tall.

He was hospitable and invited me to visit his officers' club. He explained that the army was not paid as often during the field campaigns as they were during garrison duty. Therefore he had several thousand military rubles to spend, which could be spent only outside of Russia. I took directions on how I could get to his club, while he went looking for souvenirs.

My escort[3] and I crossed a busy street used mainly for pedestrians. A few motor vehicles were slowed as we approached another imposing building. My escort pointed to a small group of Russian officers, recognizable by their insignia. There were many generals, known as "Marshall" in their rank. Several of them came up to us, and my escort explained my predicament (I had forgotten the name of the officer who had invited me to the officers' gala).[4]

"Stop!" The strong, loud order rang out in the dark night in Vienna, 1946. The venue was the flower garden leading from the boulevard to an imposing stone mansion that the Soviet Army was using for administration of Austria. I had been invited to a very special social evening at the Russian Army headquarters.

I knew enough Russian to halt when that armed sentry thrust his gun forward and barked, "стой!"[5] Asked to state my business, I explained my invitation to the party at the officers' club, by a fellow officer in the Russian army whose name I forgot but who had worked with me on the same detail to which we were both assigned as part of the Allied Occupation. The officer had to call his superior, who immediately arrived to give permission for me to attend.

My guide took me to see the entertainment: dancing, card playing, snacks and vodka, and a classical pianist. It was not at all rowdy but quiet and cultured.

At the event, many of the guests were parading[6]. The women were smartly groomed. The star performer was the internationally known pianist Emil Gilels,[7] who performed in a small theater seating several hundred. My escort offered wine and champagne. One guest was drunk. Card games were a popular pastime.

Gilels and the members of the small orchestra wore civilian clothes. The majority of men were in military dress. I was offered drinks, all alcoholic. No one invited me to play cards. I was free to wander around, with no one following me in this magnificent royal hall in a wing of the old Austrian royal palace.[8]

CWD

Notes

1. During Chuck's medical decline he continued to work on vignettes for this project, but his handwriting/printing showed the effects of his Parkinson's disease. I was not able to transcribe them until after his death. At that time I found two very similar accounts, the longer one entitled "Visiting our Allies; Russian Zone, Berlin, 1945–46", the shorter one "Two Social Events Soviet Army Style". The longer one has "Berlin" in the title, and I recall his recollections of visiting Berlin on army assignment. The shorter one has "Austrian palace" and "mansion" in the text and "two social events" in the title. Both feature a visit to an officers' club with a variety of entertainment including the internationally known pianist Emil Gilels. I have combined the accounts. My explanation is that there were two similar events. The Russian Army must have arranged a tour for Gilels to entertain officers, and Chuck caught two such events. As he told me about his experiences, he pointed to the difference between what the Russian officers' clubs offered, i.e. classical music, and what the USO purveyed. Apparently the USSR treated its officers as not only gentleman but educated and cultured as well. Val Onipko, son of an army officer (physician) was well educated and happy to discuss Russian history and literature with me.

2. He must have meant the recent fighting as the Russians moved west.

3. Where did Chuck get an escort?

4. Having found the officers' club, Chuck returned that evening.

5. Pronounced "stoi."

6. I think he means circulating.

7. This man's virtuosity was such that his reputation extended into the 21st century, when I heard a recording of his on classical radio in 2009.
8. I believe that no such elegant royal palaces were left standing in Berlin.

Medical School, Courtship, and Marriage

Chapter V

MEDICAL SCHOOL, COURTSHIP, AND MARRIAGE

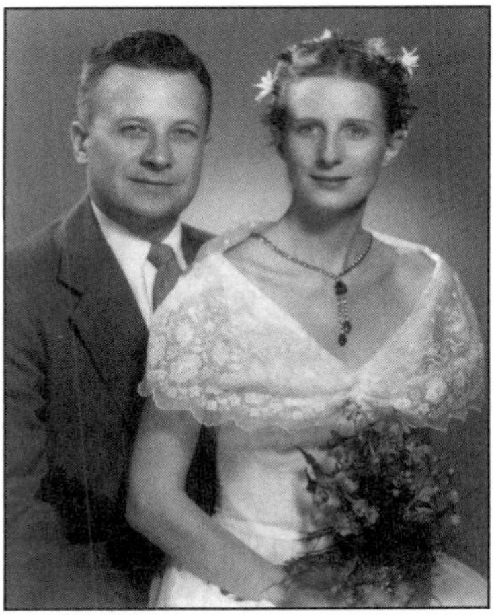

Charles and Joanne at wedding, June 17, 1950.

In the late summer of 1947, two trajectories were converging. As Chuck's future wife, I had completed my undergraduate work at Hope College in Holland, Michigan, with a B.A. *summa cum laude*, the seventh in the history of the school to graduate with a 4.0 average. Delighted to have been accepted at the world's premier medical school, Johns Hopkins University College of Medicine, I spent the summer preparing to move to Baltimore and live, with other "hen meds", in the "Hen House". Having switched in college from a pre-law curriculum, I nevertheless had a good foundation in chemistry, less in biology, minors in German and Greek (having taken four years of Latin in high school), but had been unable to fit in literature courses which I loved, not as much math as I would have liked (although my math professor offered me a scholarship). Still, I was confident that I could do whatever it took to learn, develop, and transform myself from a premed at twenty into a physician at twenty-four.

In the spring of 1947 Chuck had returned from service in the army, expecting to get married. Believing himself engaged, he was disabused of that idea by the young woman. (Later I had occasion to meet her and realized that not only was I very lucky as a result of her decision, but so was Chuck.) By summer he had been accepted at Hopkins, had made the necessary arrangements for the GI Bill to put him through medical school, and had arrived in late August, having turned thirty-one on August 12.

One September evening the second-year students gave a mixer (known in their piquant terminology as a "beer bust") for the first-year students to meet each other in our class of seventy-eight incoming students, with whom we would be living, studying, working, and evolving into physicians. (We were not, as in other medical schools, called freshmen, etc., and we were told later that, nationwide, that was the year when just one in seventeen applicants found a place in any medical school. This was because of the influx of returning veterans, applying, like Chuck, with the help of GI funding. Hopkins, however, had to accept women "on the same basis as men" or risk losing endowment.) We had eight women in a class of seventy-eight. Our class included a number of veterans, some bringing wives and small children to Baltimore. Thus our class had a considerably older mean age than the usual twenty-two for college graduation, and a span in age from two students of nineteen to Chuck's thirty-one. The lower end resulted from a few of us having been "skipped" a grade or two ahead in elementary (or "grade" or even "grammar") school, a practice of our time that even in the mid-'70s the Australians were still doing, and did with our children.

The evening of that mixer I noticed several things about Chuck, the oldest class member at thirty-one, and the only one with both Ph.D. and service time. He let us know about his recent return from the Occupation (I envied him those experiences in the army, and I felt in deference to him for his background in chemistry — M.S. in organic and Ph.D. in physiologic), and I admit that this intimidated me somewhat, biochemistry being considered the most difficult of the basic science courses in first year. (Still, I made it through without outside help, although I helped my friend Iza with the math.) One thing I noticed about Chuck that evening was his brachycephaly, causing me to think that to have a baby by someone with such a wide head would entail a very difficult delivery. (Apparently I was unconsciously thinking ahead, but in the event we had only one child with a head shaped like his father's, and the children were all, in any case, by section.) I didn't notice his limp that evening, but we were sitting most of the time.

At the convocation, we were told that, unlike the practice at most medical schools, Hopkins had not offered us a place in the class to wash out a certain percentage. They had confidence in us and intended to graduate us all. If we had problems, we were advised to seek help.

As Chuck told me later, he looked at me, and it was the proverbial "love at first sight", a concept I had always considered apocryphal. (Infatuation, yes, but how could you love anyone you didn't even know?) All he had to go on was my blond hair, high cheekbones, good figure, and animated conversation. He explained later that what he liked was my "childlikeness", in contrast to "childishness". He found me not "childish" but full of wonder, alert, and eager to observe and learn new things. Still, his love at first sight was not just a transient infatuation but endured not only the three years it took me to mature to the point of marriage-readiness but also the fifty-five years of our marriage, including the difficult times we had with our children (see *A Handful of Ashes* and *Fighting the Good Fight*).

Over the years I have realized and appreciated how lucky I was, considering the fact that in the mid-20th century intelligent girls were coached in how to hide our intelligence from men because most men, including intelligent ones, considered intelligence a male prerogative. And I knew I would need a husband of high intelligence.

Chuck disliked anatomy, considered it a waste of time for someone not oriented to surgery, and failed it the first year. After passing the test in the fall, he said, "I could have failed it again."

As medical school progressed, Chuck and I had many opportunities to get to know each other because our rotations were determined alphabetically, and my surname was Decker. We were one table apart on cadavers.

Soon he began courting me. It was apparent that he was not deterred by anything he learned about me as we came to know each other better. He illustrated the principle of showing love by doing all the little and big, kind and helpful things. He would tolerate having my best friend, Iza, along with us on picnics, plays, and lectures at the Homewood campus. It didn't hurt that he had a car, his old Studebaker, and would take us anywhere we wanted to go. Once when we attended some performance in Washington, Iza and I both fell asleep on the way back to Baltimore. Poor Chuck got lost, and we were no help but would wake up every time he passed a certain doughnut factory in his attempts to get us all back to Baltimore. He would invite me to dinner and the ballet because he knew I was relishing my first chance to attend many cultural events in a big city.

At a time when this was perfectly safe, Iza and I, after studying in the evening, would take a walk to discuss what we had learned on the ward. Then we would have a snack. Chuck knew that we often ate a kind of cupcake called Kandy Kakes, one of the line of "Tastykakes". However, as the product was labeled, we called our choice "Tastykakes". So one night Chuck told us he would bring us some, and did, but when we looked at them, we chorused, "But those aren't 'Tastykakes'!"

"Look, it says so right here," he protested, nonplussed. And so we showed him the difference. We wanted the ones with peanut butter and chocolate frosting. Sixty years later these identical "Kandy Kakes" became available in the Cleveland area, made by the same company in Philadelphia.

As he was pleading his case, he told me once, "I love you so much — I just love your blond hair."

"Well, nobody marries me for my blond hair," I let him know. So he went home to ponder that and think up other inducements for marriage. He eventually came up with a prizewinning one.

As we progressed in medical school, we often would drive Chuck's old Studebaker over to the refinery, where hundreds of lights twinkled against the night sky, where we could talk about our lives and plans for the future, and become truly acquainted. I learned of his interest in research that he was already performing in the School of Public Health at Hopkins. He was more than ready for marriage, but I was still growing up, and the question was whether the friendship and respect I felt for him would eventually blossom into love like his for me.

Finally we found ourselves in our third year, and I was still feeling too young for the commitment of marriage. I told him the story of Anne Stubblefield, a friend from St. Joseph (a twin city of my hometown, Benton Harbor) and several years older than I. She was enrolled in the classics department at the Homewood campus of Johns Hopkins. She had graduated from Wellesley, where she eventually realized that she was their "test case" of a student from the small public St. Joseph High School. She would be called into the counselor's office and asked how she was doing. Only later she realized that they must have expected her to find herself in over her depth. By the time she was doing work in Greek classics at the Homewood campus of Hopkins, she was also interested in a young man, whom her family opposed as not at her intellectual level. Her father even tried to break up the romance by working through the Greek professor, offering money for a "scholarship" for her to go to study in Athens, but Anne saw right through that and got married instead.

Finally Chuck's patience with me was wearing thin, and, knowing we were good friends and that I would want the best for him, he asked me, "If you don't want to marry me, would you introduce me to Anne?" (Anne's mother, who had met Chuck on a visit, would have loved that.) This jolted me into awareness that time was no longer on my side, and I should not let this wonderful and loving man slip away in an age when most men, even highly intelligent men, could not tolerate intelligent women, and it would behoove me to stop dragging my feet.

When Chuck realized that loving comments about my appearance did not win me, he played his trump card: "If we get married, we'll go abroad every five years." (This was a time when few people went to Europe even once, and I knew only one person, my aunt's friend Evelyn Pratt, who had crossed the Atlantic twenty-eight times.) Chuck's idea captivated me, and I told him I would call my mother to get the church. That was in our third year, with one year left to graduation.

We became engaged on April 17, and our wedding was June 17, with my mother getting the First Baptist Church in St. Joseph (in which I grew up) and doing all the onsite work, including handwritten invitations (which I considered the elegant way to go). Mother's Day came in between, and a simple Mother's Day card that, without my knowledge, Chuck sent my mother won her heart. She always loved her son-in-law. Having wished for a son for many years, she finally got a noble one.

My father was opposed to my marriage. He threatened to cut off my support for my final year of medical school, but my father-in-law-to-be, knowing that his son needed an intelligent, well-educated wife, offered to borrow against his pension to pay my final tuition. My father came around in time.

Since I have never cared for diamonds, and since, at the advice of an older artist friend in Europe, Chuck had bought for his future bride a museum piece, a belt of black silk and silver from the Caucasus, that was my engagement gift. (That artist had also painted a portrait of Chuck in army uniform for him to give to his mother. That portrait is in this volume.)

We had just two months to prepare for the wedding. I found a beautiful Swiss organdy cocktail-length dress, which I was able to wear to parties for many years, and borrowed my Aunt Bide's sapphire necklace for the occasion. I wanted none of the trappings of female submissiveness, such as a veil, or being "given away" like chattel from one man (father) to another (husband-to-be), or the usual array of attendants. Chuck's little eight-year-old nephew, Bobby, served as acolyte and lighted candles at twilight all around the periphery, and Chuck's sister-in-law, Gloria, a professional contralto, sang "Some Enchanted Evening" from *South Pacific.* During this music, Chuck walked diagonally across the church and escorted me back to the altar for the ceremony. We recited, did not repeat, our vows, which we wrote. I have never seen a wedding more beautiful.

Because of the seventeens involved (I later learned from my calculus teacher that seventeen is special for several reasons, one being that a seventeen-sided figure can be drawn with only compass and straightedge), Chuck considered the seventeenth of each month our "monthiversary" and gave me a red rose each time it came around. After several years I suggested he stop lest this custom become a burden rather than a happy expression of love.

Chuck's idea had been to take a summer job at the Center for Communicable Diseases in Atlanta, where he had worked the previous summer, and set aside some money for future needs (or opportunities), but I wanted my first taste of Europe. I pointed out that we would not have any appreciable vacation time for the foreseeable future, but we could expect soon to be earning a reasonable income, so the sensible thing would be to travel now. I was already employing a rule I later formulated: maximize the commodity in shortest supply. In this case that commodity was time, the last long vacation for several years. (This rule and others are collected in "Denko's Rules of Living" in the companion book.) And so he cashed in his war bonds, and we planned our summer in Europe.

In an age when we in this country feared the Russians (and even those of Russian parentage), we had passport problems. Mine came in good time, but Chuck's was delayed. His lawyer friend advised that he write to explain that he was not and had never been a Communist and had been offered the rank of major if he had stayed in the army. I thought that was stupid because if they wanted to think he was a spy, how would that persuade them otherwise? (When he minored in history and was a champion debater in college, someone from the FBI offered him a job. It amused me to think of this honest, straightforward man as a spy. I always said that he couldn't spy his way out of a paper bag.) Nonetheless that lawyer's strategy may have worked because Chuck's passport arrived in the final mail on our wedding day.

We headed out to New York to board a Norwegian ship that our interns and medical students group had chartered, but the Coast Guard declared it unsafe as it did not have enough fire extinguishers. We were fortunate to be staying with those friends of Chuck's, the Bouquets, and not using up our travel money on expensive hotels. Chuck and I were interviewed on television about the hundreds of students in New York waiting for a ship. To meet our need, our organization's president contacted President Harry Truman, who made available to us the S.S. *Ballou,* an army transport ship that was going over empty to bring home personnel who had earned their discharge. This ship had been used for trials of Dramamine for motion sickness because she rolled and pitched and yawed worse than any other. Chuck was seasick on the crossing but happy to be married and happy to be making me happy. I was also happy to be married and about to enjoy my first step onto European soil. As the ship ploughed on to Rotterdam, I took Dutch lessons onboard. The teacher praised my accent, which we attributed to my having heard Dutch from listening to all four grandparents speak it so my cousins and I wouldn't understand. I had never learned to speak it because my grandfather was intimidated to try to take on the respected role of teacher when I asked him to teach me Dutch.

To my astonishment and delight, the first name on the passenger manifest was that of another medical student, my high school debate partner and salutatorian[1] Art Ablin. He and Chuck struck up a lifelong friendship. The boys ate smoked eel together from street vendors (I couldn't stand the smell), and we went around together through Holland.

Europe was absolutely flat from the war, and we saw nine countries in eleven weeks on five dollars a day. We stayed in student dormitories (with cold showers), rode to Vienna with older friends in their rented car, and visited many churches and museums I wanted to see. I loved it when they called me Madame. In those days Europeans appreciated Americans. Chuck showed me places he had worked or visited in the Occupation, such as the concentration camp at Dachau, which he had visited before the ashes had been cleaned out of the ovens and the sign had read WASH YOUR HANDS AFTER WORK; CLEANLINESS IS YOUR DUTY. We stayed in the Salzburg Schloss and went to the Festival, where we saw the medieval morality play *Jedermann* performed on the cathedral steps, and heard Schwartzkopf sing in *Fidelio* before she became known in our country. The year being 1950, an even decade, Oberammergau had reinstituted its centuries-old Passion Play, for which I had secured tickets before we left home. Chuck and I laughed over how I would say, "I want to go to ___________" and he would figure out how to get us there. He took me to Lugano, a tranquil Alpine town and lake, where they were celebrating Swiss Independence Day on August 1 with the most beautiful fireworks I have ever seen. We joked that I ate my weight in wienerschnitzel that summer (many years before I began boycotting veal because of cruel farm practices). I noticed that I was learning how to travel from an expert, including such conveniences as staying at the Hotel Terminus in each city to be in the center of activity and for easy arrival and departure on trains. (Later I made sure that we took our children, not only to see the world but also to learn how to travel intelligently, as I had from Chuck.) We started collecting small countries, in this case Liechtenstein (later Andorra, San Marino, Vatican City, and Monaco). I wrote postcards to thank people for wedding gifts.

By fall we had to head back home for my mother's delicious vegetable soup and to begin our last year of medical school.

JDD

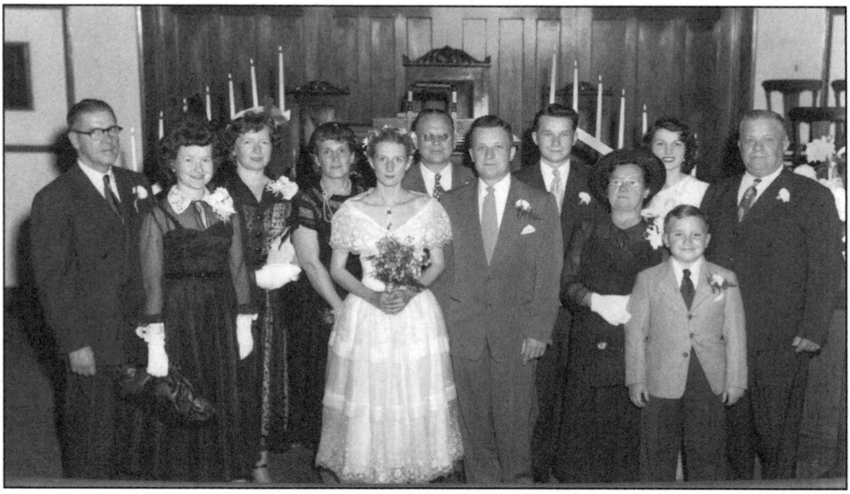

Charles and Joanne's wedding, with John and Marian Decker, Wasil and Evdokiya Denko, Munya and Paul Lyttle, John and Gloria Denko, Helen Denko Muller, and Bobby Lyttle, June 17, 1950.

Note

1. I was the valedictorian, and so was Chuck in his class. We were once invited to a dinner and Bach concert by Benedict Schneider (a cardiologist) and Genevieve Moller (a medical historian). At the table we discovered that all four had been valedictorians.

"A Friend Remembers"

I asked Iza Aldon Salman, my friend from medical school, to write a vignette because she is one of our oldest friends. She modestly declined but wrote:

> As for writing a vignette about Chuck, I don't feel qualified, but I admire your effort to commit it all on paper. I remember Chuck as *smart, friendly, easy to be with* [emphasis hers], and I am grateful to him for allowing me to join you and him on all those outings. After all, you were dating and he could have been jealous and uncooperative. Why don't you write something like "A friend remembers" and quote (and paraphrase) me? I don't have enough for a vignette.

That I have done.

Iza might have told about our picnics out at the state hospital where we studied the elderly patients and their decades-long charts. I even saw a chronic schizophrenic patient living out her life at the hospital, with a progress note by Osler.

Iza also could have told how, for fun, she and Chuck would converse back and forth in Polish and Russian, the languages close enough for understanding though written in Latin and Cyrillic alphabets respectively.

Chapter VI

Years of Training

Our final year of medical school rushed past. Chuck had acute appendicitis but in three days was carrying groceries home to our apartment. We each had a free quarter, and Chuck used his to continue his research at the School of Public Health (reference 9 in his bibliography). I spent mine at the University of Chicago and stayed with the Sandalises, who lived nearby. On my return, however, I was found to have a benign tumor on one ovary and underwent surgery. In addition to our clinical studies and our applications for internships, we had not only finals to prepare for but also boards. They were advised to take state, not national, boards. (This was bad advice because we had to get reciprocity repeatedly as we moved from state to state, and we had to pay either by reexamination or by shakedown.) We took the boards right after finals but had to review our basic sciences from two and more years back. I dreamed of some year enjoying the month of May without the pressure of examinations.

Both of us were accepted for internships at the University of Illinois Research and Education Hospital in Chicago on the near west side. It was a relief to pack everything we owned into Chuck's old Studebaker and head west. Since they had no rooming arrangements for married interns, we shared Chuck's room. (I had been assigned one in the nurses' quarters.) Intern's salary there was fifteen dollars per month plus room and board. For the next few years after our internship, we rented an apartment from a friend, Dick Young, the Anglican priest for the medical center. It was above his little chapel. Years later when I went through old checks, I found that our main expenses those years were for keeping Chuck's Studebaker running and for occasional concert tickets. When we both had the same weekend free, we would travel eighty-five miles around the south end of Lake Michigan to visit my parents north of Benton Harbor, Michigan. Usually on the Saturday night we would go to the Whitcomb Hotel in St. Joe, where very funny Jewish comedians tried out their acts before taking them on the borsch circuit in the Poconos, and I drank "pink squirrels" for the nut flavor in the grenadine. It is hard to imagine myself, after a week of work on the wards with call every second or third night, having enough energy left to go dancing on Saturday, but Chuck, even with his bad leg, loved dancing. My mother worked to feed and rest us before we had to return to the hospital on Sunday.

After a year of internship, I stayed on at Illinois for a year of pathology, but was floundering, unsure of a career or what to do next. While pondering, I worked as a pediatrician for the city of Chicago in well-baby clinics, in a private cancer-prevention clinic, and for three years in radiation research at the University of Chicago Argonne Cancer Research Laboratories (see the first three articles in my bibliography in the companion book).

By then, soon after internship, we moved to the south side, close to the University of Chicago, where we were both working. Chuck, already almost thirty-five when he received his M.D., was moving ahead as a resident in medicine at the University of Chicago. As a chemist, he took pride in the fact that while he could not save all his patients, they never died in electrolyte imbalance. He was meeting and working with people like Allan Kenyon (endocrinologist), Charlie Huggins (urologist who had won a Nobel Prize), and Del Bergenstal (who died, tragically, within a few years). From Del, Chuck learned to work with S^{35}, newly available from radiation research, for medical research, in studying cartilage in rats. Chuck always believed that, had he lived, Del would have won the Prize.

In the course of their research, Chuck went out to the prison at Joliet to draw blood from inmate volunteers for studies. (This practice has subsequently been considered unethical. I could not and cannot understand why. The detainees were paid, although not much, were not pressured, and had few other ways to earn a few dollars or contribute to society, and their doing so would be a helpful point at parole hearings.) At Joliet Chuck met Loeb of the notorious Leopold and Loeb duo who had killed a ten-year-old boy for thrills, and had been defended by Clarence Darrow. Leopold died young in prison. Loeb was the passive follower in the crime, and, although sentenced to life without parole, was released toward the end of his life. He spent his prison time working in the laboratory and assisted Chuck with his blood collection. (The story of Leopold and Loeb's crime is told in the novel *Compulsion* by Meyer Levin, the husband of Tereska Teres, friend of Izabella Aldon, my friend in medical school.)

Two radioactive bombs having recently put an end to deaths of American soldiers (and of Japanese military personnel and civilians), Chuck was the resident when Enrico Fermi was treated for malignancy and, depressed and unhappy over his role in developing the atomic bomb, gave up the struggle to survive. Chuck supported the grieving widow, Laura Fermi. Fermi's chief resident, husband of Jean Betty Clough, a friend of mine from Higman Park, was also a friend of ours in that stimulating University of Chicago society. He was the first casualty of berylliosis, which afflicted some working with radioactivity.

A more joyful patient was also on Chuck's service, the gospel singer Mahalia Jackson. When she was discharged, she put on a special concert for the medical personnel who had helped her. After innumerable encores, when it appeared that they would never stop calling her back, she marched out singing her signature hymn, *When the Saints Go Marching In.* To this day, whenever I try to make overtures to someone black, I manage to drop mention that my late husband treated Mahalia. I invariably detect an immediate surge of respect.

He was also on the service to which the chancellor of the university was admitted for his annual checkup. All the senior staff were reluctant and embarrassed to do the customary rectal examination on this VIP. Chuck, however, performed the rectal, reasoning that the chancellor deserved as good care as was given to the homeless brought in off the streets. The members of the wives' club (I was a member) and their spouses were invited to a potluck at the chancellor's house to observe (and play with) his miniature train hobby taking up the entire attic, but I don't think the chancellor remembered Chuck.

One other project Chuck took on while at Chicago: teaching himself how to invest. He credited his father with advising him to institute a savings plan of 10 percent from his first paycheck. He and his friend Bob Priest spent their lunch hours investing on paper only, buying and selling stocks with $10,000 of play money, paying commissions, studying annual reports, and honing a strategy for buying high-quality securities, often pharmaceuticals with a promising drug in the pipeline. After a year the friends began real purchases — odd lots at first. This evolved into our savings program for our sons' education and our financial future, tossing the certificates into the box, holding, and letting them have babies in the form of dividends at first, later splits. At first it would surprise me when dividend checks arrived. I would say something like, "Hey, we got a check in the mail. Let's go to the movies." Chuck would give me a disgusted look (meaning that I should have known it was coming), but we would go. Later we switched to dividend reinvestment, thus saving commissions. We bought stocks for the boys with the intention that, should they decide to pursue low-paying but socially useful careers, their incomes would be augmented. Chuck kept track of all this at the cost of about an hour a week, usually on Wednesday evening, when I was at Great Books. We had forty years of mostly bull market working for us. We were audited by the IRS several times, and once, in a hearing, Chuck fought the IRS to a draw. Before companies were required to withhold tax, while Chuck was still preparing our tax forms, we were among the 20 percent of stockholders who actually paid tax on dividends. Saving was never difficult because we did not have expensive tastes, like smoking, drinking, and high-end restaurants and nightclubs — with one exception: travel. Chuck was so good at this "buy and hold" strategy that two brokerages even offered him jobs. Our accountant said that he had had only two other clients who had used this strategy to build estates. Now this method is no longer possible, the "securities" market having become a worldwide casino.

While we were still in Chicago, a request came from the Walter Reed Army Medical Museum in Bethesda, Maryland, for Chuck's photograph (see vignette "Bachrach" and portrait on dust jacket).

When nutrition was recognized as a specialty, he was grandfathered into the American Board of Nutrition as a diplomate (see vignette "Work in Nutrition").

By the mid-1950s, Chuck secured a position as assistant professor in the Division of Rheumatology at the University of Michigan and began establishing his place in that wide-open subspecialty and one to which hundreds of thousands of sufferers were turning for help.

During our time in Chicago I had completed a classical psychoanalysis, decided on a career in psychiatry, and was accepted in Michigan's residency program, where I signed on for both the residency and a special degree they offered, an M.S. in psychiatry. To earn the latter I would attend seminars that all the residents attended, but augmented by special papers by the M.S. candidates; other credits were required in cognates (sociology, anthropology, psychology in literature, and, one of my favorite courses ever, history of science). Finally I would need to perform research leading to a dissertation. The four of us in the program would sign out to our fellows, walk across the campus for these various other courses, and have an interesting and stimulating time.

When we went to Michigan, my cousin Eunice Lampkin's husband had just graduated from Michigan's medical school. For their time at Michigan they had built a house near Dexter, which we bought. We commuted daily to work at University Hospital, following the Grand River, in the shallow waters of which we often saw standing sandhill cranes. Behind that house we had a field where, one day, I stepped on a coiled snake, which gave me a disgusted look for my clumsiness. One night I spotted a brilliant comet subtending sixty degrees of arc. I had not heard about it on the news, and I have subsequently been unable to identify that brilliant spectacle. In Dexter we were still close enough to my parents' home to use it for occasional weekends of R&R.

On another trip we tracked down a group working the Cleveland/Lloyd Dinosaur Quarry in Utah and helped them under their enormous beach umbrella. I sifted tailings and found an allosaurus tooth, which they let me keep because they always find more teeth than they can use. Chuck carted away wheelbarrows of rubble. We followed a meeting in Toronto with a camping trip across Canada to Lake Louise and the Athabasca Glacier, onto which we rode several miles in a vehicle on caterpillar treads.

All these years we had been working on my obstetrical problem. After one disappointing pregnancy early in our Chicago time and no further pregnancies for several years, I sought help from Dr. Alan Guttmacher, our obstetrics professor in medical school, who had offered me a residency. The solution he suggested was special plastic surgery performed by only one gynecologist in the world, Dr. David B. Davis, at Columbia/Presbyterian in New York. And so I underwent that surgery by that talented and compassionate physician. He solved that problem, but different problems ensued. While still at Michigan, we lost one little stillborn girl. A later preemie, John, who at two pounds was too immature to survive even in an Isolette, died the day he was born, and is buried in Ann Arbor. I had more surgery for my new problem, premature births resulting from inability to carry to term.

The time had come for Chuck to look for a new faculty position, and one was offered at Ohio State University. We were preparing to move when little John was born and died. Therefore I stayed to close up our Dexter house and, with the help of my mother, come to terms with the loss and the move. Chuck went ahead to start at Ohio State and find us a house. At OSU he began training intelligent bored housewives (whose children were launched) who wanted to do something significant, to handle, inject, and care for rats for his studies. Knowing that I needed/wanted country living with water because that was how I had grown up, and the way one grows up always feels the most like home, Chuck, like his father, trying to accommodate his wife's tastes and wishes, found a beautiful pinkish-gray stone house built into a hillside, with a dammed stream and an enormous sycamore and three acres of land at 3589 Watt Road, Gahanna, with Blendon Woods State Park five miles away. (I loved that home as much as I loved my childhood home until I was eight, built into a hillside and overlooking Lake Michigan.)

I transferred my residency to OSU with arrangements with the kind people at Michigan to finish my M.S. at a distance by writing term papers for courses I had not finished because of the premature birth. I still lacked a dissertation when I happened to be assigned a patient with seizures and severe retardation. On examining her, I noted tetanic spasms of the muscles of her face when I touched her, ordered serum calcium and phosphorus, and diagnosed idiopathic hypoparathyroidism. She responded so quickly to treatment that in two days she was playing Ping-Pong on the ward. When we were asked to present this case at medical grand rounds (psychiatry didn't usually attend), in the course of my presentation a latecomer took a seat beside Chuck and whispered, "Who's that girl presenting the case?" With his quick wit, Chuck adapted the old joke as he replied, "Why, that's no girl. That's my wife!" I used this case as a launching pad, surveyed the world literature for other cases of her condition to see whether they displayed psychiatric features, and wrote up my findings, which were published, with my chief, Rudolf Kaelbling, as a monograph supplement to *Acta Psychiatrica Scandinavica,* and hence my first freestanding "book". Thus I finished my M.S. in psychiatry.

Not long after our move, another rabbit said yes. By prior planning with my new obstetrician, I put my remaining few months of residency on hold, went on bed rest with a housekeeper/caretaker, and settled in for the eight months remaining, my only "outings" being trips to the obstetrician. Chuck offered as much help as possible, working on papers at home evenings and weekends.

It was a monotonous and worrisome eight months, and we had decided that, if unsuccessful, it would be our last attempt. I recall thinking that I would never have believed that constant reading could be anything but glorious, but despite the variety (among others I read a four-volume history of mathematics), I fantasized doing alternate days, one reading, the second active, because, of course, once the pregnancy was finished, there would be no reading days, only active days, with or without a baby.

Others helped, by visiting me. My "bed rest" did not mean, literally, me under sheets. I spent days on a couch in the family room of that strange and wonderful old house. One hot Sunday afternoon in August, friends came to visit, followed by an adorable black-and-white half-grown spaniel puppy. Once they were settled, I asked whether we should give their dog a dish of water.

"*Our* dog? We thought she was *your* dog. She followed us in."

In this way she became our first dog, Cleo, of four we acquired that way. She could open doors with doorknobs. We found homes for dozens of other dogs, abandoned at the end of Watt Road, and, in some cases, their puppies.

We finally had the formula, bed rest that permitted this fourth pregnancy to go to term, a planned section, and our eldest surviving child, Christopher, born December 20, 1960, ten years into our marriage. We carried home this perfect seven-pound three-ounce newborn, wrapped in a carriage robe, a gift crocheted by our friend Dorothy Gage, and swimming in a baby boy suit, size six months, that I sent Chuck out to buy, since I had been unable and unwilling to prepare for another possible disappointment. A snowfall had made our long driveway impassable, and we had to walk the final third. When we put Christopher into his crib, Cleo saw her role and her responsibility and positioned herself under the crib.

More than any other event — single or married, this school or that, one or other career, this continent or another — having a child changes your life forever.

Bachrach

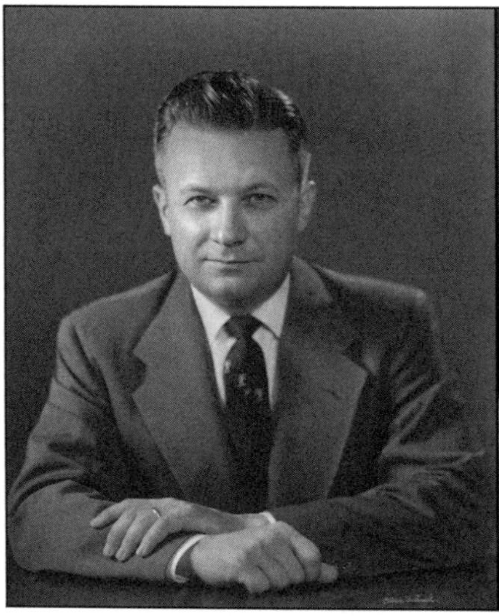

Chuck, age forty, in business suit.

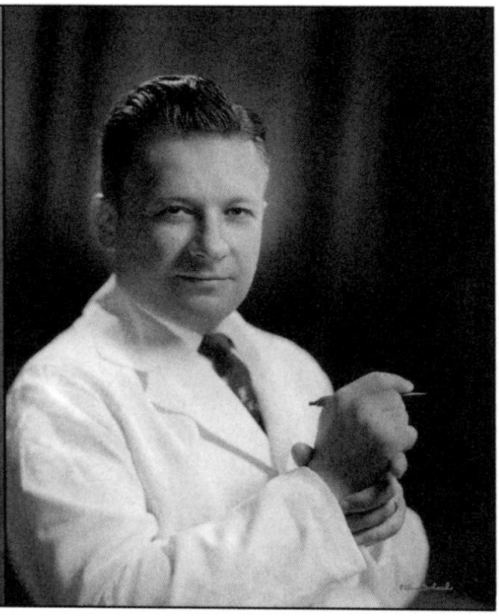

Dr. Denko in lab coat.

Early in Chuck's time at the University of Chicago, he received a letter from the Walter Reed Army Medical Museum in Bethesda, Maryland (now the Walter Reed Army Medical Center), requesting a portrait. He was told that it was to be one in a collection of four hundred who had made significant contributions to medicine, going back to Paracelsus. This was evidently a result of his work on army rations on healthy volunteers (see bibliography items 3 through 8).

I decided that this called for the finest photographer available, and that, in Chicago, was Bachrach. We had the portraits taken, one in a white coat for the Walter Reed collection, the other in a business suit for relatives.

Two Bargainers in Haiti

In our early years of marriage Joanne and I visited the Caribbean. Of all the independent countries, territories, dependencies of all kinds, we found Haiti the most interesting by being the most exotic, culturally different from ourselves, and, unfortunately after almost 150 years of independence, poverty-stricken and dictator-driven.[1]

One morning we walked from our little hotel along open gutters flowing with sewage, to the downtown, looking for sights, souvenirs, and local activity. The harbor area was the poorest we had ever seen, with shacks built on mounds of rubbish and coconut husks, and constructed of cardboard boxes and flattened gallon tins.

The activity center, however, seemed to be an open market, called the Fer Merchand from the fact that its support structure was composed of iron filigree. The many booths offered the local shoppers, dressed in bright skirts and blouses in red and blue and other primary colors, kitchen and household items, piles of shoes, dresses and infants' wear, tropical fruits and vegetables, meats with flies foraging on the surface, and colorful fish from the ocean.

We were drawn to a section featuring woodcarvings that would make good souvenirs and mementoes of the trip. After pricing the goods at several booths (nothing, of course, carried a price tag), we found carved heads with hair in the style from colonial days and entered into negotiations with the saleslady of that booth. We good-naturedly made bids and counter bids (in simple French), finally agreed on a price, and bought two. She was so pleased with the deal that she threw in a carved fish as a sign that I was a gentleman she liked to do business with.

Back at the hotel, we showed our finds to fellow travelers,

one of whom asked to be taken to the booth the next day to get one like ours. But on arrival we were disappointed to find the booth closed, curtain pulled down, not a sign of commercial activity. Puzzled, I asked her friend in the adjoining booth when she would be back.

"Ah, m'sieu, you have not heard. Madame had such a good day yesterday — she even gave a fish to the customer for good luck — and took the day off for holiday."

CWD

Note

1. Pan American, an airline that later went out of business, had offered a trip around the large islands of the Caribbean, with option to stay however long one wished at the various stops before continuing to the next. My parents spent winters in Miami, and we suggested that they accompany us. My mother, however, disliked heat and tropics, and they soon went on ahead of us. My mother said that Miami never looked good except when approached from the south. This trip was in the late pre-Castro days, and we had stops in both Havana and Camaguey, Cuba; Puerto Rico; Dominican Republic; both Kingston and Montego Bay, Jamaica; and (not in that order) Port-au-Prince, Haiti. In fact, when we flew from Port-au-Prince to clean, prosperous Kingston, Chuck made his most trenchant remark of the trip: "Haiti is the best advertisement for the British Empire."

Denko Life in Franklin County

Chapter VII

Tom Sawyer Life on Watt Road

With Christopher's birth, our life as a two-generation family was launched. My mother's visit, to help us get started, was the first of many. Whenever she came, I would move out of the kitchen, but this time she helped us transition to a family with a baby. As an only child, I was completely inexperienced with babies, having had no one to watch or practice on. Although I had worked with newborns and infants in medical school and for the city of Chicago, that was medical, not parental, care. Before the corrective surgery on his leg, as Chuck's siblings came along, he had been so severely crippled that it was all he could do to get himself around, not to mention helping with younger children.

My milk was slow in coming (because I had not gone into labor with the change in hormones, having been sectioned), but I was determined to give my infant the advantage of my antibodies. Knowing that since he weighed over seven pounds, his masseter muscles were strong enough for a good sucking reflex, I made sure that he was well hydrated with water but let him become hungry while we learned to cooperate on his first task: working for his dinner. (Helped by maternal antibodies, he had a very healthy childhood.)

Mrs. Bokros, who had worked for us during the pregnancy, continued to care for Christopher when I returned to complete my fragmented residency. She was kind and loving and always good for a malapropism. She told us that her nerves were "all in a fragile" and that she was "a nervous wretch". She seemed comfortably relaxed to me.

Between patients, I would go to the lounge and pump milk to refrigerate and take home for Mrs. B to give Cricket, as she called him, the next day. She often took him to be with her older children while she caught up on her own household duties.

Christopher was not on a good (for us) sleep schedule from the start. He would sleep all afternoon, then stay awake after his evening feeding when I would rock him, trying to get him to sleep. But every time I would lay him down, his enormous blue eyes would pop open and he would cry. I favored letting him cry himself to sleep. Actually, the pediatrician recommended this, but Chuck could not tolerate his crying and would patiently rock him until the wee hours of the morning, when Christopher would finally give up. (Now that Christopher has an infant daughter, Emily Rose, he reports that he cannot let her cry more than five minutes, just like his father.)

During this time in the Columbus area, Chuck continued his S^{35} studies on rat cartilage, saw private patients and patients in the rheumatology clinic at Ohio State, and lectured to students and residents.

Before completing my residency, I had converted our long, old-fashioned porch into an office and waiting room, where I soon began seeing a few patients, evenings, while Chuck cared for the baby. Anyone who really wanted privacy about consulting a psychiatrist really had it for a short drive into the country, since our house, at the end of the road, was even hidden from the road by the hill into which it was built. One patient in a branch of the armed services was so afraid of what seeing me might do to his career that he came under an assumed name and a different branch of service (what did I know about uniforms?) and always paid in cash. His case was so interesting that at Chuck's suggestion I later wrote him up for publication, coining the term "klismaphilia" for habituation to erotic enemas, a term that continues to be used in psychiatry (see my references in the companion book).

Another failed early pregnancy left us surmising that Christopher might be an only child. However, a European Congress of Rheumatology called for papers for a meeting in Rome; my mother came again to care for Christopher, and Chuck and I boarded ship for Europe. There Chuck presented his findings on S^{35} uptake in rats' cartilage. A representative from a Swiss drug firm, Robapharm, sought Chuck out to ask whether he would be interested in studying the effects of their product, Rumalon, in rats. He did, and the results were so compelling that Robapharm sent us to Santiago, Chile, for Chuck to report his findings and even paid for a week for us in the Chilean Volcanic Andes in the south. Chuck continued to work with Rumalon for several years (see vignette "The Rumalon Story").

I was beginning to see how we were implementing Chuck's "Five Year Plan".

My mother told about taking Christopher to a new bank branch opening with cake and punch. He evidently caught the word "bank" and, standing with hands behind him and feet wide apart, looked up at and told the manager, "I'm a bank wobbah!"

On plane trips we flew separately lest a crash should orphan Christopher. We also wrote wills, including the provision that in the event of our early deaths, Chuck's brother John and his wife Gloria would adopt Christopher.

Yet another bleeding pregnancy caused us to consider canceling a meeting (and Chuck's paper) in Aix-les-Bains, a spa in France. However, it was because that pregnancy was considered already doomed that we took the overnight train to New York to board ship, while I was still giving myself daily shots of progesterone, the only treatment thought possibly helpful, sometimes, in stabilizing a shaky pregnancy. (Trying to save the pregnancy, and successfully so, I was nevertheless living with the knowledge that if the embryo I was carrying should survive and be a girl, she might be born with a condition called adrenogenital syndrome, with its own problems, caused by progesterone taken by the pregnant mother. We were all doubly lucky, therefore, to have a live, healthy boy.) Miraculously, the bleeding gradually slowed and finally stopped. For the stabilizing effect I credited the ship's lovely rocking motion (I felt as though sleeping on a giant's breathing chest). Chuck did not find ocean travel "lovely rocking motion", but, even battling seasickness, he loved travel at sea for its resort-like features, good food, lectures, games, generally being taken care of, and arriving rested. When the captain asked me to dance, I had to explain my precarious condition.

We found ourselves in Europe with a pregnancy and a Eurail pass. Before returning home, we visited the prehistoric art cave at Altamira, Spain, the first ever discovered, before they began barring tourists because of the damage to the art from the exhaled carbon dioxide. We therefore had been privileged to see the original, not the replica they have now built. On arriving home I greeted my sister-in-law, Helen, who had been taking care of Christopher, with the news that I was pregnant again and went back on bed rest, while finding another housekeeper/caretaker for me. Six months later, on December 21, 1964, we were rewarded with Nicholas.

When I went in for the section for Nicholas, I took a copy of *Alice in Wonderland,* annotated by a mathematician, who related the story to the author's professional interest. It happened that I had never read this child's classic because when my favorite aunt, Bide, gave it to me, my mother, who preferred realistic stories, exchanged it for another. And so I finally caught up with this gap in my education. I had to explain it to the nurses. But that was trivial compared to my similar hospitalization for Christopher's birth. On that occasion I was knitting a rose-colored sweater for Sybil, our black, shorthaired dog, who got very cold when she had to go out in winter. The nurses gave that sweater a very quizzical look until I explained.

Because Christopher was so active and required such constant watching that it felt to me as if he "commandeered" time that should have been shared with his baby brother, and because we thought he would benefit by playing with his agemates, I found him a preschool at Otterbein College. I was right about his need for play. His teacher called him and three other little boys the Four Musketeers. And this gave baby Nicholas and me quiet mother/child prime time together.

Nineteen months later and after eight months' more bed rest, on July 28, 1966, Timothey, our youngest son and final child was born. All three boys were named for their father, Charles being the middle name of each.

Life with small children restricted my time in psychiatric practice, but I expanded my efforts in the direction of writing, mostly journal articles for the next few years. I also freelanced a few articles, such as a travel piece on Russia, for the *Kansas City Star,* and I wrote an article on teaching children about nature with illustrations (e.g., of Christopher and a bush duiker kissing each other through the fence at the zoo), published in *National Wildlife* in February 1964, pp. 44–46. See article quoted in companion book. (How I used what psychiatric practice and family life gave me as grist for my literary mill is told in "About the Author" in *Envy.*)

When Nicholas was not even three, at the Gahanna Community Church we had joined, where all three were baptized (with Aunt Dorothy Gage as godmother), the nursery teacher called me in to advise me that he was nearsighted. "He's a bright child who's not seeing. When I hold up a picture, he runs up and puts his face right up to it. I have a nearsighted son too — that's how I knew." While waiting for his glasses, I too recognized Nicholas's efforts to see. The day we put the heavy glasses on his nubbin of a nose, I choked back tears. He, on the other hand, danced happily down the steps from the doctor's office, and, it being Presidents' Day, asked, "Why are those dots on the flag?" He never had to be told to put on his glasses. He later told me that he had thought that trees looked fuzzy to everyone. (See my poem "Spectacles" in *Into a Mirror and Through a Lens.*) At three, Timothey followed his brother into glasses.

I had an only-girl's romantic idea of motherhood as all loving and sharing and teaching, but several potentially fatal incidents quickly disabused me of this idea and made me realize that motherhood was not the idyllic paradise I had expected. When I was the adult in charge, I found myself tense until they were all asleep at night, at which time I usually fell asleep exhausted too (see vignette "Close Calls").

When Christopher was almost eight and old enough to benefit by educational travel, Chuck submitted a paper to the Pan American Congress meeting in Mexico City. Chuck's sister, Helen, came to care for the two others. (Years later, when Christopher was with us on an eclipse trip in the Sea of Cortez, on the ship he spotted a picture of the Pyramid of the Sun near Mexico City and remembered my taking him there on the wives' excursion.) After the meeting we boarded a bus for Merida in the Yucatan to see Chichen Itza and Uxmal. As Christopher ran up and down the steep steps without handrails, I questioned the wisdom of having brought him, until he made it back down safely. We had intended to go also to Palenque, a larger, well-documented ruin, but as we approached the ticket window, they were posting a sign that the train was canceled due to flooding in the jungle.

We lived in that rural paradise long enough for Christopher to complete second grade in Westerville. When a flyer came home from school about a program sponsored by the YMCA, we thought it would be good for Christopher and so Chuck and Christopher, as Red Chief, joined Indian Guides. Thereby they socialized with other fathers and sons, visited nearby Indian mounds and flint quarries (Ohio's state stone). The group tried to teach amenities, and this included written invitations to meetings. Copying what he had seen at the rheumatology banquet in Mexico City, Christopher printed the menu for each member: Kool-Aid, cookies. Later in Rocky River, he printed invitations in dark blue marker on pieces of gray shale from the beach.

Christopher played with a neighborhood boy, running through the fields and catching pollywogs in the stream in spring. One March 29 (my birthday and easy to remember), I showed him a tangle of tiny garter snakes emerging from an abandoned duck house where they had overwintered. To this day he recalls that Tom Sawyer childhood with nostalgia and acknowledges that he had the benefit of the Gahanna experience that his brothers were too young to share. I wish they all could have enjoyed it.

Chuck had one rural experience he would have been happy to miss. I saw a snake in our basement climbing up a water pipe. When Chuck got home, I had to ask him to catch and release the unintentional trespasser, which he accomplished in a large wastebasket.

Chuck's career path was blocked at OSU, and he needed to find another appointment. This resulted in his accepting an offer to run a small research unit at Fairview General Hospital in Cleveland, where he would also see patients two half days a week and take on academic duties at Case Western Reserve University. During the spring of 1968 he commuted the 125 miles one day a week to set up his lab in his new research unit, start ordering supplies, hire a secretary and a lab technician, and find us a house. Knowing I had grown up on the shore of Lake Michigan, he found a house on a cliff overlooking Lake Erie, therefore on the northern border of the lower forty-eight, just a few miles east of the border's southernmost dip. When he showed me this house and two others, I knew it was the one and would make up, in part, for — at least substitute for — the loss of our country life near Columbus. His gentle joke about buying it was that he went to "play Monopoly" with the banker, i.e., take securities out of our box and put them into the bank's. The banker, not a man to mince words, let us know that ours was the third cheapest house on Avalon, one of the other two being a winterized summer cottage. Our savings program made possible this house, which had had to be sold in a divorce case, thus bringing the price down to $67,000, the price we paid for 21160 Avalon Drive, Rocky River, in 1968.

I liked our Gahanna Community Church, where all the boys were baptized. I was a friend of Jean Anderson, a patient of mine whom I had sent as a secretary to Chuck, and she became his gold standard. (He also gave me secretarial time of hers for my writing.) And I loved those three acres with stream and pond and our beautiful old stone house. I loved that house and property so much that if I could have, I would have moved it stone by stone. I couldn't even bear to sell it at first, so we rented it, but finally we had to sell, and I almost cried.

But, like others before us, we were driven out of Eden.

Christmas Cards

The December when Christopher was one year old, we made him a snowman. I photographed him in his sky-blue snowsuit, touching the lowest snowball with a mittened hand and looking up at the snowman's face with awe. I loved this photo, and an idea attacked my brain for the following year: to name the picture "First Christmas" (although it was Christopher's second, as his birthday was December 20), mount it on construction paper, have Chuck, whose printing was beautiful, letter it with the title and our names, and send these out as our Christmas card.

From that year as long as the boys were in elementary school, each year I took a Christmas- or winter-themed photo of one or more of the three, for use the following year. The boys were usually unidentifiable but representative of "Jederkind". One such picture had Christopher and Nicholas on a child's Yukon dogsled, being pulled by Cleo and Sybil, our dogs at the time, entitled "Mush!". I took one of the three boys, with backs to us, looking at an outdoor nativity scene with live animals. Another one used a Salvation Army man with his bucket. One showed a close-up of Nicholas's face examining the china crèche setup my aunt Bide had brought me from Provence, with a dove on the red tile roof, like those in Provence, besides the usual animals. Another one showed Nicholas in his angel costume ready for the church pageant. And there were others.

Many years after we ran out of little kids and went to commercial cards, we happened to attend a meeting in November in Buenos Aires and naturally signed on for the extension to Iguaçu Falls (with falls in Argentina but best view in Brazil) and a side trip into Paraguay. That gave me the idea of sending "pre-Christmas postcards" with, in this case, greetings from the world's widest falls. Our friends loved this, and so I continued for several more years, but I stopped when I became afraid that they might resent us for flaunting our travel. Then I got complaints, "Where are our postcards?" So I returned to them.

Finally I went to annual letters, with postcards any time of year when I had an especially interesting subject. Once I shot a solar eclipse and used that (eclipses are not hard to photograph, as one would expect).

Close Calls

I have never heard of a family of girls in which there were several life-threatening incidents. Nor can I think of another family of boys, in which several incidents broadcast the need for eternal vigilance, lest, within seconds, a child's life could be snuffed out.

But after several of these, I was never completely relaxed while the children were awake.

One early incident occurred when the Schwartzes took Timothey (at eighteen months) along with their family to a swimming pool. Timothey ran and jumped into the deep end of the pool! They, of course, fished him out. I learned of it, fortunately, after the fact.

Timothey was the occasion of another heart-stopping incident, which occurred after we moved to Rocky River. It was on one of our visits to Moll's farm, where Chuck and the boys went fishing. I was sitting with them on the pier. Imagine my horror to see Timothey tumble forward into the pond! Although Christopher relates this differently, the way I remember it is that Chuck immediately reached down into the pond and, at arm's length, caught hold of Timothey's clothes and retrieved him. I don't know how deep the water was. I didn't even have time to start diving in after him, which was what I visualized the rescue attempt would be. Thank God for Chuck's quick thinking and action. Christopher recalls Chuck's angry dressing-down of Timothey for carelessness. Such a reaction would be understandable, although not logical. (How can you blame a toddler for falling off a pier where we should not have had him in the first place?) I was too relieved even to feel guilty until later. Why didn't we think of how dangerous it would be to have our three-year-old on a dock? As an adult he told me he had been trying to see the fish.

I am to blame for another close one with Timothey. Someone

had tied a rope to the branch of a tree at the end of Parklawn, so that one could swing out over the lake and drop in. After warning him to hold on tightly, I let Timothey, at about five, swing out and back. The only possible rationale I can come up with after all these years is that I regretted the fact that, unavoidably because of Chuck's career as a research scientist, the boys could not really grow up in the country and have a "Tom Sawyer childhood" as I had had, and I kept looking for ways to replicate it. As a child, I had climbed trees and, once, an electric pole. (My father came running out in his underpants to get me down, and told the refined elderly neighbor that he would have run out naked if necessary to save me.) My friends, Nancy, Lawrence, and Streeter, and I had swung out over the hillside on thick wild grapevines as we played Tarzan, and I guess I imagined something like that for Tim. My recklessness and folly were not punished.

Once when I was quietly reading in the pediatrician's waiting room, a staff person came to tell me that Nicholas had taken the thermostat off the wall. My mother thought that was a funny one until he took her thermostat off.

Another time I found a toddler (I think Nicholas) peering over the edge of the refrigerator!

Yet another time toddler Nicholas sprinkled black pepper all over the kitchen. I believe it resulted from his poor vision. Chuck would take a deep breath, crawl in, and clean as much of the floor as possible before the next breath.

Often we are told that someone has "saved the best for last". In this case I have saved the worst for last, the one that would surely have killed my son without my quick thinking and intervention. When Christopher was four or five months old and I was bathing and dressing him on the beautiful pink marble with which we had redone the bathroom of the lovely old stone house on Watt Road in Gahanna, he was waving all four extremities, hooked the safety pin on his finger, and rammed it, point first, down his windpipe. I knew that there was no time to get help before he would be asphyxiated by spasm, and so I reached down his trachea and hooked the safety pin by the ring on its blunt end onto my little finger and withdrew it. All this before I broke out in a cold sweat. Christopher was also the child whose little feet were already in motion as I set him on the floor.

Since all these things had happened before the children were five, is it any wonder that I was never completely at ease unless they were asleep? [1]

Note

1. Unlike current practice, I believe children should have a fixed bedtime. They need regular rest. Even more, parents need childfree time for adult conversation and activity.

Christopher's Childhood

The frightening tale of Christopher as a five-month infant jamming a safety pin down his windpipe open-end first, was the first of various incidents that made me less than comfortable in caring for the boys, never knowing what event would demand what response next. (This and other crises are recorded in the vignette "Close Calls".)

When I was again at "bed rest" expecting Nicholas, one summer day Christopher asked me, "What color are rose thorns?"

"We have rose bushes right outside," I told him. "Go and find out."

To my surprise he reported that they were brown. "Go and see whether they are all brown."

His second report was "There are some pink thorns."

Knowing that the growing bush would have an abundance of green thorns, I sent him a third time, and he did return with

"There are also some green ones."

Then I had him identify the parts of the plant in the different growth stages relative to the colors of thorn.

I was happy when the boys asked questions (unless they were questions the answers to which they had already been exposed), but I always expected them to use their own senses to get as far as possible to the answer. They all became good observers and analytic problem solvers.

One happy/funny memory involves my attempt to prepare him for the birth of his sibling, who would be Nicholas. I explained that most people are a mixture of backgrounds — English, German, French, Italian, etc. — but that his father's ancestors were Russian all the way back, and mine Dutch, from the Netherlands. "This makes you, and your little brother or sister, each just half Dutch and half Russian."

The next time I heard the story, Christopher was relating it to our minister at the coffee hour. He concluded: " — and that makes me half Dutch and half Chinese!"

"Tell me more," joked the minister, looking at me and smiling.

I overheard him another time relating how he happened to be punished for some misconduct. That one ended with " — and lost all my privileges", which was my then standard mode of punishment. I didn't hear that line until forty years later, when Nicholas, Karen, Louis, and Jackson were visiting and we were on the beach. Absolutely fearless, little three-and three-quarters-year-old Jackson kept going into deeper water and bigger waves, and Nicholas kept calling him back. Finally, his patience at an end, Nicholas shouted, "That does it! Now you've lost all your privileges!" This brought Jackson back on the next wave. He called Lake Erie "Grandmama's pool" whereas Louis, at four, having seen both Pacific and Atlantic Oceans, called it "Grandmama Joanne's Ocean"! I always wanted an ocean of my own.

Living at the end of Watt Road, one day when returning home from the school bus, Christopher was followed by a lovely young mixed border collie. "Can I keep her, Mom?" he asked. "She likes me."

"We'll have to take her to the veterinarian for her shots," I told him.

"Not until after the puppies are born," the first woman veterinarian from OSU told us.

"The *what*?" I asked the doctor.

"It must have been her first heat period. The shots could injure the puppies."

"Another pregnant adolescent," I muttered.

And so we had to prepare a whelping bed by trimming down the mesh in an old playpen, and I promised to get Christopher home from school when she went into labor. But Whitefoot's timing was perfect on a Saturday morning. Eyes round with wonder, Christopher trotted back and forth with her water bowl to replace lost liquid. Finally after six puppies I thought she was finished when she fell asleep while the puppies suckled. Then another puppy fell out, in a caul, without waking Whitefoot. I taught Christopher how I saved its life by rupturing the membranes, cleaning the fluid around the nostrils, and squeezing its chest rhythmically to initiate breathing. Then I laid it beside a free nipple. Imagine waking up to find you have another infant! (See the poem "Child Midwife" in my *Mirror/Lens* book.)

In this way we acquired our fourth dog, after Cleo, the black-and-white spaniel, and Sybil, the all-black dog who came with a cantaloupe rind in her mouth and a collar almost choking her, and Kevin, a black, white, and beige border collie, who disappeared one night. (Searching the roads of Franklin County for two weeks produced no trace. I think he was taken by someone.)

I worried for six weeks about finding good homes for seven puppies, but my ad was successful. The applicants all passed my dog-adoption qualifications.

Play with Aaron

A mother would willingly take on pain, physical or mental, rather than see her child suffer. Rarely can such a transfer of pain be accomplished.

When Christopher was almost ready for preschool at Otterbein College, I was aware that he needed someone his own size to play with. Although a mother can be a reader and guide, she is only a makeshift substitute for a contemporary.

I knew that he liked and played with a little boy, Aaron, at the nursery at church, and so I invited Aaron and his mother to come one day in late August. Christopher put on his play clothes. He and I had his toys ready. We set the picnic table under the huge tree and prepared the lunch. Christopher was wildly excited, practically jumping out of his skin. "When are they coming? When are they coming?" he kept asking.

"At ten o'clock. When the big hand is on the twelve and the little hand on the ten."

But ten came and went, then 10:15, and 10:30. "I don't know what's keeping them. I'll call and find out what's the matter."

Somehow I did not get an answer, nor did I have any other way to reach them.

Christopher's disappointment was unbearable to him, and by extension to me. I felt even worse, as I could do nothing to correct the problem or assuage his disappointment. I played with him all day, but I was not a little boy.

I tried to use this as a time to prepare him for the sad reality that many other people are not as reliable about promises as his father and I. It was something I didn't like about the world but could do nothing about. While this is a lesson we all have to learn, it was sooner than I wanted to make this point to my child.

It was my first experience with dealing with the pain of my child's pain.

But soon we addressed his need to play with people his own height by sending him to the Otterbein College Preschool.

Christopher and Santa Claus

When I was a child, my mother devised the ploy of jingling a set of old sleigh bells — from when her uncle would take the children riding in his sleigh — under my window as I went to bed on Christmas Eve, to dramatize the arrival of the jolly old elf. She said I would get so excited that I would almost fall out of bed. I always liked that idea, kept the sleigh bells (I don't know where they have gone now), and rang them under Christopher's window. When he was older, he would do it for his brothers and I could watch!

Therefore when he was in first grade, and all the little skeptics disputed the reality of the saint, he was the only holdout. "I know that Santa comes. I heard the bells myself!"

But by second grade, even he was wavering. "How could Santa Claus get to all the kids in the world in one night? There must be hundreds!"

(See poem "A Child's Christmas in Ohio" in *Into a Mirror and Through a Lens.*)

JFK's Funeral Procession and Other Watt Road Stories

By Christopher Charles Denko

I've always had a pretty good memory; sometimes I can't believe it myself. But the one thing, the first thing I remember in my life was JFK's funeral procession. It must have been a very moving experience because I was only almost three. Our house in Gahanna had an old TV near an entranceway. (I don't think it was the front door but a side or back one.) It flickered its black-and-white image and my parents were crying[1] and I realized something very important was happening because I had never seen my father cry. The atmosphere of dread and gloom was pervasive — I could even feel the angst from the people on TV. I didn't really know what was going on, but I knew it was something serious.

Our house was at the end of a dead end road with a driveway about a half-mile long. People would abandon unwanted dogs here — and they would wander near there until a young boy got dropped off by the school bus around three o'clock who would befriend them and bring them home to beg and plead to let them stay. At one point we had four. Whitefoot was always kind of my dog (she was really a family dog, but she was *really* my dog). She was a very sweet medium-sized border collie, all black with one white foot. But we lived in a great house for kids and dogs with plenty of room to run. There was even an old set of dog kennels on the property[2] (we never kept the dogs there; they were house dogs) near the large garden that Pop planted every year. I would help out, but it was huge. I have no idea what we did with all the extra veggies I know we had. There was also a stream that cut through the property that was very cool for young boys to get dirty in. My friends and I would catch salamanders and such. Sometimes snakes (usually large black ones) would get into the back sort of a storage area. My mom would go back there and get them out and release them into the yard.[3] It wasn't until many years later that I realized how ahead of her time this was.

The stream, at one time, was dammed up, creating a small pond in front of the house. Unfortunately, muskrats (that's what Pop always blamed it on) ate through the dam, but I have no idea how a few rodents could eat through a cement wall several feet thick[4] and make the stream flow again.[5]

My best friend was Ozzie Adkins, who lived up the road with his large family. Across the street from them was a barn with a pond where we would catch tadpoles and play in the hay. Ozzie had been burned in a horrible fire when he was young, leaving him with scar tissue over about half of his upper torso. Years later in Cleveland, Pop was reading the local paper and asked, "What's the name of that kid you played with?" I told him, "Ozzie", and he showed me the story in which a kid in Gahanna was running alongside a riding lawnmower piloted by his brother. Well, this kid fell underneath this riding mower and got run over — and lived! He must have had the world's worst set of scars.

Another memory from that time was when we visited a local store (I thought it was a grocery store, Mom thought it was sporting goods, Pop thinks it was a combo of both)[6] and Sir Edmund Hillary was there. I must have had a soda pop or a weak coffee (Pop used to make them at the store) because I proceeded to climb Sir Edmund Hillary. He was good-natured about it and gently pulled me off.[7]

Soon after, we left Gahanna. (Many years later I would be in Columbus for a Grateful Dead show and stayed with an old friend from high school in Gahanna. It is now an entire suburb of tract housing and strip malls — nothing like little old bucolic Watt Road with cornfields and barns and ponds.)

I spent a week or two with Grandma and Grandpa Decker. They raised one child, a girl, and they didn't know much about young boys, but Grandma bought Bugles, and to this day I *love* Bugles. They are my all-time favorite snack food. I don't even remember a TV, because grandparents can *always* turn on a TV to keep the kid occupied, so I was pretty bored most of the time. There were no kids in the neighborhood, and Grandma was terrible at baseball. Grandpa was working all the time, so I never saw him. But he sure had a cool old Caddy with fins.

CCD

Notes

1. Only Chuck; I don't cry for political figures.
2. That was a horse stall, Christopher.
3. I got Chuck to catch them in a large wastebasket.
4. They dug *under* the dam.
5. It flowed anyway, over the dam, and the people before us used to ice skate there in winter, which I had hoped we could do too, but our all-around handyman/plumber, Neil Mattox, never got the dam solid again.
6. Actually, it was the Sears sporting department.
7. Hillary climbed Mount Everest, and Christopher climbed Hillary. As I have said many times, Christopher never did the same thing twice.

Pumpkin Pie

Early in our marriage, when many if not most of our medical colleagues would unwind by a day on the links, I asked Chuck whether he intended to arrange to play golf, i.e., get a membership at some club, since this was one sport he could do despite his bad leg. (He had been an archer at college.)

"No," he said, "I'd rather take up gardening, like my father. Even if each tomato costs $3.78,[1] it will be exercise for me, without fees, and right at home. The boys can help me."[2]

In Gahanna, the bottomland soil was good, much better than the hard-packed clay in Rocky River, and Chuck did produce tomatoes and peppers. One year he put in pumpkins, intending to let the boys have homegrown jack-o-lanterns.

And so that year, with a crop, though hardly a bumper crop, of pumpkins, my mother, who always loved Chuck as the son she had always wanted, decided to make him a pie out of his own pumpkins.

She did, but, whether the pumpkins were tougher than most, or whether special knives were necessary to cut them up, she practically wore calluses on her hands from the preparation. She said she would not undertake it again. But Chuck appreciated the pie for what it was, an expression of her love.

The pumpkins were too tough to carve for jack-o-lanterns.

Notes

1. One year we actually calculated this.
2. Years later I realized how much money this decision had actually saved. I met a man who spent $500 a week on his golf game.

Mensa Experiences in Columbus

One Sunday when I was at bed rest with my pregnancy with Christopher, Chuck, who was always on the lookout for ways to help me live an interesting and rewarding life, pointed to an article in our paper and said, "Here's something that might interest you." When I read about the Mensa Society, an organization for membership in which one must demonstrate an IQ in the top 2 percent, whose members were willing to be studied by qualified researchers, I snapped to attention. "Hey, that's me!" I realized. Mensa had already collected a study population for me.

Mens is Latin for "mind", and suggests thought stimulation or give-and-take exchange of ideas. This high-IQ qualification would surely bring together an interesting group of people, and they need not be in medicine, as most of our friends and acquaintances were. And so it turned out. At meetings members often disagree, but the ideas are always stimulating and worth listening to.

Therefore, even while at bed rest, I planned to pursue the organization. I couldn't dredge up an old IQ because when I contacted my high school and college for a report on my IQ, one couldn't find it, and the other wouldn't give it out, even to me. (Chuck was luckier — he got a copy of his qualifying IQ from one of his schools.) And so, after the baby was born, I had to take the test the organization offered, the Cattell, a British test, since Mensa originated in England.

We joined the Columbus chapter, where I did two questionnaire surveys. After our move to the Cleveland area, I repeated them on the Northeast Ohio chapter. My second book, *Through the keyhole at Gifted Men and Women: A Study of 159 Members of the Mensa Society,* was published under my own name, Denko, by University Microfilms International, a subsidiary of Xerox, in 1977. This book never sold in large numbers, but I received inquiries about it from Mensans in other chapters, and was asked to talk about it on one radio talk show and on the *Morning Exchange* television show in Cleveland.

Meanwhile we enjoyed the companionship of the Columbus chapter, meeting people in occupations outside medicine. At that time the meetings were scheduled to avoid the television program so popular with the members from the Battell Institute and the rest of the population, *Star Trek.* "Beam me up, Scotty."

In summer the Columbus chapter would sometimes go out for a potluck picnic at Old Man's Cave State Park, south and east of Columbus. The children could run and play, and we could rest on blankets and chat. We made friends with a family that visited us later in Rocky River and with another that we visited in Vail, Colorado.

When we moved to Rocky River, we transferred our membership to the Northeast Ohio branch (see vignette "Mensa in Northeast Ohio and Mrs. Hudson's Lodgers").

Rocky River with Children

Chapter VIII

Sixteen Family Years on Avalon

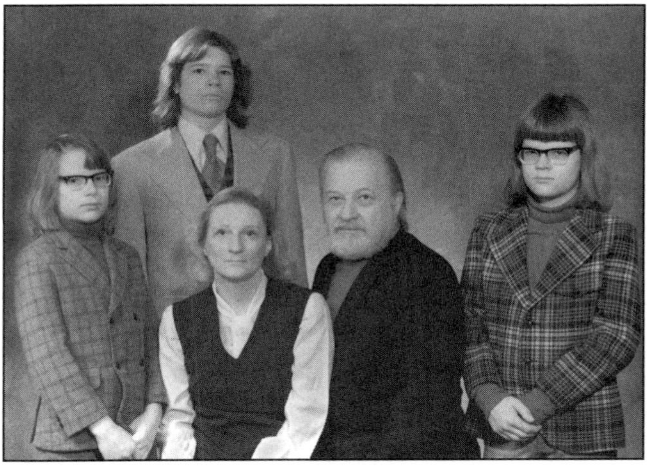

Denko family portrait: Charles, Joanne, Christopher, Nicholas, and Timothey, 1976.

Our move to the Cleveland area, with three boys aged two to eight, three dogs, and more books than the movers had ever before moved, was, like all moves, a nightmare. (Some boxes are still un-unpacked in the attic forty years later, one marked CONDENSED JUNK.) We moved in July, and we ate two-year-old Timothey's birthday cake in the new house at 21160 Avalon Drive, Rocky River, Ohio, amid boxes piled ceiling-high. The site is beautiful, on a cliff overlooking Lake Erie, a few miles east of the southernmost dip of the northern border of the lower forty-eight. Being on the lake partly made up for the loss of our country retreat in Franklin County. Describing the location, I have often told people that our next neighbors to the north are Canadian, but we've never met them.

For the summer of 1968 I had a mother's helper, a new high school graduate, who not only tended the children but also helped me learn my away around the west-side suburbs. One of my first orders of business was to choose a nursery school for Nicholas at three and a half. I visited those I had tracked down even before the move and picked one at the Rocky River Methodist Church for three mornings a week. I recall his teacher's comment later in the year that he would be an "easy" child. I took it to mean that he was docile and obedient. His being at school gave Timothey and me a little prime time alone.

The following year Timothey went to the Rocky River Presbyterian Church's nursery school, so as not to be identified as Nicholas's little brother, one problem with children too close together. (If I had had my choice, I would have liked all my children six years apart — to each his own babyhood.) When Timothey was of age for kindergarten, a Montessori School had just been opened, and I agonized over whether to send him there or to the public kindergarten. Then a light bulb went on, and we sent him to Montessori in the morning (for learning) and to the Kensington Elementary School's kindergarten in the afternoon (for socialization). He tells me that he knew how to read when he started school — he must have taught himself, or maybe it was Montessori; I never taught him — and as an adult he complained that he had been "bored" at Kensington.

The next sixteen years saw the boys through the Rocky River public school system, except for Christopher who required different schooling after ninth grade. He attended five high schools in all (see *A Handful of Ashes: One Mother's Tragedy,* under the pen name Victoria C. G. Greenleaf).

Chuck's new job was to run the Scott Research Laboratory at Fairview General Hospital, where he coordinated patient care (two half days a week), academic work at Case Western Reserve University (a half day a week), half a day in the library at the "newly arrived journals" table, and the rest of the time pursuing his research, first on the metabolism of cartilage in rats, later on metabolic changes in patients with arthritis. Having interdigitated his work in the two settings for the prior year, he was ready to pick up his research and move forward. His connections with CWRU opened up to us many university activities, such as the Handerson Medical History Society, where we reconnected with Genevieve Miller, a medical historian who had been on the staff at Hopkins when we were there. We met the librarian at Allen Memorial Medical Library, Robert Cheshire, whose first remark to me was: "For ten years I have wanted to meet the author who devised the library use study at the University of Michigan" (see my bibliography in the companion book).

An occasional trip to NIH (National Institutes of Health) in Bethesda gave Chuck an opportunity to serve on committees relating to medicine. One such was the problem of "orphan drugs", i.e., medications for diseases so rare that there are not enough patients with the disease to make it profitable for the pharmaceutical house to market the drug. He also served on a Medical Advisory Committee for the Lupus Foundation. These trips made it possible for him to get back in touch with his old friend from Ellwood City, Andy Tkach, by then White House physician to President Nixon. In fact Andy offered Chuck a job as his assistant. Tkach's wife advised against it, saying, "It's great for Andy but terrible for the family. We hardly ever see him." Of course Chuck declined because he wished to continue his tango between basic science, study of the role of inflammation in arthritis, and its pharmacology.

I was accepted on the psychiatry staff at the same hospital, Fairview General, and began juggling a slowly increasing schedule of private patients (for which I used Chuck's office) and a couple half days a week at the VA Hospital and one or another community mental health clinic, along with running the household. Chuck took on the job of provendering and cooking on weekends, although the cooking he really enjoyed was special meals for guests. (Back in the days of professional courtesy, back in Franklin County, after each baby we invited the obstetrician and his wife for a dinner of Chuck's borsch and Stroganov.) In this way he relieved me of some of the 105 meals normally consumed in a week by a family of five. Typically, on Saturday morning he would make "blinyi" (Russian "skinny pancakes", similar to crêpes). The children spent Saturday mornings with him, "helping" and learning, in contrast to when I cooked. I could work in the kitchen only with everyone else out, while I "windmilled" from fridge to cupboard to sink to stove to table and around again.

Our first September in Rocky River Christopher entered third grade and, as Red Cloud, he and Chuck transferred to the local Indian Guides troop. I don't remember Chuck's Indian name, but I jokingly called him Big Chief Thunder Cloud because he was so mild-mannered. When Nicholas and Timothey were old enough, Chuck joined with each of them. Because the father of one of Nicholas's friends, Doug Berg, lived too far away to join, Chuck took Nicholas and Doug as Indian brothers. With two "sons" in the tribe, Chuck had two pairs of fumbling hands to help with lacing wallets. As our boys grew older, Chuck was one of the father helpers in Boy Scouts, in which they all eventually earned the rank of Eagle. Chuck's and my relaxation consisted of an occasional night at the renowned Cleveland Orchestra, an occasional play at the Cleveland Play House or one or another of the many community theaters, or a trip to the Cleveland Ballet.

One winter night we all arrived home to an overheated house and discovered that the furnace was glowing and ready to blow up. Chuck crawled in on hands and knees to pull the plug. As we learned from the furnace man from whom we bought the new one, three "failsafe" devices had all failed together, as had the presale inspection.

We believed that with Rocky River's good public schools, the children should attend them and live at home, and their education would be augmented with enrichment of several types. When I learned of the Junior Nature and Science Center in Bay Village, a nearby suburb, I arranged for them to take classes there, where they eventually became "junior curators", caring for animals as they learned about them. Christopher was once assigned to plan for a visit from the blind, in which he maximized the non-visual modalities such as smell, touch, and hearing. A strong proponent of learning language in childhood, when it is easier, I arranged for a Russian tutor for Christopher and his friend, until the tutor moved away, and a French class for Nicholas one summer and a French tutor for Timothey another. I never encouraged sports, but Timothey played basketball for a couple years. The boys were all in band from fifth grade into high school, Christopher and Nicholas on flute, Christopher later on cymbals, and Timothey on clarinet, later, at their request, on baritone. Only Timothey showed particular interest in music, *asked* for piano lessons, and later attributed his loss of interest to the childish exercises. He wanted to play things like Beethoven's *Für Elise* but didn't know how to ask for it. (He is now teaching his children to identify the composers of music they hear on classical radio.) All three boys were students in Peter Pan Players and took parts in their plays (see vignette "Boys in Dramatics").

On arrival in Rocky River, we comparison-shopped several Protestant churches (my background and my preference, although after one visit, one sent us a box of envelopes before we had met anyone there), then visited Sts. Peter and Paul Russian Orthodox Church in Lakewood (Chuck's background). We joined that church when we saw the rigor of the religious education they offered, the Sunday school being run by a public school principal, and even issuing report cards! Timothey's Sunday school teacher said that when she passed out parts for Yolka (the combined Christmas dinner, performance, and party for which I eventually got the job of buying gifts for all the children, out of educational-toy catalogs), Timothey had his part learned before they were all distributed.

A couple years later, Jim and Helen Balog from the church approached Chuck with an interesting investment opportunity. They (with their daughter Mary Anne) lived in and managed a twenty-nine-unit apartment building, the Parkview in Lakewood. This building had been sold but reverted to the owner for nonpayment and was going on the market again. They hoped for new owners who would keep them on and be congenial to work with. Jim asked Chuck whether he would be interested. It was an attractive building, with a foyer with stuccoed walls and mirrors, looking like a movie set from the 1930s when it was built. (It had a waiting list of prospective tenants.)

After examining the financial records, we decided to go ahead with it. Chuck went to the bank, and joked that he "played Monopoly" with the banker again. We bought it with nothing down and quickly paid off the second mortgage to the prior owner, from rental income. Chuck having been handling our securities, and I having grown up with a father in real estate, I took on the Parkview, which was kind of fun. The Balogs were nonpareil, managing, cleaning, and fielding minor problems. Once Jim referred to "our apartment building, er, *your* apartment building", a slip that passed right over me until he corrected himself. It was a privilege to have someone who took such a proprietary interest in the building. The Balogs took care of about 90 percent of the problems and called me on the rest, including an occasional eviction or capital improvement. The books were never off by a penny. We were fortunate to have Jim, who took it as a personal challenge to do minor repairs (leaky faucets, stopped-up drains, etc.), not only in the Parkview but on Avalon as well.

At Christmastime we would have an apartment-wide potluck party, and we decorated the entryway with a cut tree with lights reflecting in the mirrors and making the foyer redolent with pine. I quickly learned that it is better to increase the rent a little each year than to increase it more the second year. Tenants could adjust easily to a small increase, and the total income was more for the building. Each summer, when the heating costs were down, I looked at the next major repair, e.g., new surfacing of the driveway. I always said that when the Balogs retired, went to Florida, got sick, died, or for some other reason could no longer run it, it would have to go on the market because there was no way to replace them. And so it happened, after thirty years of ownership, when the neighborhood and the tenant class declined, but we refused to take Title Some-Number-or-Other tenants because I didn't need to deal with the government and unreliable tenants who were not paying their way. When Helen suffered health problems and died, we sold the building with the proviso that Jim had his apartment there for life. It was a project whose time had come and gone. I tried to keep a helpful eye on Mary Anne Balog (in another apartment), and when she was evicted for nonpayment, I took in her five very nice cats "temporarily" but had to find good homes for them six months later.

Parkview had fringe benefits. For one thing, besides doing minor repairs around our own house, Jim also watched it when we traveled. Once he locked it up after we had left for Europe when I had forgotten to, having grown up without locking our doors. The apartment had a party room in the basement, which we used for our own parties. When we had taken an interesting trip, I would construct an invitation on that theme, e.g., an onion-domed cathedral for Russia, an outline map for China, and we would invite friends for a slide showing, followed by a supper at ten, catered by Helen, an excellent cook. I loved going to our own parties. People liked to be on the list for those parties, a list that included the physicians caring for our family. The ophthalmologist who took care of our two myopic boys would ask when the next party would be. Chuck called them my "soirées".

One year, Chuck asked one of his customary questions: "There's a European Congress of Rheumatology meeting in Prague in November. Do you want to go?" "Of course, submit a paper," I replied, and we went (see vignette "Chuck's Integrated Life"). This time, Christopher at nine was an excellent age for travel, but, worried about Nicholas's high myopia, we included him because I wanted him to see landmarks in the world lest his vision get worse, even though, at five, he was really too young to get much out of it.

Wanting the children to know travel of an earlier day, and because we loved ocean travel, being taken care of at sea, we crossed by ship to Le Havre and returned through the Mediterranean from Trieste. Chuck had to carry the tired Nicholas out of the early seating in the dining room. However, when we explained to entering diners that Nicholas was tired, he took umbrage, so we always attributed his condition to hunger, to the astonishment of everyone anticipating that bountiful twenty-five-course shipboard repast.

Before the meeting we routed ourselves to Brno to visit the monastery where Gregor Mendel had founded the science of genetics by studying dominant and recessive inheritance in peas, quantifying the number of pink blossoms resulting from the crossing of plants with red and white blossoms. The monk in charge was delighted with our interest and showed us Mendel's desk and garden. This linking of science, history, and geography was beyond even nine-year-old Christopher, not to mention little Nicholas. (Years later I happened upon someone's paper who believed that Mendel had "cooked his books" for the same reason that scientists have been known to do so in recent times, i.e., he was so sure of his hypothesis that he made his figures support it better than they would turn out by chance, now that more is known about statistics.)

My first experience with population pressure came in Prague, where I held one child firmly in each hand lest they be swept away in the crowds (see Christopher's vignette, "Pop's Cheap Side"). To a surprising extent, travel was not wasted on young Christopher, who, years later, commented on the castle near Prague we had visited on the wives' excursion. He said that it would appear that the emperor or whoever had been determined to bring species to extinction by bringing back a hideous collection of thousands of "trophies" to adorn all the walls, and small ones, as little as one feather, in cabinets. Christopher also remembered Piešt'any, where we had been invited after the meeting by the Czech rheumatologist who ran the government spa. He invited Chuck to return for his sabbatical.

Chuck took the children to the Russian circus in Prague (see Chuck's vignette "Day at the Circus with the Russian Commissar and Company").

On our way to the Tatras, our train stopped for a few minutes in Košice. Always one to notice billboards and the like, Chuck drew my attention to a poster of a Neanderthal skull. Unable to read the printing from the train window, we nevertheless agreed that that must mean that the local museum had one, and so, at a time when Eurailpasses allowed you to jump on and off trains at will, we jumped off, took a taxi, and saw one of these rare specimens, then caught the next train. Neither son remembers that, but Chuck did, and I do.

In Central Europe, people called Nicholas, with his blond cherubic curls, *zlaty Nikolai,* or "golden Nicholas". Nicholas developed what we thought was appendicitis in Ljubljana. I asked myself how I could ever have been so demented as to take a five-year-old to Europe. But Chuck contacted a rheumatologist from the recent congress (meetings were small back then, and most members knew each other), who directed him to a surgeon. Already on the gurney on his way to the operating room, Nicholas vomited and was cured. It was the delicious, rich (Mediterranean) seafood casserole — and he still has his appendix at forty-eight.

Ljubljana was where we took them to their first opera, Puccini's *Turandot,* which the soloists each sang in his preferred language. (We were supposed to know the story anyway.) The boys liked it when they carried the failed suitor's head on a pike.

For the return we boarded ship in Trieste. Ashore in Athens, we showed the boys the Acropolis and tried to instill its significance into their minds. It "took" with Christopher, but, back home when shown a picture of the Parthenon and asked to identify it, Nicholas replied, "Wait a minute. It's on the tip of my tongue. *The White House!*"

A dock strike in Naples gave us a day to visit Herculaneum, since Chuck and I had already seen Pompeii on a previous trip.

But when we arrived home, Timothey first turned away from me with a look of reproachful pain on his face, then couldn't stand it — ran and jumped into my arms. Helen said that the day before, he had said, "My mommy's not coming back anymore."

Back home, our family life orbited around school activities, while Chuck continued his work coordinating patient care, animal research, teaching, and learning.

Chuck and I both used ephemera to teach the children to learn and be creative, like making bird feeders out of milk cartons. In the kitchen, Chuck drew the boys' attention to stickers on bananas, identifying the countries of origin. We talked about them, and soon we had a nearby card table with banana stickers all over it. As a result, they became familiar with the countries of Central America before our trip with the two younger boys by surface down to Bogota, Colombia, for another Pan-American Congress (described in *A Handful of Ashes*).

Our move to the Cleveland area put us closer to Chuck's family in Ellwood City, Pennsylvania, permitting us to get there more frequently, for some holidays, and always before school in the fall. The reason for the latter was that not only are the prices lower in a small town, but Pennsylvania has no sales tax on clothes, so that buying there paid for the trip. Also, shopping in a small town is easier. You can park centrally and walk back and forth to visit all the stores. In a town where goodwill is more important for return custom than in a big city, a merchant who cannot supply what customers are requesting will send them to his competitor who can.

One fall when I was working on a book, for Christmas Chuck offered me a hundred hours of babysitting time to give me some "p and q" (peace and quiet), meaning that he would take the boys on several trips to Ellwood City without me. I would never have remembered this because it was so typical of his efforts to help me in my career and projects, except that twenty-five years later Mary Mularz, my friend from a writers' workshop, mentioned it because she remembered with admiration that imaginative and generous expression of love. Those trips were a win-win situation, with Chuck, the boys, and his relatives enjoying them, and me having a chance to work uninterrupted on my second book *Through the Keyhole at Gifted Men and Women: A Study of 159 Members of the Mensa Society* (see Christopher's vignette "Food Circuit").

Our first camping trip with the boys included a few days with Chuck's brother John's family in Amarillo, Texas, where the boys met their older cousins. Then we went on to Mesa Verde.

In 1972 we took a family vacation of the kind Chuck called "without slides". We traveled up and down the Alcan Highway to Alaska. We had bought a pop-up tent, a "High 'N' Dry", to attach to the top of my station wagon. Chuck and I slept in that, and the boys pitched pup tents. We camped in campgrounds with campsites of about an acre each. We had three flat tires. On one occasion, the next vehicle to come past twenty minutes later, a truck, stopped to help, although Chuck was almost through with the tire change, with all our stuff spread out over the shoulder. Like all the other dirty tourists, we bathed in Liard Hot Springs, going and coming. We also stayed every few days in a motel to get a good bath and a good rest, at the outrageous 1972 price of $80. We bought and cooked delicious fish from roadside stands along the way. At Watson Lake, we made a sign of the distance from Rocky River, burned onto firewood, and posted it with hundreds of others. On the long stretches of highway we played Twenty Questions, and seven-year-old Timothey always used either "kangaroo rat" or "lomato" (he couldn't get out the initial "t" sound) and was delighted when we guessed his offerings. Chuck, who usually won at anything like that, did not guess mine: "moon rocks". Eight-year-old Nicholas's job was writing postcards. Back home, our neighbor Betty Bucher gave me the card he had written: "We saw a snak in the rod."

In Mount McKinley National Park (now Denali) we rode the shuttle up and down the highway to within sight of the mountain for which the park is named, and were fortunate with a clear day. We stopped to watch Toklat grizzlies, brown with blond tips. While Chuck kept the little boys in camp, eleven-year-old Christopher and I climbed higher than and downwind of Dahl sheep, to the astonishment of the ranger to whom we described our adventure.

We crossed east into the Yukon over a highway like a gravel heap (I was afraid to stop lest I could never start again) to Dawson and Jack London country, where we prospected for gold on a stake the tourist bureau had taken out for tourists. But evidently the other tourists had found all the "colors". Drama majors presented readings of Robert Service's poems ("poet of the Yukon") and from London's life and works. They included the belief at the time that London had suffered a bout of scurvy over the winter, and that it was "cured" by raw potatoes and a can of tomatoes. Chuck had treated scurvy in a homeless man on Chicago's west side, and he concluded that if London's condition had been scurvy, this would not have cured it. Furthermore, three other men who overwintered in the same cabin with London, on the same diet, would have developed the same symptoms suggestive of scurvy.[1] Knowing that the London story was medically wrong, Chuck became a rheumatologic detective to delve into Jack London's life and medical history. Over several years, when his travels took him to California, he tracked down London's second wife's diary, examined London's hospitalization records, and even visited London's younger daughter in a nursing home. She was delighted to learn that Chuck had tracked down evidence that her father had not died an alcoholic death but had suffered and died from lupus, which is now accepted. The pills spilled on the floor (someone attempting suicide takes them all) had been prescribed for Jack's pain (see vignette "Jack London. A Modern Analysis of His Mysterious Disease").

Over the years there had been a series of minor misbehaviors by Christopher. Each time I worked with him, thought the issue was resolved and we had it behind us, and were ready to move on. One such incident was back in second grade, consisting of taking money from my wallet, showing it to the children at school, and lying about it. Another was the theft of a candy bar in a store with his father, who didn't see it, although the shopkeeper did, stopped him, talked to him, and let him go without calling the police. When Chuck got home, white and trembling, I told him that I wished the storekeeper had called the police, to make more of a point with Christopher. We had no way to know whether there had been other such occurrences. The incidents were getting worse, and there were never two alike. Nor did I like his associates, boys with little interest in school, while Christopher was still at the head of his class, although one teacher complained about his "attitude". While I loved him as always, I did not like him, and I was not enjoying this child whom I had worked so long and hard to have in the first place. Worse, with few exceptions, while Chuck saw some of his behavior as wrong, he did not back me up in my efforts at correction, saying things like "You weren't a boy, and you didn't even have a brother." "So?" Therefore I was left as the "heavy", trying to deal with misbehavior myself, sometimes more severely than if he had shared this no-fun part of parenthood, discipline.

Another worrisome trait of Christopher's was his impulsivity and recklessness. When we moved to Rocky River, I took him to street corners, some with traffic lights, to teach him to watch the light, if any, but also the traffic, if any, before crossing. We did practice crossings, with him making the decisions. Still, within a few years I had two calls from concerned friends. One told me she had seen him run across the railroad tracks behind her neighbor's backyard. Another reported his darting across busy Lake Road, without looking, dodging traffic. How many more such incidents were there, unreported? One December morning when we had gone on Nixon's winter daylight saving time, Christopher returned home, his face oozing blood and serum, minutes after leaving for school in the dark, having been thrown by a car into a snowbank. His injuries were minor, a cut upper lip, which, by Chuck taking him to meet the plastic surgeon at the emergency room, healed without need for revision. In cold weather it turned pink, but now is invisible. But what next? In later years he blamed me for "lack of sympathy".

"Lack of sympathy? I gave you better than sympathy. Your father and I got you a plastic surgeon to save your appearance. What about sympathy for me for having a kid who refuses to think first and places himself above the rules?"[2]

Part of my efforts to redirect Christopher included using Chuck's sabbatical to get him away from the bad influences and drop him back a grade (see vignette, "Australian Sabbatical").

After the sabbatical Christopher went into a new ninth grade at home, but our efforts to let him turn over the proverbial "new leaf" didn't work. He made no effort to make new friends, just gravitated back to the old ones in tenth grade or already dropped out. His misbehavior continued and worsened over many years. That story is told in *A Handful of Ashes,* which I wrote in hopes that it would influence our society in the direction of tightening the expectations placed on youth, but even if it could have done so, my book came too late. A short time later Timothey's behavior raised questions, and I described the problems of adolescent alcoholism in *Fighting the Good Fight,* which has been used in alcoholism and rehabilitation clinics. Both books are under my pen name, Victoria Greenleaf.

During all this turmoil, in the mid-'80s after the boys had all finished high school and Christopher was already away from home, we took Nicholas and Timothey to East and Central Africa to see the savannah animals, mainly in Tanzania, and the gorillas in Rwanda and Zaire. We camped in the Ngorongoro Crater and visited the Rift Valley where the Leakeys had made their finds. At that time Chuck's return of polio problems had not yet begun, and he was able to do everything on the trip except the four-hour climb straight (about 80 degrees) up the mountain over slippery bamboo, with our guides, shorter than I, carrying ice chests of cold drinks on their heads and, occasionally, boosting me up the mountain. Our goal was to spend an hour with the gorilla family, a silverback, several females, and their offspring. What amazed me was that the enormous silverback "babysat", letting his children climb and play all over him and suck their toes. A good lesson in paternal behavior. In this way the gorillas bought protection because our fees included money that went to their conservation program.

Our African trip was accomplished over Christmas and New Year's, and some of our fellow travelers chose it to avoid the traditional hoopla. In Zaire, formerly Belgian Congo and hence French-speaking, two charming little girls came up to Chuck, with his white hair and beard, and politely asked, "*M'sieur, êtes-vous Père Noël?*"

I considered that trip "the last Denko picnic".

In 1986 the Fairview administration finagled the "permanent endowment" of the research lab for their outpatient surgery unit and closed the research unit.[3] At that time Chuck went full-time to the university, working without pay. (This was because, for his few remaining work years after Fairview diverted the research endowment, which paid his salary, it would have been costly in money and time to move to another research facility. We always considered his unpaid research our financial contribution to medicine. Chuck's account of his career up to 1990, prepared for the international Carol Nachman Prize in Rheumatology, which he entered and in which he came in second, worldwide, is found in "Resume of Research in Osteoarthritis and Cartilage" and "Significance of My Research".

By the mid-'80s Christopher was living in Washington and had graduated from American University, having been asked to leave George Washington University. Nicholas was at the University of Pennsylvania, where he placed out of all his freshman year because of all his honors courses in high school and earned a B.S. and an M.A. in education in his four years at Penn. He practice-taught junior high school science students, and one day came to class dressed as Einstein to tell them about relativity. After graduation he received job offers to teach science, which was part of his goal, but for post-docs much later. He delayed medical school while he chose to continue working in cancer research with his friend and mentor Amato Giaccia. Timothey was at Kenyon College (a small liberal arts college) and still fighting coming to terms with his alcoholism, until Chuck finally cooperated with me on interventions and treatment programs (see *Fighting the Good Fight*).

Thus only one of the three was satisfactorily launched, soon to be working on a double doctorate on full scholarship at the University of Cincinnati. But our nest was empty.

Notes

1. Scurvy had been observed on whole shiploads of sailors, at sea for months without fresh fruits or vegetables. It was found that limes, which could be carried for months, would cure or prevent the condition, for which preventative the British sailors came to be called "limeys".

2. As an adult, Christopher was held up at gunpoint. Fortunately, I heard of it only much later. It is a miracle he lived to grow up.

3. A caveat to those wishing to leave trusts, endowments, etc., for any purpose dear to their hearts: these should include a warning that if the money is not used as designated, it reverts to the heirs or to someone else if there are no heirs.

Velikovsky Excursion

Shortly after moving to Rocky River, I met Charmaine Severson, who introduced me to our writers' group, which met for twenty-five years, until there remained too few members to have meaningful discussions. Charmaine and I happened to share an interest in astronomy, and she made me familiar with Velikovsky, a man who held the idiosyncratic view that Venus had appeared within recent human history, and that this was documented in the literature of several ancient peoples.

Therefore when Charmaine learned that Velikovsky would be giving a lecture at Youngstown State University, all four of us wanted to hear him, including Chuck and Ruth Berg, whom I had met through the school and her son Doug, Nicholas's friend.

But there was one problem: The talk was held on April 12. Chuck wanted to go with us, but he was still doing our income tax himself and making me more and more nervous that it would not be mailed in by the deadline. And so I required that for him to accompany us, he had to have it in before our little day trip, and hence before the IRS deadline. He did, and we all enjoyed the companionship of the ride out together.

On the way we stopped somewhere where they advertised Klondikes, a very good kind of chocolate-covered ice cream bar, originally the signature dairy product of a chain named Isaly's, which I encountered first in Ellwood City. Klondikes are still available, found not only in Pennsylvania but also in Cleveland, although Isaly's has been bought out. I mention this because Chuck got each of us a bar, proceeded to unwrap one and hand it to Ruth, then stopped himself and apologized, "You see, I'm so accustomed to getting them ready for the children that I just go ahead with the wrappers!"

Velikovsky was elderly and unlikely to give many more lectures. Charmaine said, "I don't know whether there's anything to his idea or not, but I wish someone would investigate it, even to disprove it, during his lifetime, so he knows he was taken seriously."

Years later, at a European Rheumatology Congress meeting in Athens, I heard an elderly rheumatologist propose an unpopular (unaccepted) theory about bacterial causation for rheumatoid arthritis. He also wanted his idea not just to drop unconsidered after his lifetime. I felt very sorry for that man, as he made his last stand. Scientists dread having their work go into oblivion, and Chuck has been fortunate in this way. (See Malemud's vignette "The Growth Hormone/Insulin-Like Growth Factor-1 (GH/IGF-1): Paracrine Axis Contributions by Charles W. Denko, Ph.D., M.D. to the Understanding of GH/IGF-1 in Regulating the Inflammatory Response".)

Grandma Wakes Up

Soon after we moved to Rocky River, Grandma Decker came to visit. One night a huge storm kicked up (Lake Erie gets tremendous storms since it is so shallow) and blew really hard for hours. The next morning it turned out that Grandma had woken up in the middle of the night, heard cries for help, and called the Coast Guard.[1] It turned out that a private boat had capsized right off our cliff and somehow she heard these poor people screaming over the din of the storm. Well, the Coast Guard got there and pulled these people out of the water. She most definitely saved those people; the waves were probably eight feet that night. If they hadn't had life preservers on, they never would have made it.

This was back when we had a beach and when Murrays' pier really was a pier. The water level of the lake is up several feet now.

Pop used to get pissed off at people who pulled up in their boats and got out on our beach. One time we came down there right when some people were leaving. They split and several minutes later I was running up the beach and stepped on the coals from their fire.

We used to have steps down to the beach, but these were pretty much unusable. It was more of a path that traversed back and forth across the face of the steep hill until you reached the beach. Landslides quickly made it impassable. We usually took the Buchers' stairs — they had stairs but no beach — we had beach but no stairs. By the early 1980s Pop had a beach wall put in to protect what was left of the cliff. It was voted best beach wall on Lake Erie by a bunch of engineers. It totally saved the cliff and now it[2] is gradually growing in, filling up with small trees, whose roots will protect the cliff.[3]

CCD

Notes

1. Actually my mother, whom I had given the bedroom on the lake side, banged on our door and said, "I heard cries for help coming from the lake." I had the local police number in my head, we had a bedside phone for our occasional patient call in the night, so I got right through to the police. Their response was "So *that's* where they are!" Help arrived in three minutes. They raced down the ravine just east of us, sirens screaming and red lights twirling, and hauled out seven terrified, dripping people as a result of my mother's quick action.
2. The trough behind the wall.
3. When we bought the property, the steps, made of railroad ties, were very good. One bad storm had destroyed them and taken many trees from the hillside. This had stopped trespassers. We decided to have a seawall put in instead, at the then enormous price of $25,000. It was said to be the best on the west side of Cleveland.

The Easter-Egg Hunt

The spring after we moved to Rocky River, our family was invited to a family Easter egg hunt at the home of one of Christopher's classmates. With a large yard, with trees, shrubbery, garden plots, and grass, the host family had planned cleverly to offer three areas with graduated difficulty for finding the eggs. Christopher and Nicholas were in age-appropriate groups. The youngest age group, those under three, looked for eggs arranged like oval pastel polka dots on the grass, right in the open. Timothey, who would be three in three months, was the oldest in the toddler group.

When the starting bell rang, those younger than Timothey stood around wondering what to do, while Timothey immediately began raking in eggs with both hands, emptying and refilling his pail in the open grass area.

His older brothers brought home numbers of eggs comparable to the findings of others in their groups, making, with Timothey's, a total of ten dozen. Fortunately they were pullet eggs, but still that week I had to think of all the hard-boiled egg dishes I had ever heard of, to make our way through all those eggs: creamed eggs over rice, potato salad, egg salad sandwiches, deviled eggs.

Shoelace Tying

When Timothey was two and seven months, he was able to tie his shoelaces. It was not without a struggle. He would chew on his extended tongue, wrap the lace around the appropriate fingers, and when it fell apart, start all over, but he would finally accomplish the task. I made a movie of this, with the date in the background, and I expect to find that movie when I clean my "office". The only thing Chuck ever questioned my use of money for was the use of an entire roll of film ($5 before developing) for little Timothey's accomplishment.

Nor was that the end of it. When we went to Ellwood to buy school clothes for the boys, the shoe store personnel (owner Edelman, his wife who kept the books, and a salesperson or two) were so impressed to hear of Tim's achievements that they gathered around to watch his performance. Mr. Edelman said that only half of five-year-olds entering school are able to tie their shoes. This is no longer a test of development (like the ability to pick up Cheerios), because of Velcro fasteners.

Treasure Hunts

Several years after we moved to the Cleveland area, World Publishing left (and later returned). In anticipation of the move, they had a marvelous sale: beautiful coffee-table nature books for five dollars, children's books for as little as twenty-five cents. Some of the latter were imperfect, with, for example, the cover put on upside down. Anyway, I went to the sale several times to lay in supplies of books for various purposes such as future gifts. It was my treasure hunt.

Meanwhile, Christopher got the idea of making treasure hunts for his younger brothers. He wrote clever clues in the form of riddles or plays on words. One such was something to the effect of where you would meet Santa Claus, i.e., up the chimney. I gave him the World books to use as prizes.

Recently I found a book that Nicholas, at seven and a half, used as a treasure-hunt prize for Christopher. He had seen me inscribe, on the corner of the flyleaf, a book I gave someone. So he inscribed in the corner:

To
christop-
her from a tr
egere hunt from
nicholas
jluy, 9172

Those World books were win-win trophies.

Day at the Circus with the Russian Commissar and Company

In the late 1960s I had been invited to present a paper at the World Congress of Rheumatology convening in Prague. During that period the victorious allies strove to demonstrate their close friendship. Their organizational leaders wanted to show off Czechoslovakian recovery from the ravages of World War II. Therefore they permitted the almost unheard-of presentation of the great, the fabulous Moscow Circus in a non-Communist venue.

I wanted to take our two sons, Christopher and Nicholas, and the near-teenaged daughter of a friend. (Joanne went to the opera.)

At the ticket booth, in a lighthearted tone and my best Russian, I said, "I want four of your best seats."

Guess what — I got them! They were in the center of the main section, two or three rows roped off, level with the large stage. The stage held an ice rink on which several large brown bears darted back and forth skating, actually successfully playing ice hockey! I wondered who helped them put on their skates.

Looking over my right and left shoulders, I saw that the rest of the roped-off section was occupied by Russian military officers with their shoulder boards jutting out. They were smiling amiably, and it was plain that the Russians had been instructed to be on friendly terms with the locals. I talked with several of them in broken Russian and English, and I noticed their stainless steel teeth.

As intermission approached, the buzz of conversation suddenly quieted. The Russian commissar and his underlings (including one woman officer), with their painted ladies, had arrived, and it turned out that we had been given their seats. It appeared that this had been done intentionally to embarrass the Russian contingent. The circus came to a halt while all eyes were on how the Russians would handle the sticky situation. But the Russians were not to be outdone by the Czech pranksters. The commissar immediately took in the fact that an American and three children were enjoying the clowns' tricks. He held a quick consultation with the ushers, while the Czech locals were obviously enjoying the discomfiture of the Russian officers.

But, not to be outdone, the commissar quickly turned the situation to his advantage by asking for four more chairs to be brought and inviting us to join their group. The locals recognized that they had been "hoist on their own petard", and the circus continued with the excellent acts for which they are noted.

By the end of the circus, the Russians had thawed, shook our hands cordially, and wished us "*do svidaniya!*"

CWD

Christopher's Writing

Christopher had a marvelous fifth grade teacher, Mrs. Fran Kemp, who had the children write and illustrate a book, which she helped them bind, using cloth they brought from home. Christopher was too young, of course, to have read Melville's masterpiece, *Moby Dick,* but the movie had been out and even shown on television. Christopher's novel idea was to write the story from the point of view of the whale. I found, for the binding, some material with a blue pattern that might suggest ocean. The result was that Mrs. Kemp selected him to attend a "Young Writers' Conference" for schoolchildren. That book is in Christopher's memorabilia, which I plan to put into his daughter's legacy box.

When asked what he wanted to become, Christopher said, "A writer." By this he meant a penman. Truly, his writing and printing were beautiful, and some years he printed our Christmas cards for me.

After our experiences with Mrs. Kemp, I made sure that his younger brothers were also in her class. She said that children in fifth grade show tendencies in one direction or the other, the humanities or the math/science direction. Christopher's was definitely literary, while his younger brothers were stronger in math and science. When Christopher was beginning to show oppositional tendencies with Mrs. Kemp, she tried to redirect him with various strategies. Admittedly a bad speller, she had him correct her spelling. She had the children give her a report card, and his impressed her with its accuracy.

From the *Moby Dick* story I conceived the idea of having each child write a Christmas story each year, for use as their gifts to grandparents.

As an adult, Christopher once said to me, "I think I'm meant for something great."

"If so," I replied, "I think the area would be literary, but you should be working in that direction already because writing for publication is an acquired skill, and you need all the years to acquire it that you can get. If one of you three should get me to Stockholm, and it should be you, it would be in literature."

Enrichment for Our Sons

It was my belief that our sons should experience a variety of enriching experiences, although I knew they would not, could not, continue in all of them. When they were in elementary school, I took the attitude that the ordinary curriculum should be supplemented in any way possible. For example, I did not consider band, which was optional, an option. With or without any musical talent, they could learn to do several things at once besides how to play a particular instrument: read music, keep time, follow the conductor, and be exposed to the band music.

Therefore Christopher and Nicholas took up the flute, and Christopher later crashed the cymbals in the marching band. Timothey began with clarinet, and later, at their request, changed to baritone. Having begun in fifth grade, by ninth or tenth grade they had had five or six years' musical experience. And Timothey even *asked* for piano lessons.

Another supplementation was the Lake Erie Junior Nature and Science Center in Bay Village, where they were taught about nature and, in return, helped with animals' care and feeding and became "junior curators". Christopher was once asked to plan a tour for the sight-impaired that would maximize use of the other senses.

Both Indian Guides, which they did with their father, and Boy Scouts offered outdoor experiences, and their nature-center work counted toward what they were expected to do for Scouts projects. Our early family trips with the boys were oriented around the outdoors and nature. These included camping trips to the Southwest (Mesa Verde, Grand Canyon, Joshua Tree), up the East Coast to Prince Edward Island (*Anne of Green Gables* country), up the Alcan Highway to Alaska, home via the Yukon (Jack London country that interested CWD to pursue his Jack London medical studies), and the International Peace Park (Waterton Lakes and Glacier).

Our church gave our boys good instruction in Old and New Testament.

When the children were in elementary school, an independent local group called the Peter Pan Players offered drama classes. In line with my efforts to find others to enrich my children, I sent them all to these classes. When Christopher was about to enter the highest grade at Peter Pan, he had misbehaved badly in Australia. That caused me to tell him that his punishment would be not to attend the final year of Peter Pan. When the teacher learned about this, she told me that they had picked a play with him in mind for the part of Peter Zenger, a Colonial printer who fought for freedom of the press. So, of course, I had to relent. For his costume, I had a friend make his Colonial jacket, attached aluminum foil "buckles" to a pair of my black Daniel Green corduroy slippers, which he wore with my white knee sox, and bought a tricorne hat from Williamsburg. I can still visualize how he took his bow with the two leading ladies, one little actress holding each hand.

When Nicholas and Timothey were in the earlier grades, a play was chosen called *The Tiniest Heart,* referring to playing cards. Each of their teachers wanted our son for the role of the Ace, but it was given to Timothey because of course he was smaller. They wore sandwich signs for their card character. It also is a lovely memory.

Nicholas was involved with drama in high school and college. In high school, Nicholas, Joe, and Mary were friends and had parts in all the plays, including *West Side Story, The Elephant Man,* and *Shadow Box.* After his junior year Nicholas went to the summer high school Speech Institute at Northwestern University[1] and had a once-in-a-lifetime opportunity to play Shakespeare, Caliban in *The Tempest.* I flew to Chicago to see it and attended the cast party. When Bob Santo, the drama teacher, announced a trip over the Christmas break to New York to see plays, I saw no reason for high school students to go straight to Broadway — we have good theater opportunities in Cleveland, including many excellent community theaters — and so I did not send him on that trip. As a result, when the call came for drama students for walk-on parts as "the bad boys from across town" in the professional production of *A Child's Christmas in Wales,* he was sent for that and spent Christmas vacation "walking on" and going almost every night to a cast party given by one or another well-to-do theater supporter.

Years later Nicholas told me how lucky we were that like his father he couldn't sing. If he could have, he would have gone into theater, with all its uncertainties of getting work, but he could only act and dance, and for professional theater, you have to be able to sing too.[2]

Nicholas graduated from high school with the school's record "grade point accume" because he went to school to learn, not to get the highest grade point average, for which you need to limit yourself to honors courses. Every year he won the woodworking award, and the home ec teacher commissioned him to make her a butcher-block table. He also made Mary a jewelry box of Philippine mahogany lined with velvet, and I bought him the mahogany for another one for me. Dramatics, debate, and speech also did not offer honors grades, but he and Mary and Joe excelled in these and went on to state meets.

At the University of Pennsylvania, Quadramics, the dramatics organization, was Nicholas's only extracurricular activity. He constructed a stage set to float in a swimming pool, the setting for Stephen Sondheim's version of Aristophanes' *The Frogs.* Nicholas directed *Amadeus,* which was the first student production in Philadelphia ever to receive mention on local television. Chuck and I flew out to see these performances.

Notes

1. Which I also had attended after my junior year.
2. True, we would have worried about the uncertainties, but I have wished his scientific career would have left time for an occasional role in little theater.

Australian Sabbatical

By 1974 Chuck had earned a six-month sabbatical. He had two invitations: to take it in Czechoslovakia with a friend who ran a government spa or to take it with Michael Whitehouse, who worked at Australian National University (ANU), the best of several new post-WW II universities, in Canberra, the capital. Chuck had met Michael in Columbus, the Whitehouses had visited us in Rocky River, the men had corresponded, and the Whitehouses had gone on to Australia. Several advantages were inherent in the Australian invitation: a new country and continent, the use of English for all of us, and, most of all, the reversal of seasons. The reason I preferred the latter was my hope to get Christopher away from several undesirable friends and drop him back a grade on his return, by his not having completed the equivalent of ninth grade there because of their school year being out of synchrony with ours. We had questioned the wisdom of Christopher's early entrance to first grade, and this would partly undo that. I realized that the little boys would move ahead regardless of the partial grade they did in Australia. My scheme worked for the two younger boys, but not for Christopher, who, on our return, gravitated back to the same undesirables. Nevertheless, the experience was an adventure for all of us, the chance to live in a foreign capital, observe life there, and return home with a new perspective. We had to leave Whitefoot, our only surviving dog, in Chuck's lab (because of quarantine in Australia).

Our 1974–'75 adventure began before even leaving the States. We camped across the Southwest, and this offered the chance to show the boys the Painted Desert, the Petrified Forest, and the Grand Canyon. Time constraints and the little boys' age precluded their taking the fabled trip down Bright Angel Trail on a mule. I hope they can do it someday. The final night before embarking, we camped at Joshua Tree National Park. Helen Meis, a former patient of Chuck's, then living in Los Angeles, had an extra car space in their condo and let us leave the station wagon there. With twenty-seven suitcases we boarded the *Oriana* for our twenty-day crossing. The crossing was so leisurely because of days at several ports, the first of which was San Francisco. We took the boys to see the coast redwoods at Muir Woods. The next was Oahu, and, as luck would have it, the day was December 6, Pearl Harbor Day. Chuck took the boys to the ceremony at the sunken *Arizona* at Pearl, while I spent most of the day at the Polynesian Cultural Center. This institution is an example of one thing serving several purposes: Brigham Young University has a branch on Oahu to make higher education possible for the citizens of the many islands of the Pacific. They established a confluence of six villages representing six Pacific cultures; the students are given a chance to work at crafts in those villages, as a payment for tuition, while visitors like myself could observe and compare the cultures.

The next day ashore was in Fiji, where a band on the pier welcomed us. We stopped in Auckland, New Zealand and visited their museum where we saw a skeleton of their extinct dodo.

The children could play in the playroom and even eat Aussie meals there, baked bean sandwiches. This was the first time for any of us to cross the equator, with all its King Neptune frivolities — throwing raw liver at one another and pushing people into the pool. My moment of greatest excitement came one dark night when on deck I identified two hazy glowing oval patches in the sky, the Greater and Lesser Magellanic Clouds. With arms extended I could cover them with my thumbs, and so I called them the giant thumbprints of God. Also the unimpressive Southern Cross, so beloved by denizens of the Southern Hemisphere.

Another enjoyable feature of the trip was my meeting Lorna Curtin, wife of the Australian ambassador to England. At a Scrabble party on shipboard she recognized that, though rusty and out of practice, I would be a good opponent, and so we played a tournament across the Pacific and each won the same number of games. She was better, however, and always won by several points, while I would squeak through with one or two points. We later visited the Curtins in Sydney. Their son suffered a malignant melanoma, and Chuck's input helped his treatment.

Finally we arrived in Sydney harbor and were met by our host, Michael, who drove us to Canberra. The first news was bad: they wanted to put us into a "staging flat" but only temporarily, then into faculty housing. That would have entailed a move, which I opposed, especially when I saw the comfortable facilities for graduate students and others with relatively short time in Canberra, many with young children, in a more convenient neighborhood. We persuaded them that the staging flats met our needs, being close to the elementary school where many of the diplomatic personnel's children attended. A public high school was available for Christopher.

But first, we had timed our arrival to coincide with Christmas and their summer vacation. (One of their songs went, "You know it's Christmastime when the red fern blooms".) I inquired how Aussie children spent their vacations. For Christopher I found a drama group, into which he was accepted, given a part, and traveled to perform in the outback. I found him a Boy Scout troop, and the boys went hiking in the Blue Mountains. For the little boys I found a day camp at a park, where one of the play devices was a pulley on a wire, for gliding down a slope. It was called a flying fox, the name given to one of their bats. The real "flying foxes" looked like pieces of newspaper swirled by the wind about the night sky.

Despite Canberra's excellent public transportation, it immediately became apparent that we would need a car. The secondhand one we bought had the typical sun-damaged finish, making me think of it as sunburned. For a couple weeks it took three of us to navigate with it, one on the controls, one on the map, and one (Christopher) yelling, "Keep left!" Chuck immediately noticed that Aussie men typically drove the one family car to work, parked it for the day, and drove home, while their wives shopped at the butcher shop, the greengrocer's, etc., on foot, and staggered home laden with provisions. I drove him to the university each day and used the car for errands. A trained observer who always noticed everything, Chuck also commented on their male sports orientation, with football fields and cricket ovals, and even croquet, it seemed at every block.

We found a nearby Methodist Church whose lovely minister and family were very cordial and invited us to events. (One of their six children, a daughter, was making trouble for this family as Christopher was doing for us. She was also in the drama group. (People from New Guinea that we met in that church were just one generation away from cannibalism.) In return for their hospitality I volunteered to take the third grade religious education a day a week. I did anything I felt like and usually discussed one of the parables. The children in their uniforms were very polite; they all stood up when I entered the room and didn't sit back down until I was comfortable.

It had never crossed my mind to practice psychiatry in Australia, but psychiatrists were in short supply, and they reached out to me, so I made an effort to get credentialed. I met almost all the requirements, lacking only my original diploma from Hopkins, which was safely stored in our attic in Rocky River, in a place where Jim Balog could never have found it. An affidavit from my medical school would not do. Therefore instead of seeing patients, I joined the bushwalking wives' club and saw an echidna (one of the two monotremes, i.e., egg-laying mammals) disappear into a cleft in a tree. Our whole family saw the other monotreme, the platypus, with not only a duck-like bill but also a poison glad in its hind foot), but only its head as it swam, like a beaver, in the lake in Canberra. Within a few miles of Canberra we saw many kangaroos and koalas munching eucalyptus leaves up in trees. We saw also the emu, Australia's large flightless bird, which shares space opposite the kangaroo on Australia's emblem.

Realizing that six months would go by very quickly, I immediately instituted a "one sightsee a weekend" policy, which included the typical pioneer household in Canberra and the astronomy station at Tidbinbilla. We saw one of the four extant copies of the Magna Carta (1215), kept in temperature- and humidity-controlled inert gas, delineating for the first time, they said, [1] a right for women, the right to recompense if someone killed a woman's husband, thereby cutting off her support.

Although our friends expressed concern that we did not enroll at least Christopher in private school (as they did their children), I was not expecting the disparity between public and private schools, which had not yet reached our country. I took all three to the neighborhood public schools. I gave the schools the boys' birthdays and told them to place them wherever that qualified them. Christopher was put into "third form", equivalent to our ninth grade. The first day of school Timothey came home and said, "Guess what! They sent me from second grade down the hall to third!" A little later Nicholas came in and announced, "Guess what! They sent me upstairs to fourth grade." (Back in Rocky River that fall they stayed in those new grades.) Thus Australia, at that time, was not reluctant to have children skip a grade. When Australia's minister of education visited the school, he asked me how I compared it to ours back home, and I told him about the "skipping". (In a small country — it was eleven million then — most of the educated people know each other and can sometimes, I believe, have influence of a kind I feel we lack in a much larger population.)

Over a long Easter weekend we saw one of the marvels of Australia, the highest on my list, the Great Barrier Reef. We took the train north along the coast, visited Brisbane's horticultural gardens, and proceeded north to Cairns, where we crossed over to Green Island, one of the main tourist sites for seeing the reef.

The glass-bottomed boat didn't help much because we rocked so much with the waves, but I was enthralled with the life we could see by just walking on the dead reef (in protective shoes because the coral could cut our skin and cause bad infections), not primarily fish in the shallow waters but lower life forms, pink sea cucumbers that looked like blobs of bubble gum and vivid cobalt-blue starfish.

We visited Mensans we had contacted beforehand. They told us they had a carpet snake living under the house, and, with no screens in the window, I slept restlessly. In Mackay we met people we are still in contact with — Mila Hoagland and her family, a Dutch physician who left the Dutch East Indies when they were lost by Holland, and established a family practice in Australia. She and her husband took us into the outback (see Chuck's vignette, "A Visit to Abo Country"). Mila took us to a place where we could see living coral extending, opening and closing their polyps as they fed from the nutrient-rich ocean water, and retracting into their strong sheaths when startled by our approach. Another stamp collector, like Chuck with his interest in stamps with maps on them, Mila specialized in stamps with sea life, which Australia issues in abundance. (When I travel, I look for such stamps for post cards to her.)

As we returned south toward Canberra, we stopped at Townsville, a city with a record rainfall, twelve feet a year. They had a plague, this one of toads. As we walked down the main street, we had to avoid stepping on them, and as we looked through the showcase window of the automobile dealer, we saw them hopping under the new cars.

I went alone to Melbourne one weekend, and one of the Mensans took me to Phillip's Island to see the "march of the fairy penguins", who come home from the sea to their burrows at sundown, at such a narrow strip of beach that they could fence it off so visitors could watch from the other side of the fence but not disturb the smallest penguins. Another Mensan took me to a forest where the lyrebirds construct bowers during the courting season (but we were not there at the right time). What fascinated me, however, were what he called vegetable fungi, a fungus that had grown on a plant and had become a cast replacing it.

Our other long trip was to Alice Springs and Ayers Rock. We took the train to Adelaide in the south, then up the center of the continent, past now-wild camels that had been imported in hopes of using them in the desert. In Alice we saw one of the problems of the aborigines, wholesale alcoholism. We then took the bus to Ayers Rock, which glows at sundown and is a religious site for the aborigines, the home of "Rainbow Serpent". Nevertheless, we all climbed it, including Timothey, using the chain pegged to the steeper parts of the climb. At eight, he was the youngest that day. Here we saw our second Australian plague, a plague of mice, presumably marsupial mice, although I didn't check that out. We would unintentionally catch them and have to open the door of the motel room to release them (see Christopher's vignette, "Ayers Rock").

We made friends with the Australian Mensa locsec Don Laycock (see vignette, "Don Laycock and the New Guinean Languages").

Chuck's work at ANU included the effect of copper on arthritis (see Chuck's vignette "The Alcusal Story").

As the time came to leave Australia, we returned to Sydney, visited the zoo, where we saw the tree-climbing marsupial from Papua New Guinea, and boarded the *Oronsay,* a sister ship of the *Oriana.* On this run there was a lovely elderly Jewish woman from Rhodesia (about whose fate I have worried when that colony was broken into Zambia and Zimbabwe), with whom I played Scrabble. One remark of hers stays with me to this day. She commented that I was "greedy". I felt a surge of resentment, opened my mouth to protest, but then realized she was right and closed it while I pondered. Then I agreed that I want many good things for myself and my family, but not at any cost to others, so there must be a less pejorative word for it, maybe "ambitious".

The stops were the same as those outward bound. On Fiji, however, I was able to attend the typical South Sea Islands hotel's nightclub act, with someone walking on glowing coals. The waiter who seated me also invited me to his home island, which I had to decline, regretfully. The only additional stop on the return voyage was Vancouver, where we took the boys to Stanley Park and the collection of Northwest Native American totem poles.

On disembarking in Los Angeles and picking up our car, with thanks to Helen and Herschel Meis, we wanted to get home, but not so quickly as to miss opportunities along the way. I had read about the bristlecone pines, recently discovered to be older even than our redwoods, and so we detoured to Inyo County in eastern California. There we visited the Methuselah Tree, found to be 4,789 years old, in the Ancient Bristlecone Pine Grove in the rain shadow on the dry slope of the White Mountains. Windblown and sand-scoured, these trees struggle for existence, sometimes growing almost parallel to the ground. One strategy for their longevity is to sacrifice large parts of their wood, with the result that as much as 90 percent of the tree's volume is deadwood. Nevertheless, the living portions sprout tufts and pinecones, able to reproduce. As an adult, Nicholas told me that when I explained to the boys what we were about to see, he inferred that, being so old, these trees would be even bigger and taller than the Coast Redwoods we had taken the boys to see at Muir Woods when the ship stopped in San Francisco. Ancient they certainly were, but not gigantic, and they could survive where there was too little water for other trees.

We had left our affairs in the capable hands of the Balogs while we were in Australia. Besides paying the bills, they held our other mail, except for one Christmas card with a lot of handwritten message visible through the envelope. They forwarded that card from the Otts, whom we had known from our Mensa days in Columbus. They told us that they were lodge caretakers at a company's R&R ranch near Vail, Colorado, where they were free to have guests during the week. I had written to them, explaining that we would be delighted to stop on our way home from Australia.

That was where our sabbatical adventure ended. They drove us by Jeep high up into the mountains. One comment made by Joe, a headmaster in a boys' school, was that Timothey might be our brightest child. His observation leading to this was that he had watched Timothey size up the problem of riding a bicycle. He ended up propping it against a light post, mounted, and rode off. Timothy has since told me that he already knew how to ride a bicycle, but the problem with that one was its size.

And so we arrived home with most of the summer of 1975 ahead of us and a wonderful collection of family memories binding us together.

Note

1. Just a few weeks ago I learned that this was a solipsistic claim by the Brits, who often fail to recognize any contributions other than their own. In a book *Sprezzatura: 50 Ways Italian Genius Shaped the World* [*sprezzatura* means the art of effortless mastery] by Peter D'Epiro and Mary Desmond Pinkowish, I read that well over a millennium earlier than 1215, in the Twelve Tables of Roman Law, a woman who absented herself from her husband's home on three consecutive nights each year could avoid some of the legal strictures of marriage. Later, under Justinian's Code, rape, even of a female slave, was a crime punishable by death. Of course if the master did it, it was probably not considered rape, but his right.

Ayers Rock

We lived in Australia from late 1975 into '76. I was thirteen or fourteen.[1]

Pop took the family to Ayers Rock, the world's largest free-standing single rock (Sebele in Swaziland is #2). It was a three-day train ride through the Australian outback (I'm pretty sure we got on the train in Melbourne, but maybe Adelaide.)[2]

When we got there we rented a Mini Moke, one of the world's smallest cars, and to this day I have no idea how we all fit in it.[3]

Alice Springs was the nearest town of any size to Ayers Rock so we stayed in a hotel there.[4] At the time, there was a plague of mice. These things were *everywhere*. When you opened and shut your motel door, two or three would get crushed in the weather stripping. At night when you walked in the dark, you could hear waves of mice fleeing from your approach. For fun the little kids in the area would go out after school and with heavy flip-flops whack mice and hang their bodies from clotheslines to see who could kill the most.[5] (When I was in the Louisiana bayou one time, my guide told me that the area was being overrun by nutria, basically large water rats. He said that a bounty was put out on nutria. I said, "Well, how many are there?" He said, "How fast can you pull a trigger?" That's how this was, millions of mice.[6]

The first night we were there, I was picking at my food (it was terrible). I said to Pop, real quietly, "This food is terrible." He said, "Yeah, worse than at home." It was the *only* time in my life I missed my mother's cooking (sorry, Mom).[7] Only much later in life did I realize that the mice had gotten into the food, and that's why it was so bad.

It was the first time in my life that I had seen a plague of anything. Years later on the Gulf Coast at the Crystal River, I was checking out manatees and saw hundreds of thousands of hermit crabs on the beach. Also, leaving the Sumava Mountains in Southern Bohemia, we hit a stretch of mountain road (very deserted except for our car) and thousands and thousands of frogs or toads all over the road for about ten to fifteen miles. I have no idea where they came from or why they were on the road in the Sumava Mountains.[8]

Mom said there were lots of frogs in Townsville or Cairns (in Queensland), but I don't remember them that much.[9]

CCD

Notes

1. Born December 20, 1960, he turned fourteen shortly after our arrival in December 1974.

2. Actually we took our first train from Canberra, our home away from home, to Melbourne, another train to Adelaide, where we were entertained by Mensan friends of friends we had made in Canberra, then finally boarded the third to Alice Springs. That was through the desert where camels roamed freely. They had been imported in hopes of using them for travel and transport, as in Arabia. It didn't work out, so now the camels make it on their own.

3. It was the only time I have ever bought special insurance for a rented car. This was fortunate because a piece of gravel shattered the "windscreen", the shards of which dropped into my lap.

4. And finally got to the Rock by bus where we stayed in a motel.

5. I called it an "honest-to-Old-Testament plague".

6. These mice were not placental mammals like ours but marsupial mice, like the other Australian mammals, but I didn't think to dissect a dead one.

7. I do the absolute minimum in time and energy to put out the required nutrition because I find it such a boring and distasteful burden. This frees up time to do interesting things. Chuck was the only one who gained weight, but he had access to the hospital cafeteria.

8. Chuck and I saw hundreds of frogs hopping on the road one wet night in Arkansas, but I wouldn't call these a plague, just an abundant hatching.

9. It was Townsville, and I believe they were toads from the sugar cane fields, but nothing like the mice at the Rock. In a country noted for desert, Townsville had a display at the railroad station showing where they were on the annual rainfall of twelve feet!

Christopher doesn't seem to have been impressed by the Rock itself. Tourists gathered at sundown, when it took on a fiery glow. The following day we climbed it, with hundreds of other visitors. Later we were taken to some of the caves at the base with aboriginal art. The locals considered the Rock sacred to the Rainbow Serpent and did not appreciate how we tourists overran it and disrespected it.

Australian Aboriginal Art

While in Australia, we made a point to encounter and learn about their aboriginal population (derisively called *abos* by the English-descended locals). We visited Alice Springs in Central Australia, which is considered their capital, where we saw evidence of their high alcoholism rate, and on to Ayers Rock (see Ayers Rock vignette).

In a small shopping mall near our staging flats (where we spent our entire six months) was a small aboriginal art shop run by

Rohan, a woman who had lived with and even undergone ritual adoption by some of the aboriginal locals. She had aboriginal buyers around the country who knew the art she wanted and would send shipments of aboriginal work. "It's like Christmas when it comes," she told me.

Their paintings, usually on bark, were highly stylized and symbolic, with channels with sharp bends, not naturalistic curves, representing watercourses, water being very important in the desert. The colors were desert tones and black, from natural pigments. Certain artists were well known, and their work in demand by museums. But as the artists aged, they all developed cataracts from the desert sun despite their dark brown eyes, and experts could detect the decline in their work. Although I did not have a feel for these, I picked out several to bring home to Rocky River.

I was more interested in their decorated objects for everyday use. I don't think the children ever got the hang of throwing the boomerang. Our didgeridoo is a decorated trunk of a small sapling hollowed out by burning. We were never able to inhale through the nose and at the same time exhale through the mouth, blowing on the end to produce a constant tone, which the locals could do for hours.

The most interesting things I bought from Rohan were a pair of kurdaitja shoes, i.e., shaman's or witchdoctor's shoes. These shoes are made of emu feathers and human hair, rolled on the thigh of the woman making them, to make a strong fiber. They are oval-shaped, the same at both ends, held on by an ankle strap. This makes the prints the same at both ends, so that the track does not reveal the direction taken as the shaman goes about his duties, which might include murder. These were said to be of "museum quality", but Rohan had no buyer but me. When we got home, I mounted them under glass in an effort to protect them, but they evidently contain tiny insects, so I am taking them to a professional. When I would show them at our Australian soiree or on other occasions, asking people to guess what they were. The most frequent guess I got was "birds' nests?".

A Visit to Abo Country

Abo is Australian for "aborigine", a term applied to the natives who occupy the central desert of that country.[1]

During the mid-seventies our family spent my sabbatical at the new, post WWII ANU (Australian National University) in Canberra, A.C.T. (Australian Capital Territory), situated on the east coast. We took a vacation by train to Queensland (partly to see the Great Barrier Reef) and stopped in Cairns, a moderate-sized town serving the sugar industry, where we were entertained by the family of Dr. Mila Hoagland, a family practitioner whose family had left the Dutch West Indies when the Dutch gave it up.[2] There in a small park was a large artificial pond housing a marine crocodile, the largest of its kind at twenty-four feet long, and a fearsome creature.

Our friends drove us on to the Atherton Escarpment to a small town somewhat deserted, and on to the desert where an enormous rock jutted out of the sand, about a hundred feet high, a half mile long, and a quarter mile broad on ground level. The lower part of this rock was covered with painted figures representing animal and human characters. Each day the setting sun was reflected in brilliant colors.[3]

The habitation of the natives was a primitive one, a windbreak of various plants and sheets of building material. Several such structures each surrounded a fire, and each fire was surrounded by men, women, and children in casual attire, lounging about, as were several dogs. Several white men were chatting nearby. One answered my question, "We are the Flying Doctors of North Australia providing medical care to these people. Would you like to see more about them? We are flying out tomorrow." My curiosity was abated, and I said no.[4]

CWD

Notes

1. The term is no longer considered a polite way to refer to these, the true "locals" of Australia, but when we were there, it was in widespread use.
2. Cairns being north of the Tropic of Capricorn, it was in the Tropics. I remember a comment of Mila's, similar to complaints about winters everywhere: "We have cold winters here — I have to put on a sweater!"
3. This was like a small version of Ayers Rock.
4. A similar offer came when we were in Alice Springs and it had to be declined because we had no one to leave the younger children with, and the doctors' plane wouldn't hold all of us. I would dearly love to have gone.

Grammar

As Christopher proceeded through Kensington Elementary School, I noticed that the teaching was pretty vague about grammar (for which, a hundred years ago, we named "grammar schools"). When I talked to the teachers about this lack, their response was on the order of "Oh, we deal with that as it comes up". Which is not how one approaches a complex subject.

Needless to say, there is much too much grammar to learn in such a slapdash fashion. If these children ever heard about nouns and verbs, they certainly never made it to tenses, participles, gerunds, infinitives, and moods. And so, as with everything else I felt they should know, I took matters into my own hands when the younger two were in so-called middle school. One summer we devoted the first hour of every day to the study of grammar, with diagramming. Since they had some idea of the parts of a sentence, we rushed over those and quickly got to the participles, infinitives, and gerunds. "No, in this sentence 'skiing' is a participle because it modifies the noun, i.e., 'We saw the boys skiing down the hill', that is, they were the 'skiing-down-the-hill boys'. In this sentence it is a noun, made from a verb and therefore a gerund, and subject of the clause, 'Skiing is great fun, but swimming exercises every muscle.'" They fought my grammar classes and were not always quick to get down to work. I was trying to teach the "work first; then play" principle. "If you had started when I told you to, you'd be ready to go swimming." By summer's end, they had a fairly good grasp.

That fall Timothey began French in seventh grade. A month into the school year, he told us, "You know, Mrs. Morrow used to ask, 'Class, who can tell us what an infinitive is?' but now she just says, 'Timothey, tell the class what an infinitive is.'

I believe that there is no other way to understand the structure of language as good as studying a highly inflected one, and so I made sure they each got the two years of Latin still offered at Rocky River High.

When Nicholas, Timothey, and I climbed to see the mountain gorillas, on the way down, when we were euphoric with accomplishment, Nicholas made a complicated remark in which the subject and verb were at a distance from each other and not in agreement, and I pointed it out to him.

"My mother always does that to me too," said our guide. "It makes me so mad."

"You should appreciate it and be grateful," said Nicholas. "They should have taught you that in school and didn't."

Years later I heard Timothey correct his daughter Madeleine's

"Me and So-and-so did this or that."

When Timothey was in psychiatric residency, he told me, "My attending likes it when we talk about words, and I tell him about grammar. After rounds, of course. And he says how lucky I am to have a mother like you."

Units of Measure

When the two younger boys were in middle school, one came home with an assignment to list all the units of measure he could think of, besides the well-known English and metric units.

So the four of us sat around the table thinking up such units: watts, ohms, coulombs, faradays, pascals, calories, Ångstroms, light years. "*Li,* a Chinese measure of distance, is a word Scrabble players use", I told the boys.

"My father used to talk about *versts,* a unit of distance in Russia," Chuck commented. With a twinkle in his eye, he added, "Ask your teacher if he knows what a millihelen is."

I bit. "A millihelen? I never heard of that. What's a millihelen?"

"Beauty sufficient to launch one ship — mine."

Ellwood's Food Circuit

When we were kids, once a month Pop[1] would take us to Ellwood City to visit the Denko relatives.[2] Back then we had both grandparents,[3] Aunt Munya and Aunt Helen. Munya[4] lived in the house on Glen Avenue with Grandma and Grandpa where Pop had been raised. This was one old house. And, although it was cluttered, it was very welcoming. Plus, we got to watch TV (cartoons, and other kid-friendly fare) that we couldn't watch at home.[5] So going to Ellwood was a big deal. We also got to eat candy, something verboten in Rocky River.[6]

One thing I noticed about Ellwood was how many people knew Pop. We couldn't walk down the street without "Hey, Doc, how are ya'?" "Hey, Chuck, long time." "Dr. Denko, where have you been?" *Everyone* knew Pop.[7]

Everyone knew Pop. (Just like his Dad. When we went to Grandpa's funeral, half the town showed up. They were pouring out the doors of the church waiting to pay their respects.)

The first place we always stopped was the Sinclair station owned by the Italian guy Ralph DiBlasio.[8] We would gas up from the trip, and Pop would catch up on the latest talk around town. This guy really liked Pop. I think he liked the fact that even though Pop was a doctor and lived in the big city far away, he would still buy his gas right there in Ellwood and be interested in the goings on around town.

Sometimes we would stop at the National Lunch on Main Street. This place had not changed since 1944. With its long countertop and bar stools, we would line up and order the specialty, chilidogs. Now I haven't had a chilidog in twenty years, but I remember those as being exceptionally good. Everyone in there knew Pop too. They would ask about Cleveland, but they really liked to talk about Ellwood. Pop would always humor them.

Pete Gaydosz owned the largest hardware store in the world. It was located across the river (the Connoquenessing Creek – *JDD*), in the part of Ellwood called "Homewood". Maybe not the largest in terms of size, but largest in terms of quantity of product. This guy had everything. It was the kind of store you went to even if you didn't need anything. You would go there and see things and realize, "Oh, yeah, I *need* one of those." We got things ranging from extra keys made to full-blown archery sets, from fishing poles to wool socks, from garden tools to shoelaces. You name it ... If this guy didn't have it ...[9]

After shopping for some time we would all be hungry for pizza bread. This was found only across the river, near Pete's hardware store. At ten cents apiece, I don't know how they made money (maybe because we each got two or three). Little pizzas made on bread slices — who would have thunk it? It doesn't sound all that appetizing, yet they were awesome.

So after a full day of shopping and eating, we were always just in time to return to Grandma's for a huge meal of whatever she spent all day in the kitchen preparing. The food was universally delicious, but it was never possible to eat enough to keep everyone happy. "Have more, have more, you're a growing boy." "What, you don't like? You only ate three, what's the problem?" "Just one more, it's good for you!" Sometimes it's hard to say no to Grandma, especially when she's making me a meatball I can't refuse.[10]

Koneč![11]

CCD

Notes

1. I tried for years to get Christopher to call his father the more respectful "Dad".

2. Those visits were not the "once a month" he mentions but timed to weather, vacation, and other activities, or to relieve me. I am happy that Timothey has adapted this idea to relieving Patricia on Saturdays by taking Madeleine and Charles Michael to Patricia's parents' home or bringing them to visit me when they have time enough.

3. Actually all four, but the Decker side in Benton Harbor, Michigan, was much farther and therefore harder to arrange to visit, and more often my mother came to us.

4. Widowed the day Christopher was ten, 12/20/1970

5. I always said that in Ellwood they probably didn't know the television had an OFF switch.

6. Instead of the incessant sugar input, like that of all their contemporaries, I allowed them to have candy one day a month, "Candy Day", which Chuck honored by bringing it home to them. They all made it to their teens with perfect teeth, and into middle age with beautiful teeth and little need for repair.
7. Chuck and I both laughed over the time a fellow, wanting an introduction, greeted Chuck with "Who's this? Your wife?"
8. When I get to Ellwood, I still make a point to fill up there and tell the new owner to convey my greetings to Ralph.
9. Denko visits to Ellwood produced an uptick in the economy.
10. I can visualize the scene, having visited many times. As my fork would be approaching my mouth, Munya could contain herself no longer but inquire, "How do you like my meatballs?" She even asked Cleo, our dog, how she liked the meatballs. Once in excitement Cleo wet on the carpet. To my apology, Munya replied, "It's only a small carpet!"
11. "Finally" or "The End" in Czech.

One reason Chuck loved to go to Ellwood, without me, sometimes, was that I tried to keep his weight down at home. There nobody had to try to stuff him. He really cooperated.

Pop's Cheap Side

Pop was always doing things that my friends' parents didn't do. He would rinse out the tomato sauce can with water to get the last little bit; he would reuse paper towels (after drying them out), and bags and plastic always got used again. Sometimes it was embarrassing, like when my lunch sandwich bag was in the newspaper delivery bag instead of a nice new sandwich bag like all the other kids'.[1]

He always drove secondhand cars even though as a doctor making 60K/year in the seventies he could have afforded a new car.[2] My father drove the white Rambler *forever* because it refused to break down. Then came the '69 Cutlass Supreme (gold-colored, two-door). At first it was a used car,[3] but by the time I was fourteen or fifteen it was very cool because '69 Cutlasses with 396-cubic-inch engines were *very* cool with fourteen- and fifteen-year-old kids (my buddies) in high school.[4] So suddenly Pop was a lot cooler both to me and to my buddies. Actually, whenever any of my friends met Pop they generally thought he was OK, which, when you're fourteen or fifteen, *no one's* parents are OK.

But I digress.

When I was eleven or twelve (1972 or '73) we went to Dearborn, Michigan. I think Pop had a conference and took the family.[5] As we came down the main drag of town from the highway, it became apparent that a gas price war was going on. The prices were drastically lower than in Cleveland and were getting lower the closer we got to the center of town. Since we had driven from Cleveland, the tank was near empty, and Pop was excitedly talking about the gas prices and how it was a great deal and on and on (just as he does today). Finally when the price hit twenty cents/gallon, Pop couldn't take it any more and he pulled in to fill up. He was gloating as the young man filled the tank.[6] Pop was so happy, until two blocks farther down the price dropped to eighteen cents and Pop went ballistic.

So here's a guy making good money freaking out over a two cents/gallon savings in a maybe twenty-gallon tank tops, making it a maximum forty cents cheaper. I couldn't figure it out, and I wasn't brought up during the Depression either.[7]

Even better than that: We were in Prague in '69[8] and went to the local outdoor market to pick up souvenirs. Pop wanted to get change purses. On the outskirts of the market the change purses were 7K (Czech koruny). We kept going. A few more rows and the price was 6K. A few more rows, 5K was too good to pass up. We loaded up and got six or seven. As we were leaving, we saw 4K change purses, and again Pop went ballistic. When Czechoslovakia gained independence in November 1989, the exchange rate was 45K/$1. I feel fairly certain it was some constant exchange rate during the Communists. So a 1K saving on six or seven change purses amounted to 6 or 7K/45K/$1, approximately eighteen cents U.S. I guess it was the principle more than anything else.[9]

Now, I don't take it as seriously as Pop, but I still wash out the last of the tomato paste with water, I reuse bags, I recycle. (My parents used to recycle in the '70s when no one knew what recycling was.) I also bargain with the marketplace people (no matter what country), but I generally don't freak out over a 6 or 7K loss. I've learned to take everything more in stride, because raising my blood pressure the way I know Pop's must have gone up just doesn't do me any good.[10, 11]

P.S. Later on that same trip, we were in the mountains near Starý Smokovec, and I saw an old man putting pepper into a huge shot of vodka (it looked like a small glass of water). I said, "Pop, Pop, that guy is putting pepper in his water." He tried to explain it wasn't water, but since we *never* had alcohol at home, I didn't know what he meant.[12]

CCD

Notes

1. Too bad that it was only recently that I saw and procured for myself a T-shirt that said: "Embarrassing my children; just one more service I offer." Your father and I could have both worn one of those.

2. This is incorrect. With just two exceptions, we always bought new, inexpensive cars and ran them until they got expensive and troublesome to keep up. One exception came before

Christopher was born. We needed two cars. My father's vision precluded driving, and so my parents had one extra car that they gave us. The other exception I learned of from Timothey while working on this project. He said he remembered hearing his father say he had bought a second-hand car from a colleague at the hospital.

Chuck wanted the car that would transport the kids and me to be in safe running order. I distinctly remember an Oldsmobile station wagon I bought. For some reason Chuck favored the Chevy across the street. But I went back and bought the Olds because the salesman had told us he had had heart trouble, had to give up heavier work, and was given a chance at selling cars. He seemed nervous and in need of a success. Worried that he might despair and even commit suicide, I gave it to him. There was not much difference between the two wagons anyway.

When I would buy a new car, the salesman was always disappointed to see me get out my checkbook to pay for it since he had expected to sell me a lot of credit. It was not until Chuck was in decline that I caught on to the idea of saving the first year's depreciation in value by buying a good, late-model Volvo. Chuck had totaled two Volvos due to problems with depth perception, both bought new, and suffered only a scratch, and this persuaded me of the safety value of the make. Once when I had a car in for servicing, I told the mechanic that my purpose for a car was to get safely from point A to point B, not for status. He found that such a remarkable attitude that he kept repeating that line back to me every time I came in.

Christopher no doubt got his idea from the fact that we wore cars out and got a new car, for cash, only when the upkeep became time and money costly.

3. Maybe that was the one from the hospital friend.

4. I didn't know any of this. What was the make of a Cutlass? Was that that Oldsmobile?

5. This was when we had decided that the time had come to take the children to Henry Ford's Greenfield Village.

6. This was before self-serve, because we never paid the surcharge, although I noted that with one technologic change, millions of jobs were suddenly gone.

7. If you had been, you would understand.

8. Christopher, check out this "cheap guy" who takes his children traveling, including to Europe when they are in elementary school and to many other places, camping to Alaska, to Mesa Verde and the Grand Canyon on the way to a sabbatical in Australia.

9. One of his father's interesting economies that Christopher forgot was that Chuck would mix two or three kinds of cereal instead of buying the advertised "multigrain" product.

10. And you don't have children to educate. Well, now you have little Emily Rose.

11. When Chuck filled out the questionnaire I gave Mensans for my book, he made the point that he enjoyed handling money better than most, including many on welfare.

12. As you can see, travel is not wasted on the young.

Timothey's Thin Skin

Recently Timothey told me how unhappy he was as a young child. Some nights he would even cry himself to sleep. He was not able to give me a general reason for this.

He did have several specific complaints about how I had treated him in childhood. For example, since I thought little boys' pants hanging low in the crotch very unattractive, and since they wouldn't wear belts, I made elastic suspenders, to be worn under the shirt so as not to show, but to keep the pants up at waist level. While Christopher and Nicholas didn't like this, I never got any serious objection from them. But with Timothey, once when playing tag, someone tore his shirt, saw the suspenders, and made fun of them. Similarly, I had the children bring home their used paper bags from lunch (I interpret this as my being a woman twenty-five years ahead of her time), and the little herd animals ridiculed this too.

Another idea I had conceived when I had two boys with birthdays within five days of Christmas: to give books for the birthday and toys for Christmas. So I extended this idea to Timothey, but unfortunately his birthday was July 28. Again, when kids asked what he got for his birthday, books were not a praiseworthy gift in their eyes.

I told him I am sorry I contributed to his unhappiness with boys who couldn't appreciate any deviation from standard.

Like each of his older brothers, Timothey had two birthday parties, one at seven and one at eleven. When the boys were seven, we had the old pin-the-tail-on-the-donkey contest and dropping clothespins into a milk bottle. The older kids went to a movie. No clowns or magicians.

Thirteen-Year-Old at Sea

The summer when Timothey turned thirteen Chuck gave a talk at Erasmus University in Rotterdam and had other business in Switzerland. Since Timothey had been too young for the earlier transatlantic crossing with Christopher and Nicholas (and Nicholas was really too young to get much out of it), we decided to take the two younger ones on this trip, again an ocean crossing.

We took a bus to Montreal, where we boarded the Polish ship *Stefan Batory* (the only ship at the time with a five-star dining room) and enjoyed a 1000-mile cruise down the St. Lawrence before even heading out into the Atlantic. We passed the brilliantly lighted Quebec at night, and in the Gulf of St. Lawrence I saw an enormous pod of a hundred or so whales, but didn't have time to call the others, and nobody announced it over the PA. Halfway across, on July 28, when the ship acquired a teenager, they made a fuss over Timothey, with not only a card signed by the entire staff of ship's officers, but a cake with sparklers, and the band playing a Polish equivalent of *Happy Birthday.* I sent a press release home, and the article that came out in the west-side paper identified Chuck as a psychiatrist.

We disembarked at Bremerhaven and used our Eurailpasses to head south to Switzerland. But, able to disembark and reembark on the train at will, I suggested we spend a few hours in Bremen, reasoning that they must have a statue of "The Town Musicians of Bremen". They did. Everywhere you turned was another representation of that popular children's tale. In Basle, we took the boys to the zoo to see Przewalski horses, the horses bred back to their wild forebears. (I have recently read that their line is now running free in their original home of Mongolia.) The boys hiked in Liechtenstein while Chuck and I rested. We also visited one of the most popular tourist sites in Europe, the attic where Anne Frank and her family hid, where a Japanese mother in formal attire was patiently helping her five-year-old son sign the guest book in Kanji. We returned home on the Russian *M. V. Lermontov.* Timothey signed up for chess, and Nicholas and I sang and danced *Kalinka.*

The Lost Cat

One unseasonably cold November evening, I picked up Timothey who was taking classes at our local nature center and serving there as a junior curator. He came to the car with a half-grown black-and-white kitten in his arms. "She was at the back door where we were making animal rations. I fed her. Can't we keep her? Look, Mom, she's already spayed. She has a scar, so somebody cared for her and she's just lost."

"But what about Whitepaw? I don't see how we can work with a dog and a cat. I'm afraid you have to take her back."

And he did, reluctantly.

Immediately I regretted it. That night I kept awakening in my warm bed, thinking of the kitten in the cold Metroparks.

The next day I told my friend Gerry Thorrat I had made a mistake, and together we went looking for the cat. We circled around all the roads several times, and parked to explore paths on foot, but that day and the next we were unsuccessful. It was like the proverbial needle in a haystack.

On the third day Gerry suggested that if she were a cat, she would follow children returning home from school along the edge of the park. As we circumnavigated the periphery, we encountered a postman making his deliveries on foot. And so we asked whether he had seen a black-and-white kitten.

His face fell. "Is she yours?" he asked. "Yesterday I spotted her huddled against a tree trunk. I caught her, put her in my car for warmth while I finished, and gave her my sandwich. She was so hungry she almost swallowed it whole. My cat died recently, and I thought she could be my replacement for my little Cleo. But if she's yours — "

"No, no! We're so happy she found you and a home." And we told him our story.

Gerry, who found me unduly cynical, reminded me, "There are many good people in the world, and we and the cat have found one of them."

Pot Luck Suppers

All through the boys' school years I loved the PTA potlucks because the women outdid themselves to show off their culinary skills. I developed a strategy of being nearly the first in line and then falling in again at the end. Chuck once took his borsch and was annoyed because instead of taking a taste test, they would take a large bowlful to try, and then throw it out. On the other hand, twenty years later a woman who had evidently not thrown out the borsch came up to us at a little theater, introduced herself, and praised Chuck's PTA offering.

Recently I received a note from the mother of an Indian Guide in Christopher's tribe, thanking me for helping her son, a teacher, by discussing how he was teaching literature. The mother added, however, that when their adolescent daughter had died unexpectedly on a vacation trip, Chuck had in condolence brought her a tureen of what she called "purple borsch". It is, of course, beet red.

I eventually got into the habit of taking deviled eggs to any potluck because I was the only one in Ohio who made them "right", with vinegar, and members of whatever organization always reminded me to bring those good "narcissus eggs" (white protein, yellow yolk, and rusty red paprika).

When they were in middle school, I would arrange to sit with Nicholas's English teacher, from whom we always had such favorable feedback, to discuss literature.

"I have never heard as good a presentation on Jack London, from adult or student, as Nicholas's, and the slides were so interesting."

"I didn't know he gave a talk. He must have borrowed my slides. On the trip we talked about *To Build a Fire,* as we were facing my mother's death. What are you reading now?"

And we went on to talk, as always, about books.

The Car Thief

The summer when Nicholas was fourteen and Timothey almost thirteen, I happened to have tickets to a summer concert at Blossom, when Chuck was out of town. I invited Donna, a nurse from our ward, intending to take her and her teenaged daughter and our two younger boys, but Nicholas had been asked by his Scoutmaster to accompany him to Scout headquarters downtown to make arrangements about a large campout. That left the four of us, and Donna offered to drive.

After a lovely concert, Donna dropped Tim and me off in our driveway about 11:30. To my shock my car was gone. And so was Nicholas! I sent Timothey to bed before he knew anything was amiss. The Scoutmaster told me the arrangements had had to be postponed, and he had no idea where Nicholas was. He offered to go look, but I told him to wait while I made calls. The hospitals reported no such admission, and the policeman at Rocky River headquarters said, "Lady, kids do this all the time. Does he know how to drive?"

"No, he's just fourteen," I told him.

"He'll be back soon," he tried to reassure me.

As I was hanging up the phone, the amber revolving lights of a tow truck moved up the driveway. I saw Nicholas get out his wallet to pay for the tow.

There must have been lightning darting from my eyes because while I was questioning the tow-truck man about where he picked up the car (it was at Nicholas' friend's home), the garage man said, "Don't be too hard on him, lady. He's awful scared! Your transmission is giving trouble."

"He has plenty of reason to be scared. I know about the transmission and have an appointment for servicing," I told the man, and added to Nicholas, "Wait for me in the kitchen."

After a long pause, I confronted my son. "You stole my car!"

"I'm awful sorry, Mom. I know I shouldn't have."

"And if my car hadn't been giving me trouble, I wouldn't have found out, which is what you planned on, and there's no telling what your next malfeasance would have been."

"I'm sorry, Mom," he repeated.

"And another thing—where did you learn to drive?"

"From Chris's *Sportsmanlike Driving* book."

"Do they call it 'sportsmanlike' to drive a stolen car?" I screamed.

"I guess I'm grounded," he admitted.

"Until we leave for Europe in six weeks. Go to bed."

As he walked past me on his way out of the kitchen, he silently kissed me on the cheek.

To the best of my knowledge he honored the six weeks of grounding.

Academic Challenge

For many years Cleveland has had a quiz program for competing high school students, called *Academic Challenge.* It is open to juniors and seniors, who try out to be on the team, and schools can compete only every other year. We had watched the program for years, and had sung out the answers to many of the questions, but doing this from the comfort of a living room is vastly different from doing it under hot, bright television lights.

Nicholas hit the year when he was a junior, and Timothey was captain as a senior.

I had told them that win or lose, they had made me very proud just to be on the team, and the stress of competing against another team could adversely affect the outcome. Both their teams won, and Timothey's went on to win an escalating contest newly announced in his year.

When Christopher was at Grand River, they had planned to send him to *Academic Challenge* also, but by the following year he had left to go to another school.

One thing I noticed with both the younger boys' contests: There was always a segment with questions from the Old Testament (not New Testament, to keep it fair for Jewish contestants). Each time the competing team and the other contestants on our team were clueless, whereas our sons knew all those answers, thanks to the teaching at Sts. Peter and Paul Russian Orthodox Church Sunday School.

Don Laycock and Papua New Guinean Languages

Several years after our sabbatical we received a letter from Don Laycock, whom we had met in Australia, where he was president of the very active Australian Mensa. This linguistics specialist in the languages of Papua New Guinea, where a fifth of all the languages of the planet are spoken, is collecting words and making dictionaries of languages, some spoken by as few as a couple hundred speakers, before they are lost. In the letter Don told us he was planning a trip around the world, stopping to lecture various places on his way to England. He asked if we would put him up for a few days in Cleveland. In return, he offered to "sing for his supper", i.e., give a lecture for whomever we wished. For some reason we had not received his letter until after he had left Australia, but he had listed his stops, and so I sent copies of our welcoming letter to all of them, so that at least one would catch him. We connected, and Chuck and I took off separate days to show him around Cleveland, the Art Museum, the Natural History Museum, and our European-style West Side Market, but the Cleveland Orchestra was not performing at Severance. Resting on a bench in one of the art museum galleries, he and I talked about our respective sadnesses. His wife had a bizarre psychotic illness that the doctors had not been able to help, and we were at the peak of our troubles with Christopher, who was by then no longer living at home.

The younger boys loved it that Don let them stay up to see Benny Hill, a British comedian whom I would not have let them watch. They were impressed when Don showed them his initials after the article on New Guinean languages in our *Encyclopedia Britannica.* I liked for my children to have opportunities to meet and interact with various adults. Don admired my filing system — between the balusters of the banister.

Meanwhile, before his arrival I had had time to plan one of my soirées in the Parkview party room, inviting our friends to hear his lecture.

I remember his discussion of "pidgins" and "creoles", each a kind of language based on an older language with acquisitions in vocabulary and grammar from other languages. (Chuck said they sounded like "casseroles".) Don also explained that there is nothing definitive about our eight parts of speech. Other languages have others, e.g., in some there is found a "postposition", similar to our "preposition" but placed *after* the noun or pronoun it locates. These New Guinean languages also have a way to alert the hearer that a question is coming. This is similar to the Spanish use of the upside-down question mark at the beginning of a sentence, but the New Guinean designation is a verbalization because of course their languages are not written. We also indicate a question by our rising pitch at the end.

Mensa in Northeast Ohio and Mrs. Hudson's Lodgers

When we transferred our membership to the Northeast Ohio Branch, our experience was at first less positive, partly because one prominent clique consisted of several women who were not only obnoxious but functionally so stupid that, according to Margaret Barlow, our blind member, "They must have cribbed to get in." For a time we attended many monthly meetings. Mensa policy was not to pay speakers, but this rarely made a problem because speakers often said that they enjoyed having a look at us and seeing how highly intelligent people played. I went to Dallas for one AG (national annual gathering), where I gave a slide presentation about our recent experiences in Russia.

I made friends with Margaret, who taught the educable mentally retarded (EMR). She enjoyed *movies,* and she appreciated going with me because, while she could follow most of the story by her ability to distinguish voices, I would whisper precisely the visual clue essential for following what was going on. She was the woman who suggested Christopher's Eagle project: tape recording books for children in schools for the blind.

Several years after our move, the Northeast Ohio chapter split because of the distance for alternating meetings between Cleveland and Akron, and the increasing size of the membership.

A fringe advantage of having the Parkview was that on occasion smaller groups — SIGs, or special interest groups — could meet in its basement party room.

Eventually I had calls from a member looking for an apartment. We rented her one, but this produced trouble: a man, interested in her but evidently rejected, shot at her through the window. Feeling responsible for not only her safety but also that of other tenants, I hired a detective to keep watch in the driveway for a week until the crisis seemed over.

Later this same tenant asked me to run for "loc sec" ("local secretary", British terminology and equivalent of president). I refused for a while because I knew I would be running unopposed, and it was the year for our chapter to host a regional gathering (RG), which I would have to chair. I finally agreed, reasoning that this would be a new learning experience for me. My board picked the 1940s for our theme for the RG, but avoiding the war. For entertainment I engaged a singing group from the Clague Playhouse to do a medley of songs of the era, with changes of hats and other atmospheric props. The RG was well attended and very successful.

I was defeated for a second term because, I believe, I was trying to promote using our smarts to do something of social value in addition to fun and games. I had in mind taking on the tutoring of kids in seventh or eighth grade who were in danger of dropping out in a year or two. I got nowhere with this idea.

As I walked out of that meeting, I commented to someone, "I lost an election, but I won my freedom." Being loc sec had taken a lot of time, despite the fact that I had a very good board, the first all-female board in our chapter. Fifteen years later Adelaide Jaffe (a member who had won $28,000 on *Jeopardy*) observed that I had been their best loc sec, having delegated all the jobs, with deadlines. I attributed our success to the high quality, motivation, and responsibility of the board.

One attractive feature of Mensa was its special interest groups. The one that Chuck and I enjoyed was Mrs. Hudson's Lodgers, a Sherlock Holmes group similar to the international Baker Street Irregulars (named for the nine- or ten-year-old street urchins who did odd jobs portering, pilfering, and living by their wits, that Holmes used for his eyes and ears on the street), but without the stringent examination for "investiture". Monthly meetings were fun, often including quizzes, games, talks on subjects Edwardian remotely related to the stories in the canon. When Dwight McDonald was chair, the highpoint of the year was an all-day meeting with several invited speakers, usually college professors with subject matter relevant to Edwardian England. (I love to be lectured at.) By dinnertime we would convene attired as characters from the canon. For the men this was easy. There were many British officers, naval personnel, upper-class British types, tradesmen of many kinds, even the Dalai Lama. My friend Charmaine Seversen dressed her husband, Allen, as a "poulterer" in carpenter's apron with chicken feathers loosely glued on. The members would arrive as these characters and maintain the persona through the evening. For women it was harder. Not only were there fewer female characters in the canon, but they were also less distinctive, thus harder to portray. One year I went as the dancer Ireney Adler, in my ballet recital costume complete with tutu. I won the plaque that year, probably because I could be identified. I don't remember what persona Chuck took on for the Sherlock Holmes evening, but when we attended the Boar's

Head and Yule Log medieval dinner, he wore his academic gown to which I had attached gold astrologic symbols, thereby converting this chemist into a medieval alchemist.

When Dwight McDonald could no longer run Mrs. Hudson's Lodgers, the Stetaks (an architect and a pharmacist couple who had taken the exam and been "invested" in the original Baker Street Irregulars) kept it going. It struggled on for a while but eventually fell apart.

High School All-Night Parties

As our boys were graduating, many high schools attempted to combat drinking after the senior prom or graduation by having the parents put on an all-night party. This involved skits, songs, dancing, and funny performances of all kinds.

Of course Christopher did not graduate from Rocky River, and I was ashamed and afraid to be seen around the high school in case people there would know the reason. Nonetheless Nicholas came four years later, and Timothey a year after that, and Chuck and I became involved in their all-night parties, which Rocky River parents put on after graduation. Only Chuck met with the group that wrote the variety show, so I could have those free afternoons. This was also because I have no talent for humorous writing, didn't know the popular songs they were parodying, and felt I would not be a contributing member.

In the organizational meetings Chuck was fighting booze references and even, in Timothey's class, one mother's wish to appear topless onstage, which the committee didn't permit. Nicholas's parent committee had been more conservative.

In one skit a line of us with rolled stockings did the Charleston as we twirled our beads. One teacher, whose strict (good) teaching methods for honors English made her a good target for satire, was Mrs. Gratar. I danced onto the stage as Mrs. G, whom everyone recognized, and that performance was so popular that I was asked to repeat it for Timothey's class.

One mother commented, backstage, "The main thing is for my daughter to be happy. Don't you agree?"

"Not quite. Most important is for them to be virtuous. If they can be happy too, that's a bonus."

Beaver Island

The remarkable thing about my childhood was the fact that I grew up in the country on the shore of Lake Michigan, and, attending a country school with fewer than a hundred pupils in nine grades, I was practically tutored. I have always felt sorry for city children. Before I married, I fantasized creating a similar environment for my children to grow up in, with a country school like Lafayette to attend. Still I knew that with a scientist husband, we would need to be within daily commuting distance of a university where he could pursue his research. Our house at the end of Watt Road, with its dammed pond, though not perfect, was something of an approximation, but we had to leave it. Living on the cliff above Lake Erie was an attempt to recreate the water part, but it entailed city living. I could not give my children what I had had.

An alternative might have been to vacation each year in a spot similar to where I grew up. When we lived on Watt Road, I recall going out to look at farms, with land and a house, to use as a weekend retreat, but they were not on a Great Lake, we could not be a part of the community, and the project of getting the farmhouse ready even for weekends was daunting. Besides, for vacations I found this a non-solution because I wanted vacations, summer and other, to meet my plans for exploring the world with the family. The "country living" remained an elusive fantasy.

Then my friend Anne Morrissett invited us to her summer place on Beaver Island. I remembered seeing Beaver Island on the map in my Michigan civics book when I was in elementary school. The dotted line from the mainland to this island in the northern end of Lake Michigan meant that there was ferry service. For many years I had dreamed of going there someday, and my chance had come.

Our first trip was in our old recreational vehicle. It happened that we picked up Nicholas at Northwestern University's summer High School Speech Institute (after I had made another trip to see him perform as Caliban in *The Tempest*). We circled the southern end of Lake Michigan and headed north, camping near Holland, and finally reaching Charlevoix in time for the ferry. Entering Paradise Bay, the finest natural harbor on the Great Lakes, is impressive, and so was the short trip across the island to Donegal Bay to Anne's summer house.

Then I heard her story. Her family, consisting of the parents and six children, three adopted and three by the other method, had come for the traditional two-week summer vacation for many years. Then they decided to build their own place. Marion, Anne's husband, was found to have cancer, and so for his last summer she pushed through her project of building a house with a central living area and two wings of several small bedrooms each.

But Anne had farther-reaching plans. She had bought several acres with the hope of getting her friends to buy off lots and build their own houses, with the intention that her friends would be up there with her.

This came close to meeting my old hopes. Beaver Island is now more like Higman Park, where I grew up, than Higman Park is like it now. While I could not make our boys younger, if we had a house up there, it could be a Denko retreat — and so it has become. Our "summer place" is winterized with electric heating. It is most accessible for the Pittsburgh Denko family, and this year, 2011, I am delighted that Patricia, Madeleine, and Charles are spending the entire summer there, living and playing with the local children. It is my hope that the other Denko grandchildren will also have opportunities to taste country/lake living on Beaver.

And that's not all. Seven acres on a dune facing Lake Michigan and the setting sun were divided into two parcels. I bought the first, with a basement in place that grandfathered me into building a house there. When the other half went on the market, I got my check to the tax collector half an hour before it would be auctioned and bought it. I am now protecting the basement and planning a family (siblings and children) vacation home. It is part of the evolving Denko trust on Beaver Island.

The Reduced Denko Family

Chapter IX

Reduced to a Two-Member Family

When Timothey went off to Kenyon College, we moved on to our Denko version of the "empty nest". I had expected that at this juncture Chuck and I would be able to pursue our careers with no more diversions at home. Chuck could have longer hours at the lab, if he wished, and did, on the whole, because, when the boys were not living at home, the serious problems we faced did not consume many hours every week. But, unlike many empty nests with the fledglings flying and self-sufficient except for financial support during schooling, we had two of the three who were precarious. Waiting in a doctor's office, I chanced upon an article in *People* about the Terman lifelong study of gifted children. As the women in that study were approaching retirement age, the most contented were those with a career and no children; those with children were still trying to "fix" them. I wasn't the only one.

Those years were not without trauma. Christopher's delinquency had escalated. While I had been attempting to correct his increasingly wide swings from normal, Chuck, believing his lies and making excuses for him, was clearly in denial. Chuck was a weight obstructing my efforts and dragging me down rather than a collaborator in my attempts to stop Christopher's chaotic and delinquent behavior. The legal system, with its endless use of the least restrictive tools in its armamentarium (probation, school for boys with social problems), also believed Christopher's lies and blocked my endeavors to contain him until he could be redirected. It reminded me of running up the stairs, trying to catch a track runner (see *A Handful of Ashes*). Years later Christopher volunteered, "You were the only one who knew everything I was up to. Nobody else did." He was wrong. There was more going on than ever reached me. But he was right about one thing: he had everyone but me bamboozled.

We had consulted a psychiatrist in Australia who believed we were covertly encouraging and enjoying his misbehavior. We consulted another one back home. Christopher ended up in juvenile court and was sent to a boarding school for boys with social and behavior problems. That school did not accept him back the following year, although he was on the dean's list and planned for their Academic Challenge team. Even this did not speak to the judge. After an abortive effort at a residential correctional institution, he was sent by the judge who believed his lies to live with his Uncle John and family in Texas.

I decided that my life would no longer be held hostage to Christopher's, with his random returns home, like a cyclone. When he needed something (like money), his father would give it to him without question. I told Chuck that if he let Christopher in, I would leave. These events had a wakeup effect: Chuck was finally no longer in denial. I credit him with taking on, for the next few years, ongoing contact with Christopher, who had gone to live in Washington where he was taken to court by George Washington University and expelled. He finally graduated from American University (see *A Handful of Ashes*).

Chuck would visit Christopher two or three times a year, taking his younger brothers along in the summer (see Christopher's humorous vignette "Summer Fishing, Sort Of"). Chuck's involvement may have been a lifeline that kept Christopher in touch with the mainstream and on his way back to a semblance of normal living.

Our parental challenges, however, were not over. Timothey, at Kenyon College, was obviously a practicing adolescent alcoholic. But Chuck had learned. He cooperated with me for several years, in the two interventions, two hospitalizations, and six-month halfway house, while Timothey finished college and went to live with Nicholas in Philadelphia (see *Fighting the Good Fight*).

Soon after Fairview General Hospital closed its research unit, Chuck went full time to Case Western Reserve University, without pay. Those were his most productive years, as he pursued his belief that osteoarthritis is not a result of "wear-and-tear" but a metabolic disturbance (see the vignettes "Resume of Research in Osteoarthritis and Cartilage" and "Significance of My Research").

One year Chuck asked his formulaic question: "There's a Scandinavian Rheumatology Society meeting In Reykjavik. Do you want to go to Iceland?" I did, and we did, but the timing was bad, just after the end of the school year at Kenyon. Our plans were all made, tickets bought, and hotel reserved, when Timothey came with a request. He explained that his friend had a summer job at Kenyon but was not allowed to stay on campus until the summer term began. "Can Tom stay with me for a few days and save the cost of a trip back home to Florida?"

I had a rule of long standing: when Chuck and I were both out of the house, no friend of either sex was allowed on the property.

"Timothey, I like to see you help out your friend. I just wish it were when your father and I were home. Do you think you and Tom can abide by the rules?"

He thought he could. (I had forgotten that you can tell when an alcoholic is lying by the fact that his lips are moving.)

Before the meeting we saw the geothermal phenomena for which Iceland is noted, like Yellowstone, including Westermann Island and Geysir, the geyser for which all geysers worldwide are named. In fact as our bus arrived in Reykjavik from the airport, a sign alerted us to a day trip to the "black glacier", on only that very day of the week, and so we changed our trip to Geysir, which could be any day, and headed off to the south shore to see the glacier covered with ash.

Returning home, when we arrived at the Cleveland/Hopkins Airport at 5:00 a.m., there was no sign of the boys, who were supposed to pick us up. When the taxi dropped us off at home, the scene was one of destruction and chaos with the boys drunk and asleep amid empty beer bottles. I sent them to bed. In the morning I contacted the other boy's mother, got him out of the house, and supervised Timothey's cleanup efforts. We did not arrange another intervention and hospitalization at that time because Timothey said he planned to live with Nicholas and work. Chuck took Timothey, his clothes, and his stereo to Philadelphia, where there were a number of lost jobs, no help for Nicholas even with food money, until Nicholas had had enough. (I reminded him that I had not asked him to take Timothey in.) Finally, one evening Timothey overheard a couple walking on the sidewalk under his window and realized that the things he really wanted out of life — a family, a profession, travel, i.e., life like the one he had grown up with — were incompatible with alcohol and would require the Twelve Steps.

It was his apocalypse. He called his father to ask him to bring him home, and, with the help of Barbara Craver, the former intervention worker, we set up a long-term hospitalization in an alcoholism unit in Milwaukee,[1] followed by a halfway house.[2] As Timothey was working in a hospital lab, he watched the white-coated medical students and began to analyze how to climb out of the hole he had dug. He secured a letter of recommendation from a Kenyon professor who recognized his giftedness beneath the alcoholism, went to a medical school admissions office, asked what to do to make himself a welcome candidate for medical school, and followed their advice about which courses to repeat and which to take for the first time, such as embryology, which he had skipped while getting a truly liberal education, taking philosophy with the philosophy majors (and making friends with Garth Vant Hul, who went on to study international law and is now running CARE in West Africa), French Revolution (with the history majors), and advanced calculus (pulling down a B while drunk). He worked on getting back on a medical track without our knowledge or advice or intercession with the admissions people, and when he was accepted at two medical schools, he picked the University of Cincinnati, where, it happened, Nicholas was already studying. Soon Timothey was giving talks at the VA Hospital on "Life after Alcohol". He evolved a life with his mother's specialty and his father's type of academic career. He is now a clinical professor at Western Psychiatric Hospital, University of Pittsburgh, working on several depression studies, heading up a multi-site project, and has become credentialed to administer electric shock therapy, more frighteningly called electroconvulsive therapy, though they stop short of a major seizure. Like his father, he takes his family, when possible, on work trips (see *Fighting the Good Fight*).

Crises from Nicholas were fewer and time-limited. Still in high school, he totaled two automobiles within ten days in alcohol-related accidents. Somehow, until years later we did not know about the alcohol, and neither did the police.

Long hoping to attend an Ivy League University, Nicholas was accepted at the University of Pennsylvania, where he placed out of all freshman courses as a result of his honors courses at Rocky River High. Therefore in four years he earned his B.S. plus an M.A in education. His only extracurricular activity was Quadramics, the drama society. He acted, made a stage set to float in the swimming pool where they produced Sondheim's version of Aristophanes' *The Frogs*, and directed *Amadeus*, the first student production ever to receive comment on Philadelphia's television news. We flew out to see these performances.

Later, Beth Waldman, his girlfriend, told us that, realizing that alcoholism was in his future, he stopped drinking. During college and after graduation he worked under Amato Giaccia, his friend and mentor, on a Milheim Cancer Research Grant at the Wistar Institute in Philadelphia, then went to medical school at the University of Cincinnati on full scholarship, where he earned the double doctorate (like his father's) and on to academic work in radiation research in oncology under Giaccia, at Stanford University, rising to assistant professor. Later he suffered non-Hodgkin's lymphoma, now in remission with the help of Timothey's peripheral blood stem cells (see vignette on his life in the companion book).

Those years were punctuated by the inevitable deaths of our parents. My mother went first, at the unseemly early age of seventy-one, with a wildly malignant colon cancer. We had asked her whether she wanted to spend her remaining time with us, but who needs to be incapacitated in a house with active boys? She stayed with her sisters in Kalamazoo, who said that she rallied a little each time I visited. Then Chuck's father, with complications from a broken leg from being hit by a car. Then his mother, peacefully, in her nineties. And finally my father, from Alzheimer's, for whom I had to travel to Florida to have him declared incompetent and arrange for a Florida guardian, John Butterwick, his stockbroker, and settle him in a nursing home. He said funny things, e.g., "When you've been married five hundred years as I have". My parents' conditions required my involvement and my travel back and forth tending to their needs, as their only child. Chuck's sisters were able and willing to make decisions for their parents, conferring with Chuck.

A few years later Chuck lost in rapid succession a younger sister (Munya) and younger brother (John), both from cancer of the colon.

In the early years of our marriage, when you could just go to a window and buy a ticket, or look through our travel agent's book of sailings to find which ships would get us to a meeting and back with time to spare in the vicinity of the meeting, Chuck was the experienced traveler who would plan how to bring it all together. As time went on, however, we would receive travel brochures, sometimes from our numerous alumni organizations (together we had attended half the Big Ten universities and a handful of private schools) and sometimes from eco-travel groups. I began by consulting him about these, but I noticed that he would lay aside the brochure to "think about it", so I started just telling him I was sending in the deposit, since I did not know how long I could count on his (or my) health to hold up. In this way we were the first signed up with the University of Michigan for one of my lifelong dreams, to set foot on the continent of Antarctica, which I had spotted on the inside cover of my orange geography book. That trip happened in 1986 within a couple weeks of when we achieved another goal of mine going back to my days at Lafayette School: to cross paths with Halley's Comet, which I had read about in a children's encyclopedia and calculated when would be its next "apparition" in its seventy-six-year-orbit (see my poem "The Visitor" in *Interlink*). In Antarctica Chuck was able to do everything but climb the volcano and swim in its warm effluent on Deception Island.

Chuck and I were planning a trip to the Galapagos Islands. The timing was perfect for Nicholas to go along, between his semesters. "Your brother would have more fun if you went too," I told Timothey, with his new hospital lab job, "and so would we, but I'm not inviting you because you haven't been on the job long enough to ask for time off even without pay, even if they'd give it to you. Succeeding on the job has to come first." Timothey told us that he had told his supervisor we had invited him, but he had declined because they needed him at the lab. She told him she too was saving for a Galapagos trip.

In my innocence I thought that getting hired would be the end of my son's work-related problems. All he would have to do would be to do his work. What could be simpler? Evidently another aspect of life that Timothy had not learned during his years-long hiatus from the real world was that you must follow the instructions of your superiors, regardless of whether you like the instructions or the superiors. As the old joke goes, "The boss may not always be right, but he is always the boss." Stories Timothey told us made it obvious that he was antagonizing his supervisor. I brought this to Roger's attention. "He must be coming off sounding arrogant. What in the hell does an only recently recovering alcoholic have to be arrogant about?" Roger reminded me that Tim's personality and self-esteem had taken a beating, from which, also, he would need to recover.

Another time, when Chuck did not want to leave his work, I took Nicholas to Madagascar, primarily to see the lemurs, but an unexpected bonus resulted from the spectacular lizards. I also caught a glimpse (Nicholas was down the trail) of a cicilian, a wormlike legless amphibian, exuding a puff of bad odor as it vanished down its hole. On that trip, in a museum in the Comoros, another exciting sight was a mounted specimen of the ancient fish coelacanth, thought to be extinct for millions of years, but recently discovered by fishermen. On Aldebara we saw more giant land tortoises similar to those in the Galapagos, and we floated with manta rays over the coral lagoon.

When Nicholas and Timothey were in medical school in Cincinnati, instead of paying rent they each bought a house, Nicholas, a century house, two floors of which he remodeled and rented to cover the mortgage payments, and Timothey, a Victorian "painted lady". They came home for vacations. One Thanksgiving we had a potluck, with the Balogs and their daughter Mary Anne and her fiancé, in the apartment party room. I took the stuffed turkey and gravy, and games our boys had liked to play as kids, such as Don't Spill the Beans. I commented how much I enjoyed watching them enjoy that, and Nicholas added, "It's fun for me now that Tim has grown up and can lose without crying."

Later I took Timothey ("recovering") to Borneo, primarily

to see orangutans in the wild, where he said, in a tone almost of awe while he was criticizing the childish, bad behavior of a tour of school children, "I feel so privileged to cross paths with these 'men of the forest'." The proboscis monkeys were another delight as they jumped forty feet from their daytime trees into the river to cross to where they spent the night. In mangrove swamps we watched mudskippers, fish using their buckling fins as legs to crawl ashore with oxygen-laden seawater in their gills for breathing (see my poem "Mudskipper" in *Interlink*). On Borneo's Turtle Island we saw mother turtles laying eggs and eight-week-older turtlets hatching from their shells, climbing up through the sand, and returning to the sea. We carried them in buckets past the predatory gulls with their eyes on hors d'oeuvres (see poem "Maternity Ward on Selignan Island" in *Interlink*).

In 1991 our natural history museum offered a shipboard trip[3] to the Sea of Cortez to see a solar eclipse lasting a second short of seven minutes (just a few seconds short of the longest possible solar eclipse when all the variables are just right). This eclipse was in the saros (family) of eclipses eighteen years and some months apart, going back to the one in 1919 in Africa, in which astronomers confirmed Einstein's hypothesis of the curvature of space by the bending of light from a distant star. On this trip we took Christopher, who by this time had burned out the worst of his delinquency. At the event, with all the excitement and screaming and the glory of the vision itself, he became a "shadow chaser", going, whenever possible, with us or on his own, to see other eclipses. The passageways on our ship on that trip were decorated with pictures of Mexican attractions, and I was delighted that Christopher pointed out the unidentified photograph of the Pyramid of the Sun and recalled having been taken there at age eight.

By this time I had devised a requirement: when we took a son or sons on a trip, they were to eat with us at night, so that we could "catch up" on their lives and interests as well as the day's activities. There were even exceptions to this. On one trip that flew us past Angel Falls in Venezuela, the world's highest, falling like a diaphanous scarf off a *tepui* (a high, narrow mesa), I encouraged Timothey, by then a medical student, sometimes to sit with the young ship's doctor. At our table, when a fellow passenger introduced himself as Dr. Thomas Weller, Chuck asked whether his brother or father at the University of Michigan, had won a Nobel Prize in the 1950s. "Shh, shh, shh," the man whispered. "That was me, but I don't want it to get around the ship." We promised to keep his secret but told Timothy to meet and talk to him. Tim got him to sign a medical text for work he did on malaria. It was not until the flight home that we divulged his Nobel Prize to Timothey.

Several years later, Christopher, considerably subdued, went with Chuck and me when we saw an eclipse off Curacao, another in the Black Sea (with Timothey also that time), another in Zambia (with Nicholas's wife, Karen, and Christopher helping with Chuck's increasing disability), including a trip on the Edwardian blue train, Rovos Rail, to Victoria Falls, and another with just the two of us after Chuck's death, on the Sudan border in Egypt (including the antiquities along the Nile). Having traveled with his work, mostly in Eastern Europe, Christopher volunteered that he had never experienced more friendly people than the Egyptians. On eclipse trips we were lucky, never clouded out.

When the famous "Little Red Ship", the *World Explorer* (originally the *Lindblad Explorer*), about to be retired, was repositioning from the Mediterranean to the Amazon run, they decided not to cross empty but offered a five-week trip describing a huge letter "J" down the South Atlantic from island to island along the mid-Atlantic Ridge, then west to South Georgia and the Falklands.

Chuck and I boarded in the Canaries (see vignette "Travel around the Edges"). We visited the Cape Verde Islands (off the bulge of Africa, active in the slave trade); Ascension (where American pilots refueled in WW II and the saying was "If we miss

Ascension, my wife gets a pension") (see my poem "Ascension Island Land Crab" in *Interlink*); St. Helena (where Napoleon spent his terminal exile); Tristan da Cunha (the world's most remote inhabited spot, with 300 inhabitants and five surnames, a philatelist's paradise); South Georgia with Shackleton's grave and thousands of king penguins, as well as albatross nests, where the enormous chicks exercise their wings for an entire year before taking their make-or-break flight) (see my poem "Royal Albatross Chick" in *Interlink)*; and finally the Falkland Islands (where decades after the Falklands War, many fields were fenced and marked with CAUTION signs for live land mines). (See CWD's vignette "Special Rheumatology on Tristan da Cunha.")

During his full-time years at Case Western Reserve University, Chuck was able to continue his work on the biochemistry of rheumatologic disorders. There he was eventually recommended for the rank of full professor but was told that he had exceeded the age limit, to his and my disappointment.

From 1987 until his death in 2005 his major achievement was demonstrating osteoarthritis as a metabolic disturbance.

Notes

1. Milwaukee is known as a town with twice as many breweries as churches.

2. Timothey's halfway house was within blocks of where Jeffrey Dahmer was doing his cannibalistic thing with young men. Fortunately none of us knew about Dahmer until later.

3. On this trip I had an unforgettable conversation about world problems with a NASA scientist who happened to be black. He said, "God help me, I had hoped AIDS would solve the African population problem." And I replied, "God help me, so did I, and I'm a physician."

Letter from Timothey

8-6-90

Dear Dad,

This is a letter I've been intending to write for some time, and I hope it coincides somewhat with your birthday.

I first somehow got onto this train of thought in super-group at Milwaukee Psych, and my addictionologist was crying at the end. It went something like this:

My Dad always found the time to do things with me that I liked and he really didn't like. He'd throw the football with me, throw the tennis ball to me, take me fishing, watch football with me: the Steelers & Penn State — he'd even get Mom to let us watch the whole game. And I just pushed him away. I remember him coming to our intramural basketball game against the faculty, and I'd rather talk to my silly girlfriend. I'd lie to him, and he always kept coming back. He never gave up on me. He drove to DC twice to get me into treatment. When I'm a father, I want to be just like him.

I guess that's somewhat abbreviated, but I hope the message is there.

Love

Timothey

P.S. I don't want Mom to be hurt by omission, so maybe not letting her see this'd be a good idea.

The only part of Timothey's letter that was hurtful to me was that Timothey thought I would be hurt by his male-male love for his father. I am delighted that he appreciates what his father did for him.

Summer Fishing, Sort Of

For a few years running, Pop and the boys and I would get together for a late summer fishing trip. This was back when the RV was still working, probably the mid-'80s. The first year they picked me up in D.C. and we headed north into Pennsylvania (you know — God's country).[1] I don't know how or why, but we ended up at Raystown Lake near Altoona. This was an Army Corps of Engineers project, and it created the largest manmade lake in Pennsylvania. The fishing offshore was terrible. We found out later all the big ones were out far and deep.

But we had a good time setting up camp and wandering around and even fishing a little. I think Nick had been in school a year or two, and Timothey was about to enroll [in college. *JDD*]. So this was sort of their last hurrah before going back.

We stayed up late at night, sitting around the fire and discussing everyone's plans for the upcoming year. The guy on the site next to ours was waiting for a group of friends to show up for the weekend. He had so much food and bar, he was only too happy to help us out in exchange for a little conversation. But I guess that conversation[2] either got very animated or very late because Pop came out of the RV at one point yelling and blustering about getting to sleep. "God damn it! How are you going to catch fish if you stay up all night?"[3] Well, as I said, the fishing was dismal, but Pop was right so we packed it in. Driving back to D.C. was pretty rough the next day, but Nick and Tim helped out. The next time we went on a fishing trip (Kelley's Island with Billy Pflueger, scion of the Shakespeare Company making fishing equipment), when Pop came out to yell, we told him we were going night fishing, and he was good with that, albeit grumbling all the way back to the RV.

CCD

Notes

1. Here Christopher is referring to Chuck's abiding rootedness in the hills of Western Pennsylvania. Although I didn't mention Michigan one percent as often in conversation as Chuck did Pennsylvania (and when he would, for example, compare something in Chicago to something in Ellwood, I would point out that comparing Chicago in the '50s to Ellwood in the '30s was beyond the usual "apples to oranges", more like "hot fudge sundae to T-bone steak"), whenever we drove up US23 under an enormous sign across the entire highway welcoming us to Michigan, I would always announce to the car, "Now we're entering God's country."
2. Now he's talking about the group of men talking into the night.
3. As if they were there mainly to catch fish — and I never heard him swear.

Christopher's Dutch Genes

When people try to decide which parent or other older relative children resemble, I usually have difficulty seeing the comparison unless it is stark. John Butterwick, my father's broker, said that Christopher's large, barrel chest reminded him of a solid Dutch burgher, but that he didn't look particularly Dutch in the countenance.

After not having seen Christopher for several years until his early twenties, I was presented with a photograph of him in cap and gown walking toward the camera. I gasped at my reaction to my father's return from the dead!

Later, when Christopher was home for Christmas in 2000, he was wearing a reddish-brown moustache. I happened to be sitting on his left, and when he turned his head for me to get a three-quarter view of his face, I had a reaction like a *déjà vu*. It was as though I was looking at the father I remembered from my childhood. I mentioned to him this striking resemblance.

Then he told me about an experience he had had while doing business and visiting friends in Amsterdam. A friend of Christopher's friend looked at Christopher and said, "Yep, that's the one! He's the spittin' image of the Rembrandt painting at the museum."[1] The man was referring to a prior conversation in which the mutual friend had told his friend that Christopher could have sat for the painting

Note

1. We discussed whether it was a character in *The Night Watch.* I see similarity in a self-portrait of Rembrandt.

Medical Airlift

In the summer of 1999, I received a desperate call from Christopher in Prague, where he was part owner of a "lounge" called The Marquis de Sade. It was like our neighborhood bars, where, because of the tiny living quarters, people meet their friends in the evening. (I had a friend who was traveling in Czechoslovakia check out the lounge, unbeknownst to Christopher, and she said that despite the name, it was like many others around the city.) When a flood put part of Prague under water, Christopher housed the homeless there and in his apartment.

Christopher related that John, a friend of his from the States, had been visiting and, not understanding the traffic signals, had walked in front of a car, which had thrown him many feet, causing him to land on his head. He had been taken to their premier hospital, which I later learned had originally been a military hospital and therefore was oriented to trauma victims. John was unconscious, and they held out little hope for his recovery, but, as I later learned, they had trephined his skull, i.e., removed a portion of the skull in order that as the brain swelled from the trauma, it could swell outward, relieving pressure, rather than downward to the base of the skull, where pressure would destroy the vital centers at the base of the brain, causing death. A trauma physician in this country told me that this lifesaving procedure had been given up in this country for patients like John because the results, while lifesaving, most often leave the patient in a vegetative state, and whole wards are full of them.

When he called, Christopher's request was for his father to find a specialist, perhaps from Germany, to evaluate possible help for his friend. While his goal was to save his friend, the Czech physicians had already done that, and the question was what to do next.

For several days, while we were calling back and forth to the Czech physician and to our local trauma center, deciding what to do, every time the phone rang, I thought it was probably news of John's death.

Nevertheless, what we worked out was to airlift John to the level 1 trauma center at Metro Hospital in Cleveland. This necessitated flight of a plane equipped for medical care, with physician and pharmacist, to Prague, transport of John by ambulance to the Prague airport, and flight to Cleveland (with one refueling stop), then transport to Metro Hospital by helicopter. Through all this he survived.

After a couple weeks, John opened one eye.

By this time long-term survival seemed possible, and the best judgment was to get him back to his home area in Washington, D.C., and into the care of their Medicaid people. Three weeks later, when Christopher visited, John's eyes followed him around the room, and he said rational, distinguishable syllables in farewell, "Good-bye, Chris".

After his brain function slowly returned, a plate was implanted over the trephination to protect the brain. Months of rehabilitation followed. Finally this man, who would have been given up as hopeless in this country, was alive and well, except for certain signs of brain damage, such as irritability. (Aren't we all irritable sometimes?)

Occasionally John sends me a letter. He has undergone a religious conversion. He has also suffered leukemia, from which he is in remission, and is now reading philosophy, Hegel, Chris tells me. (I find Hegel very difficult.) While Christopher doesn't believe he understands much of it, his recovery is, nevertheless, a medical miracle. Christopher recently told me that four physicians in the Czech Republic and eight in D.C. said John wouldn't survive.

Chuck and Waratah

Once when the boys were away at college and Chuck and I were home alone on a Sunday afternoon, Charmaine Seversen, a friend from a writers' workshop (and I might add a very good literary critic) came over unexpectedly. She seemed charmed with how she found Chuck rolling around on the floor with our dog at the time, Waratah, named for an Australian flower. He always thought that at least young dogs should live in families with children for this kind of play. Anyway, he sometimes made up for their absence.

Later that afternoon I asked him to make tea for us, Charmaine being a British tea drinker, and he did, returning with three cups of tea, a plate of cookies for Charmaine and me, and a plate with a couple cookies on one side for him and several dog biscuits on the other for Waratah. He didn't seem to understand why that should amuse Charmaine and me.

Having mentioned Charmaine, I wish to include an experience

of hers that should not be lost, even though not relevant to either Waratah or our lineage.

One snowy night a woman telephoned Charmaine, an author and poet who taught an evening writing class, to ask her help in writing a poem about an experience that had both enraged her and caused her to suffer unbearable grief. The woman's daughter had made a suicide pact with her drug-dealing boyfriend, but only the daughter went through with the suicide. Charmaine put her off until the following day, but that night the woman committed suicide, bereaving her husband and son. Charmaine said to me, "Instead, I should have gotten her to you."

My reply: "She should have killed the boyfriend instead. No jury would ever convict."

Charmaine's experience reminded me of a similar one of mine. I was asked to interview a man who had applied for a job on our team at the Argonne Cancer Research Hospital of the University of Chigago. I told him quite honestly that he was overqualified for our job, and it would be best for both of us if he found a job better related to his skills, and we found a different technician, because if we took him on, he would soon look for a job using his talents better. Although this was not a time when jobs were hard to find, that night he committed suicide.

Gabriella Mistral's Home in Vicuña

I was satisfied with one solar eclipse, the marvelous 1991 eclipse we saw for a second under seven minutes from shipboard in the Sea of Cortez, and had not intended to attend another. However when the Museum of Natural History offered another eclipse trip in November 1994, with a visit to the international observatory high in the Chilean Andes, I signed on because of an added inducement: They offered a pre-eclipse extension to Easter

Island. I found it hard to imagine getting there any other way.

A remarkable feature of the trip (besides Easter Island, the eclipse, and the enormous telescopes high in the clear, cold, dry air of the Chilean Andes) occurred because thousands of visitors were converging on the eclipse from all over the world. Transportation was complicated, with little air transport and poor roads. In fact when I returned to Chile from Easter Island, after the eclipse I learned of German tourists who had planned my identical schedule of flights, leaving Easter Island in time for the eclipse in Chile, but Lan Chile had bumped them, destroying their intelligent travel plans and depriving them of the eclipse experience. I determined never to use Lan Chile again.

Back on the mainland, we witnessed the eclipse high in the Andes, almost on the Bolivian border. We were billeted at an army barracks, where we were given the bunks, and the recruits slept out on the mountain. Then, between the eclipse and the observatories, we were on a bus when I happened to notice from the printout that we would be going through a town named for a member of the camel family related to the llama — the small town of Vicuña. This town's name jogged my memory from having read the poetry of Gabriella Mistral, the first South American Nobel laureate in any category, back in the mid-20th century. This was the pen name of a poet who wrote poems about children and who lived in Vicuña.

I beckoned to our guide. "David [pronounced Dahveed], I see we're going through Vicuña. They must have a bust of Gabriella Mistral in the square or some other recognition. Can you take us to see it?"

"You've heard of Gabriella Mistral?" he asked, so excited he almost fell off the bus.

"I've read her poetry in a bilingual book in the original and English translation, put out by my school, Johns Hopkins University Press."

"I'll do better than show you a statue. I'll take you to her home, which is preserved in what is now a post office." When we got off the bus, I heard the astronomy-oriented members of the group muttering such things as "Why are we stopping here?", "Why are we going to a post office?", and "Who the hell is Gabriella Mistral?"

My answer to that one was, "She won a Nobel Prize. Have you?"

The postmistress in charge of the memorial showed us the poet's and her mother's former living area, with snowy white linen on the narrow cots, and another room with school desks like mine from my three-room country school, where she had taught a handful of children, a role she assumed without pay.

As we continued our journey, David and I discussed her poetry, including her best-known poem, in which she described children holding hands, stretching across the narrow valley from one mountain to another. I told him also about the poems I was writing about the mother/child relationship, and he was pleased that I offered to send him copies of some of mine.

But the story did not end with this charming addition to the fall eclipse trip.

On New Year's Eve the telephone rang, and a voice said, "This is David."

"David? David? Oh, David!" I exclaimed. "You're calling from Coquimbo?" And so we chatted and reminisced, and he thanked me for the poems I had sent, which he had shown his English professor at the University of Coquimbo.

Our Buddhist Hermit

Early in the 1990s, my cousin Eunice Noordyke Lampkin, who also is a travel aficionado, happened to mention to me that she had been trying for ten years to get someone to go hiking with her in the Himalayas, but all her takers thus far had been men.

"Well, you've got a woman now," I told her. We invited Chuck immediately, but he declined to accompany us.

And so we were off to the Taj, Fatehpur Sikri, Shwedagon Pagoda in Yangon, Myanmar (formerly Rangoon, Burma) with its seventy-six-carat diamond at the pinnacle, and other points east, the highpoint being a five-day hike in the Himalayas in Nepal. We had sherpas who took down the camp each morning, put thirty pounds each on their backs, and went jogging along the path, passing us and having lunch ready when we arrived. We even had a girl sherpa, who, when her day's work was done, would sit near the fire and knit baby clothes for her infant back home. Eunice and I had the distinction of having our "loo", a square canvas arrangement with a pit, stolen from us one night and waking up to have no facilities on the bare ridge. But I digress.

One bright day, as prayer flags fluttered, our guide asked whether we wanted to visit the hermit.

"Of course. We came to be educated. Who and where is the hermit?"

As we climbed almost vertical stone steps wide enough for their tiny feet, that we had to ascend sideways, I asked myself, "How do you have an audience with someone who speaks only Telegu, or something?"

In his one-room shelter atop his mountain peak, our host sat in lotus position, clad in saffron and with shaved head. Surrounded by piles of manuscript, he greeted us in Oxfordian English. He explained that he was writing textbooks for Indian children to learn English because they had no future without it. He was supplied with his necessities by the school in the village we would pass through at the end of our hike.

After our return home, my cousin, a music teacher, collected and sent the hermit hundreds of pounds of educational materials for ideas. She never heard whether they arrived. I did hear back from our guide in Srinagar, to whom I sent several money orders to help him and his family through the troubles with

Pakistan. He asked me to find him a job in America. One of several reasons I couldn't was that his specialty was ancient Indian musical instruments. Remarkably, the money orders got through to him. His address reads:

Firdous Ahmad
c/o Aftab Ahmed Bazaz (Cloth Merchant)
Shop #5 Sarsyed, Market Wazirragh, near A.S. College
Srinagar 190088, KHR INDIA

Since Eunice planned the trip to India and liked five-star hotels and took a long shower each morning, I got into the habit of reading the English-language newspaper that was slid under the door until she was ready for the day.

One day I read about gang warfare in the streets, but these were not gangs like ours. These gangs were composed of men who had been born with undescended testicles. (The newspaper called them some kind of homosexuals, but that would not be our classification.) They would be forever infertile because their condition, which must be corrected in childhood, would never be treated in India (at least among the masses), as it is, in a relatively simple surgical procedure, in this country. (Of course they don't need any more fertile adults in India.) Therefore, having no prospect of marriage or a normal adult life with a self-sustaining occupation, they had no choice but to live together, taking in young boys with the same disability. To earn a living they threatened/bribed parties and weddings to pay them not to crash the party and embarrass the guests. Apparently two gangs were fighting over turf.

When our guide arrived, I showed him the article and asked for comment. He blushed a deep purple and looked the other way. "Come on — I'm old enough to be your grandmother, or, in India, your great-great-grandmother." He seemed neither willing nor able to shed any more light on the subject, but later, on our hike in the Himalayas, we met an American doctor who knew of and confirmed this practice.

Two Indian woman physicians in our country denied ever having heard of this solution to this problem.

A Visit to Greenland, Country of Strange Superlatives

Several years ago our family and I were fortunate to visit the strange country of Greenland (current name in Inuit is Kalaalit Nunaat). The name for the country is different and unusual just as the harsh physical environment is very different from that of Cleveland, Ohio. A giant ice cap covers nearly the entire country, which is the size of Texas and contains fewer than 100,000 people.

One morning our little group docked at a village in the southern part of the country. After strolling about, we sat in the park, where the locals came to study these visitors and tried to demonstrate their fishing skills. I was looking at their hands for evidence of arthritis, and they seemed happy to have this attention paid to them.[1] After we left, my son Nicholas said, "Dad, it's good that you aren't a urologist."[2]

CWD

Notes

1. They were delighted with the attention of being examined, smiling broad, toothless grins. It made their day.

2. Chuck was never far from rheumatology. He thought about how certain behaviors or occupations would put special demands on joints. Once we won tickets to see the Riverdance group from Ireland, mostly women but with a leading male dancer,

Michael Flately, who danced in tap/toe shoes, and whose dancing involved coming down on his toes, sending shock waves up his body. Our tickets (in return for a donation to the local public television station) entitled us to a reception with the dancers after the performance. Instead of shaking hands with Flately and moving along in the line, Chuck asked him how his back was holding up under this punishment and together they estimated the life in dance this man might expect. Another time Chuck took the two younger boys and me to see a Jewish comedian whose performance included balancing on one foot on a ladder, twirling rings around the other ankle, and juggling several balls during his jokes. After the performance Chuck shook his hand and gently pulled on his fingers to test their flexibility, while the boys vanished, embarrassed, into another part of the room.

One reason we took Nicholas and Timothy on this trip was that, in addition to seeing Greenland, medical lectures on shipboard were offered for credit for our ongoing medical education to keep our licenses updated, and the boys could attend these too. They were on the topic "Medicine at the Extremes". By this was meant extreme cold, desert conditions, high altitude, and ocean depths. The course was given by a professor the boys had in medical school.

Originally our tour had included Baffin Island, which attracted me for wildlife, including narwhales.[1] On this trip we were unable to get to Baffin Island at all because the ice had never broken up, although it was already August. Therefore our tour kept us entirely around Greenland and included several formerly unscheduled visits such as to that retirement village for elderly fishermen, an enormous improvement over the old method of setting the elderly adrift on the ice. From the ship we saw at a distance a huge whale, which our marine biologist said was a "blue whale" and the first she had ever seen. That is the largest animal that has ever lived on planet Earth and twice the size of the largest dinosaur. Near an abandoned mine we were shown Precambrian rock that is the oldest on the surface of our planet, going back 4.2 billion years, almost a third of the way to the Big Bang. By zodiac we cruised at the base of a cliff where thousands of kittiwakes were nesting. We saw the bodies of a family that had mummified naturally in a cave 500 years ago. We were taken to Disko Bay, the outlet of the fjord down which the glacier moves sixty feet a day, and large numbers of icebergs are calved. In 1912 one of them had a rendezvous with the *Titanic.*

Note

1. These tusked whales had always intrigued me. After Chuck's death I joined a group camping at the upper end of Baffin Island, where we saw hundreds in the bay too shallow for their enemies, the orca, but rich in Arctic char, their, and our, favorite fish. They even had a gam, a whale party, and stroked each other's tusks at what would have been midnight if they had had a night. We stood watching in our nightgowns.

In the Wake of Odysseus

When the travel brochure arrived from the University of Chicago for a trip following in the wake of Odysseus from Troy around the eastern end of the Mediterranean back to Ithaca, I got on the phone to reserve, having hoped some day to see the ruins of Troy. The story was that all Chicago's spaces were taken, so I called the shipping line. Their word was that they no longer had any of the cheap cabins that we always favored, so I told them we would have to decline. So, not to have an empty stateroom, they compromised. "We'll give you one on the upper deck at the same price." Nicholas had plans to go hiking in Wales, but Timothey was free, and I managed to get him into a shared cabin.

We assembled to board ship in Istanbul. It became apparent that the tour included participants from the University of Minnesota, the University of Chicago, and Harvard, and the buzz was that John Updike was in the Harvard group. "How do you make conversation with Updike?" the women were asking each other.

"Well, one thing you don't say is 'I just loved your book' — he's heard that," I told them. "I think I know what I'll do."

My chance came sooner than I expected. In our cabin (since it was in first class, and the captain didn't know we hadn't paid the first-class rate) was an invitation to the captain's table for dinner that night.

At a lull in the conversation I said, "Mr. Updike, you'll be interested to know why I've never read any of your books." It was not quite true, but necessary for what followed.

This got his attention. "What, what, why?"

"I lead a Great Books Discussion Group, and we read only dead authors, so you'll be happy to know you don't qualify." General laughter.

The following day we reached Troy, eleven or so cities built each on top of the last, with the Troy of the Trojan War being, as I recall, Troy 8.

Other sites on the trip were identified with, e.g., the cave of Polyphemus, the Cyclops, and Circe's Palace. A classicist from Harvard and an art historian from Chicago lectured to us. A day ashore in Nauplion on Father's Day gave Timothey a chance to buy his father a T-shirt with the Hippocratic oath in Greek. We went ashore at the summer villa of Tiberius, an art connoisseur who commissioned art of sadistic and bloody events from mythology. On the sculpture showing Odysseus running a burning pole into Polyphemus' (the Cyclops) only eye, Chuck noticed rheumatoid arthritis in the fingers (see vignette "Did the Model for Polyphemus Have Acromegalic Arthritis?"). When Chuck drew our attention to this, Updike became enthusiastic and said, "Yes, Denko, write it up!" Another fascinating stop was at the shrine of Tiresias, the oracle, through whom Odysseus asked for advice from his deceased mother and heroes in the underworld. In preparation, the suppliants were given no food for several days, just wine, and deprived of sleep. By the time they heard the oracle, they usually couldn't remember the riddles in which the oracle spoke or figure them out if they did.

Whether the sites represented places where Odysseus actually stopped was irrelevant, but the ruins where Tiresias held court resembled a damp basement.

Monarch Butterflies in Mexico

In February of 2000, after Nicholas and Karen had been married the previous summer, we invited them to go with us to see the wintering monarch butterflies in the Santa Rosaria Preserve in the Trans-Volcanic Mountain Range west of Mexico City, in the state of Michoacan.[1] After arriving in Mexico City, we were given a day to acclimatize to the altitude before heading out to the monarch area by bus. One of our small group happened to be the woman who had headed the team developing Viagra. She knew that the medication was sold over the counter in Mexico and was interested to learn what they charged for it, so we sent Nicholas, who was perfectly willing to buy a trial supply. It was naturally much cheaper than in the States.

We stayed in a tiny charming hotel with fireplaces in many rooms, and went by truck out to see the butterflies. On the monarch wintering mountain billions of butterflies hung from the trees like draperies, but, not in hibernation, they had to feed and find water for hydration. Thus there was a constant river of butterflies down the mountain about twenty feet above ground level, and back up during sunlight hours. On the mountain itself, the air was full of butterflies on the wing, and they would alight on people, especially those who wore red. Karen (a photographer of pets and children since becoming allergic and unable to work in the cancer research lab) and I were clicking memories constantly. I told Nicholas and Karen, "I hope that after my death you will remember with happiness this day we shared."

From our guide we had learned of the butterfly research programs, including banding them in the States and Canada with the hope of retrieving a miniscule fraction of the bands, from wherever they rested or died en route or in Mexico. (Several years earlier Chuck and I had, in fact, taken a day trip with the Natural History Museum, to the Toledo area to swish our butterfly nets and affix bands to the leading wing edge, to identify place and date of the butterfly resting on its southward trip. An earlier year, while driving Timothey west on Lake Road to his class at the nature center in Bay Village in September, I was amazed to see dozens of monarchs heading south, about fifteen feet above the ground, also on their migration to Mexico.)

We were asked to buy up any of these bands that were offered, with a view to sending them on to the researchers. While a visitor for a couple days would have little chance of spotting a banded butterfly, the locals, including guides, both official and unofficial, were aware of the bounty offered (in pesos and, of course, in preferred dollars, the going rate being a dollar a tag). Nicholas and I were together when a local offered to sell us four such bands, which we were happy to buy so as to have them sent on to the lepidopterist at the University of Oklahoma.

When our group gathered in the truck to return to the hotel, we were handed out our box lunches, including cans of fruit juices with a tiny teardrop-shaped opening under the protective tape.

As we were sharing experiences, Nicholas got out the four bands to show our tour friends. (I would never examine something so small and valuable in the bed of a truck, in the open, with gentle breezes, anywhere, in fact, except in a room with walls and table, for fear of losing them. But Nicholas was intrepid.) Soon he announced that he could find only three, and I chided him, too late, for his recklessness, but as we continued with our lunches, a strange look crept over his face. He wiped his tongue with a finger and produced the fourth band, which had somehow found its way through the tiny orifice in the juice can, floated on the liquid surface, and washed back out of the can and into his mouth, rather than clinging to the inner surface of the can and being lost to science.

Karen always said that Nicholas had a talent for completely legitimately making the world work for him. A good example was the time he saw that a flight was overbooked in San Francisco, offered to take a later one, was given an upgrade to business class, as well as a later free flight, by running caught up in Chicago with the flight to which he was supposed to transfer from the original one, and arrived in Cleveland on time.

This happy vacation occurred several years before Nicholas's luck changed, with his terrible adversity in the form of his non-Hodgkins lymphoma.

Note

1. The Mexican abbreviation of Mich. on license plates and signs attracted my attention because it is the literary abbreviation for my home state of Michigan, MI being only the postal service abbreviation.

Chuck's Fund of Information

Drawing on Chuck's fund of information, the geographic facts of which he attributed to his instruction in geography in high school and at Geneva College, he and I once played a "game" to see how close he could come to the populations of foreign cities. He was remarkably close with European cities, less good with cities on other continents. Also, we were once invited to an evening with Charmaine and Allan Seversen to play Trivial Pursuit. However after half an hour it became apparent that Chuck kept getting everything right, giving nobody else a turn, so we quit.

When we crossed on the *Stefan Batory* to Europe, part of the ship's entertainment was a quiz game, with many questions targeted at persons of Polish descent on this Polish ship. Chuck was in it until the final question, at which point I concluded that he would be eliminated when they asked, "What is the name of the estate where Chopin was born?"

To my astonishment, he produced a mangled (admittedly by him) version of *Zelazowa Wola,* to their also great astonishment that someone without Polish connections could come this close. They awarded him a beautiful green woven woman's belt as prize.

Years later when we were in Poland with People-to-People, I skipped one of our meetings with local physicians and managed to get out to Chopin's birthplace while Chuck was conferring with Polish doctors about medical ethics.[1] In an alcove where Chopin's mother actually gave birth to the composer, the Chopin Society keeps a perpetual memorial of fresh flowers.

I pointed out to the guide that Poland can claim three C's: Copernicus, Curie, and, of course, Chopin.

Note

1. We learned that the cost of platinum drugs precluded their use in ovarian cancer, leaving no effective treatment for women suffering this disease in Poland.

Exploring Chuck's Ancestral Homeland

Chuck spoke Russian as a first language. What he had learned at home he called "peasant Russian", but he went on to take literary Russian at Penn State, which of course facilitated travel in Russia.

Our first visit to the USSR was in 1983, when the European Congress of Rheumatology met in Moscow, and Chuck gave a paper. However, their program for wives was so good that he skipped many of the sessions to visit, e.g., Dostoevsky's parental home in a hospital where his physician father cared for the poor. They showed us little Feodor's toy horse on rollers with a pull-string. They took us to Lenin's dacha in the country, where they showed us Russia's early telephone. On our sightseeing excursions, the other wives were impressed because I knew just enough Russian to transliterate Cyrillic, street signs, for example, and I knew that what looked like "pectopaw" was really "restaurant".

We took a post-Congress extension to Leningrad, where I nagged until our guide [1] finally was able (after numerous excuses, such as "only groups of five, not four or six" or "only on Tuesdays, not Wednesdays") to get us to the basement of the Hermitage to see the Scythian gold collection. (They made us, including Chuck on his cane, run around three sides of that enormous museum to enter at the correct entrance.) Peter the Great, in the early 18th century, had his archaeologists use state-of-the-art methods to excavate burial mounds on the north shore of the Black Sea, dating from about 500 BC. I was impressed with the delicacy of the goldsmithing, e.g., fine quills drawn out on a tiny hedgehog. I also noticed a chariot with angels hovering over it, which I attributed to Zoroastrian influence, since I had read that their religion was the first with angels. Always the rheumatologist, Chuck spotted a gold bowl with an engraving of a shaman examining a patient with evidence of rheumatoid arthritis. The medicine man was wearing what we call a "stocking cap", a sign of authority. He was palpating the patient's ankle through a boot, and the patient was wincing in pain. His hands grasped a staff and several finger joints were swollen. This combination goes with rheumatoid arthritis. Chuck pursued this in correspondence with the Hermitage, for permission and a photograph to include in a short article. Chuck's colleague, Charles Malemud, is working to get this published posthumously. (Chuck's vignette is "Arthritis in Scythian Art", and his paper is "Rheumatoid Arthritis in Scythian Art".)

I had long hoped someday to travel the Trans-Siberian Railway.[2] For a long time one needed a reservation about eighteen months in advance. Therefore when Johns Hopkins offered what I expected to be the better half, the eastern end from Vladivostok to Irkutsk, and my friend from St. Joe, Anne Morrissett, who had wanted to travel with us, was going with her son, Roger, and suggested that we travel with them, I jumped on the idea. I was right about the eastern end, meadows of wildflowers naïve to pesticides. In Irkutsk a solar physicist, Aleksey Golovko, showed us his observatory, and tour members much more knowledgeable about astrophysics than I were astonished at the first-class work he was doing with primitive equipment.

We were a day late flying on to Moscow[3] due to flight problems. On the extra afternoon in Irkutsk we were taken to their geology museum, a small, crowded facility packed with specimens, many of which, the docent explained, had been sent back by visitors as representative of their areas of origin. I had interesting specimens from my native area, Berrien County in southwestern Michigan.

Once covered by an inland sea, the beaches yielded a harvest of fossil crinoids that we called Indian beads. Fulgurites came from the dunes. These are naturally occurring glass (the only other kind besides obsidian), caused when lightning strikes a tree growing in the dunes, transmitting the heat down through the root system, fusing the sand surrounding it, making tubes with glassy smooth interiors and crumbly sandy sheathes produced as the heat rapidly dissipates.[4] Because of the fragility and because I didn't trust the Russian postal system, I was reluctant to send these, and unless I knew someone who was going there I had no way to get them to Irkutsk, until several years later. (See vignette "Chuck's Polio Disability".)

With our policy of not repeating in our travels, I had no reason to expect ever to be back in Irkutsk. A few years later, however, when a boat trip around Lake Baikal (the world's deepest, in central Siberia) was announced, I suggested to Chuck that we could this time do the western end of the Trans-Siberian to join the group. He had had a hankering to get to the Pushkin Museum in Moscow to see and photograph a replica of a Roman sculpture of a warrior, the model for which had been so carefully copied that it showed arthritis (which would have precluded the individual from being a warrior in real life), so I arranged for two extra days at the beginning of the trip. For the first day I wrote to the Pushkin Museum. Although I had had no response, they let us in despite it having been the wrong day or something. I can still picture Chuck toiling up the long double flight of enormous marble steps with a handrail so wide I could hardly span it with my hand, to get to the sculpture, which I photographed. (Both Timothey, in his vignette, and our friend Blaise Levai in his, commented on how Chuck's determination to climb stairs was a symbol of his indomitable will.)

On our second extra day we were met at the hotel in Irkutsk by the physicist we had met on the former trip, Aleksey Golovko, whom Mrs. Betchart had asked to take us out to the geology museum with our gifts, a place very difficult to reach by public transportation or even by taxi. They were happy with our gifts from Berrien County, Michigan, fulgurites and fossil crinoids. They had us make out identification cards with our names as donors. Aleksey also wrote poetry, his with an English side-by-side translation. I sent him a copy of my mother/child poems, but a copy of his never reached me.

Then we were ready for the lake tour. With an ornithologist, a geologist, and a piscitologist aboard, the land excursions were led by our guide, Victor Kuzevanov, a mathematician and botanist who ran the Irkutsk greenhouse with its collection of Siberian plants. The wildflowers were lovely. We could not see their freshwater seals in the wild because of a storm, but we saw them ashore, in captivity, where they were being studied.

My mind-boggling memory was seeing a stromatolite. We think of fossils mainly as calcified bones from animals, but there are others, leaf imprints, footprints, and the stromatolite Victor showed us. I had seen globular basketball-sized fossilized colonies of bacteria on a television program from Australia, and I somehow concluded that their stromatolites were unique in the world. On the shore of Lake Baikal the stromatolite Victor showed us was a stony column. I was in awe of its tremendous age, 2.1 billion years!

Unfortunately, Chuck missed the shore excursions of this trip because we had to "walk a plank" to get ashore; he did not feel stable enough, and there was no way to help him. This trip being promoted to scientists, Chuck and another elderly scientist, even more disabled, stayed onboard and chatted while the rest of us explored. I wish he could have seen that stromatolite. Chuck was good at appreciating what he could do and see, and, with the store of knowledge he took, he usually saw and recognized more than most tourists.

That very fall we tour members received a letter from Mrs. Betchart asking for help for Victor's greenhouse. The Siberian winter was so cold, even for Siberia, that its plants were endangered. He needed both electric and gas heaters, and so we sent the money required to save his collection.

Another Scandinavian Rheumatology Congress was held in Tempere, Finland, and of course I agreed, Finland being the only Scandinavian country we had missed. Poland and Finland being separated only by a narrow arm of the Baltic, with an overnight ferry, I suggested that we plan a three-country tour,[5] to include Byelorussia to visit Chuck's surviving cousin Vera and her daughter, Valery, in Brest, and Poland, to visit Cracow, a medieval city untouched by World War II. While there we visited the Jagellonian University, one of the very old European universities (1364). Actually it was established by King Casimir III, who died before he could get it rolling. A few years later King Wladislaus Jagiello took up the project and devoted his revenues from the salt mine (royal perks) to the project. His queen, Jadwiga (herself probably illiterate; why did nobility have to learn to read when they had servants to read for them?), sold her jewels for the university. Here my sources diverge. One says the proceeds made possible the enrollment of 203 students. I recall being told at the museum that her money from the jewels went to endow a chair. In its museum we were shown the book in which Copernicus was matriculated, and his tuition paid. *Plus ça change, plus c'est la même chose.* And we went on to Oświęcim (the arrogant Nazis called it Auschwitz).

Chuck's cousin and her daughter lived in Brest, just over the Polish border at the same latitude as Warsaw, and the point of entry of the Wehrmacht in 1939. We entered by train from Warsaw and were held at the border for several hours in the middle of the night because we didn't catch on (until we were talking it over with friends at home) that they were waiting for their bribe, until they gave up on us as hopeless and waved us through. In Brest a park commemorated their heroic month-long stand against the Germans, with stones marking events of their resistance, including the Russian hospital from which patients emerged with hands in the air and were gunned down. We took Chuck's relatives along to visit the Russian national park about fifty miles north of Brest, adjoining a similar Polish park across the border, where we saw some of the last remaining European bison (see Chuck's vignette re Germans burning his family's village: "Denko Relatives in Russia").

We took the overnight ferry from Gdansk (Germans call it Danzig) to Helsinki. To get to Gdansk, we took the train north from Cracow and had to change in Warsaw (see vignette "A True Polish Joke"). After the meeting we flew home over Greenland, which was a glorious glittering ice sheet on one of their few clear, sunny days.

On our Black Sea eclipse trip we spent half a day in Kiev, Ukraine, and heard terrible tales about the girls being taken and sold into slavery in Turkey, as late as the early 20th century.

Our niece Madeleine Denko Carter, who is in frequent contact with her Greek relatives on her mother's (Gloria Denko's) side, has also been in contact with the Belarusan relatives and hopes to visit there, as does Christopher, but even now travel in Russia is difficult.

Notes

1. This guide was very knowledgeable, with excellent English, but she made one mistake. I told her I had a patient who was afraid to travel to Russia for fear they would throw him in jail, since he was homosexual. "Oh, no, not if they're not a citizen," she said. My look told her I had caught the mistake but would say nothing.

2. The Russians are understandably proud of the history of this railway. It was the second national railway system, France's being one year earlier. It is wide-gauge and extends over eleven

time zones, although the entire system runs on Moscow time.

3. When we refueled in Ekaterinburg, we were asked to disembark with our carryons. Because they rolled out a long stairway onto the tarmac, I asked if Chuck might remain, which they permitted. I went into the terminal, and, foolishly thinking we would just return the same way, I left my purse, with ticket, passport, dollars, rubles, etc., with Chuck. Inside I realized we were expected to reboard. With fifteen minutes I had to get my papers from the plane. Analyzing my plight, I looked for a young woman in uniform, who would probably speak English. It worked like a charm. She got someone to escort me back to the plane.
4. When I was in high school, my English teacher took me to the home of her friend whose hobby it was to roam the dunes looking for these glass casts of root systems, string them with wire because of their fragility, and bring them home to hang from the rafters of his basement.
5. It was actually four. The congress arranged a day trip to Tallinn, Estonia, a medieval Hanseatic League city.

A True Polish Joke

The way we were able to see so much of Europe was that there were many international rheumatology congresses, and by getting to the meeting we could spend more time in that region, before or after. Chuck would come home and say, for example, "Do you want to go to Athens?" or "Do you want to go to Aix-les-Bain?" and I would say, "Of course. Submit a paper."

One day his question was "Do you want to go to Finland?" and my reply was, "Great! That's the last of our five Scandinavian countries, and we could use it as a time to see your relatives in Byelorussia."

After flying into Warsaw, we took the train to Brest, met Vera and Valery (Chuck's cousin and her daughter), returned to the southern part of Poland for our Krakow adventure, and headed north to Gdansk for the ferry. We had to change trains in Warsaw and board our commuter train at a ninety-second stop in a suburb. At that time Chuck used a cane and got around well enough to be carrying his small suitcase and a briefcase with slides for his upcoming talk. I hurried ahead to try to get us seats on the crowded train, when, to my shock, I heard Chuck's frightened voice yelling something I couldn't understand. I rushed back to the car behind the places I had found, as the train pulled out and found Chuck on the floor! Teenaged muggers had knocked him over, robbed him, and disembarked before the train pulled out.

Fortunately he was not hurt. Together, with the help of bystanders (actually "bysitters") I got him up and to our seats to assess the damages, physical and financial. It so happened that these Charlie Chaplin-like clowns had left the currency of various countries and had taken only his travelers' checks, which we were able to get replaced once we got to Finland.

"But, Chuck, what were you yelling? I knew your voice, of course, and I could tell you were in trouble, so I rushed right back, but I couldn't make out what you were saying."

"I was trying to call for help in Polish."[1]

Note

1. Chuck's effort reminded me of a cartoon I saw years ago, of a swimmer floundering and yelling, "*Au secours! Au secours!*" while an observer on shore tells his friend, "He's either a Frenchman or an awful snob." Chuck was not Polish and was as far as you can get from being a snob.

Special Rheumatology on Tristan da Cunha

When the *World Explorer* repositioned from the Mediterranean to the Amazon, requiring crossing the Atlantic, the planners realized the wastefulness of crossing empty, and so they came up, for the first (only?) time with a crossing that described a huge letter "J", following the islands of the mid-Atlantic ridge south, then west to the Falklands, taking five weeks. When there were no good lectures about the places we would be visiting, just spending hours on deck scanning the horizon and talking to other passengers provided a vacation at sea (see vignette "Travel Around the Edges" regarding how by advancing our starting date by two days I gave us a day in Madrid to see the Prado Museum and another in the Canaries to visit another island and hear their "whistling language").

The island of much interest to inveterate travelers (because it is accessible only by ship, having no landing strip, and is five days by ship from the closest human habitation at the southern end of Africa) is Tristan da Cunha. Alert, as always, to anything rheumatologic, on Tristan da Cunha Chuck talked to the British consul about how young men on the island suffered back troubles which had been found to be caused by carrying excessive loads down the mountain. He even examined some of the patients. He hoped to write a letter to the editor of a rheumatology journal about this occupational arthritis, but this was one idea that never made it into print. The following is his experience:

When you were a child, you probably wondered where in the world was Tristan da Cunha.[1] It is a small country in the South Atlantic. On a recent trip from one island to another down the mid-Atlantic Ridge in the South Atlantic, we visited it. It is now somewhat politically important, having been a part of the British Empire and a stopping-off point for water on long ocean voyages. It is now free but retains close ties to England and has regular connections by ship.[2]

We found it to have a unique rheumatologic problem. The footpaths are narrow and rocky. Cattle roam free until they are needed for meat, at which time they are slaughtered on the mountainsides. After butchering them, the young men carry the quarters down the steep hillsides, bracing their footsteps so as not to fall, until reaching the small settlement.

Many young men developed severe lumbosacral pain, difficult to control despite use of pain-relieving medication prescribed by the island physician, along with physiotherapeutic measures. This back pain and stiffness created a serious problem requiring a diagnosis. The nearest specialist for referral was several hundred miles away, in the country of South Africa. By the time patients reached South Africa, the sea trip and rest had provided relief. X-ray and blood studies relieved their worst worries about joint-destroying arthritis. When the consulting physician learned that these men were accustomed to carry on their shoulders a quarter of an ox down steep mountain paths, or half a wild sheep, which might weigh 300 pounds, the prescription was clear: cut up the meat before starting down the mountain. The results confirmed the analysis. Denouement: When I saw these men some months after their new program was in place, they were willing to have me examine them for joint function. They had a normal range of motion with normal muscle power and no joint tenderness. They returned to carrying meat (in smaller pieces) with no recurrence of symptoms.

CWD

Notes

1. Only, I might add, if you were a stamp collector or old enough to have been taught geography as CWD was, in high school and again in college. As he had explained to me, stamp collectors were all aware of this tiny country with a few hundred inhabitants, and stamps were one of its two main industries, the other being fishing.

2. It was settled by shipwreck survivors and there are only five surnames.

Chuck's Final Years

Chapter X

HIS FINAL YEARS

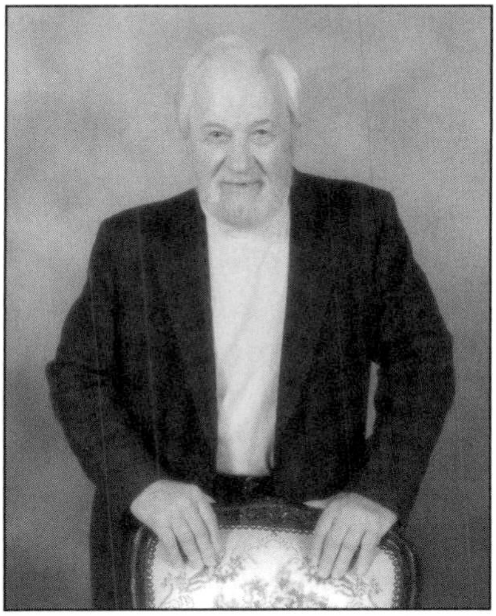

Charles Denko, Ph.D., M.D., at age seventy-five.

In the late 1990s, Chuck at eighty-four was experiencing increased difficulty walking due to weakness of his left leg, which he interpreted as caused by recurrent polio. At first I thought he was wrong because such recurrence usually happens about thirty years after the primary attack, and he had had polio at age one. He was probably right, and if a recurrence had to happen, he was fortunate that it waited more than eight decades. In any event, the onset of Parkinson's disease, with its problems in gait, complicated the picture. He never showed much tremor, but mild rigidity in the arms, and the mask-like facies characteristic of Parkinson's, making it difficult to talk, smile, or laugh due to muscle rigidity. This was identified first by our son Timothey, an astute clinician. During the years when these symptoms were creeping up insidiously, when we traveled, it was good to have a strong son along to help Chuck get on and off buses, trains, and planes.

Soon after Nicholas and Karen were married in 1999, we took them along to see the monarch butterflies wintering in Mexico. Chuck could not climb the mountain to where the butterflies hung like draperies in the trees, as he could have done a few years earlier, so he waited as far as the truck could take us. (See vignette, "Monarch Butterflies in Mexico").

In the summer of 2001, Chuck accomplished two eco-trips. The first was to Africa for an eclipse on the summer solstice in Zambia (see vignette "Travel Around the Edges"). In the late summer he brought me the brochure about a trip through the Northwest Passage by the Russian icebreaker *Kapitan Klebnikov,* and wanted to go. It was his last eco-trip as it turned out. We flew to Resolute in the Northwest Territories of Canada's Arctic. After we boarded ship, the captain and the ship's doctor came to our cabin to advise against it for Chuck, but he was able to persuade them that he could manage—and did. He had only one small accident. He was thrown off his seat in rough waters, struck his head on the locker, and required several stitches in his scalp. As long as the ocean was ice-covered, the passage was very smooth.

We went ashore to where Franklin's ill-fated expedition had wintered. We saw polar bears and walruses on ice floes, and were taken ashore to see foxes and geese in great numbers. Chuck enjoyed going to the "north pole", meaning magnetic, where the compass went wild. They landed us by zodiac or by helicopter, making special helicopter trips with Chuck, who could not walk on the rough and pitted tundra, so that he could see these animals and snow geese from the helicopter. He felt affection and kinship with the muskoxen, pointing out what he called their "social conscience" when he saw the protective ring they formed around their juveniles. By a coast guard regulation our ship was not allowed to enter American ports (and we went ashore by Zodiac in northern Alaska) because the *Klebnikov* did not have cough shields over the buffet service. Therefore the trip was planned to disembark in Providenya, Russia, from where we would fly home. Our trip ended in mid-September 2001 (see vignette "09/11/2001").

During these years Chuck continued working, although it was becoming increasingly difficult. After I worried for many years about his lateness after his late-afternoon rounds, the feared call came from Lakewood Hospital. Chuck had rolled his Volvo by hitting a parked car, due to loss of depth perception. The police found him hanging, unhurt, from his seatbelt, and I found him chatting with the nurses in the emergency room. (This was not his first accident. About six months earlier he had totaled another car, but somehow I had assumed it was a one-of-a-kind accident and did not terminate his driving, although Christopher said I should have. And Christopher was right.) On the second occasion, Chuck never protested my taking his keys. For a time he worked mornings, taking a taxi to the university, and I would pick him up at noon, an hour's roundtrip in light traffic.

When this schedule became too difficult for him, Charles Malemud, Chuck's colleague (and former student) came to our house to work with him and organize his data for publication. Malemud is still working on publication of Chuck's final paper, on the evidence for rheumatoid arthritis in the engraving on the Scythian gold bowl in the Hermitage Museum in St. Petersburg (see vignette "Arthritis in Scythian Art").

Years earlier when stairs had become harder for him, we had had a stairway elevator installed. In anticipation of future need, we had the garage made into a bed/sitting room and bath. Our builder, Ken Spero, even tracked down a certain kind of commercial flooring which, at the university, Chuck had found the easiest to walk on, without slipping, with the help of his cane, later walker. In March 2003, I stopped practice. Helen Balog had died, Jim was in decline, and so was the real estate market. We sold the Parkview with the understanding that Jim had lifelong tenancy in their apartment.

I found a home health agency that supplied several foreign-born men to help with Chuck, mostly professionals (sociology professor, dentist, gastroenterologist), unable to work at their profession here. Then Jonas Jasaitis, with degrees in sociology and pedagogy in Lithuania, worked with Chuck until the political situation made his return home feasible. The final home health aid, Val Onipko, a physician trained in Ukraine but without license to practice here, had worked in family practice and forensic pathology before bringing his family to this country to give his daughters a better start in life. He was a marvelous helper and friend, and offered many excellent suggestions to improve our day-to-day care of Chuck. Although he had never known Chuck as a complete person in his prime, Val loved him like an uncle[1] and promised to stay as long as I needed him, before finding work better suited to his medical training. When I took him along to help Chuck with dinner at the Cleveland Astronomical Society, and elsewhere, I introduced him as Chuck's nephew, as a way for him to feel comfortable about his role. Everyone immediately warmed to this intelligent, reserved, gentleman (I use this word rarely and deliberately) and commented on how fortunate we were to have him. When Chuck did not need help, Val worked on an M.B.A. by distance learning from the University of Colorado in Denver. (After Chuck's death, he worked in the pharmaceutical industry, monitoring drug studies in hospitals.) Val helped me make Chuck's final years as good as possible.

He and I took Chuck many places. We went to a great blue heronry in the nearby Cuyahoga National Park, where from the car we could watch the birds bringing in twigs to renovate their nests in preparation for the return of the females. (I told one of my patients about this phenomenon, and her witty comment was "She was probably nagging him.") We went to Caesar's Creek, a water conservancy project, where the Corps of Engineers lets visitors prospect for fossil trilobites, and they say one trilobite is found on average per hour. (Val found and gave me an incomplete trilobite. I hope to go back to spend more time and find several to leave my grandchildren.) By this time Chuck cared less where we took him than that I was with him. We took him to a Russian Orthodox monastery in the hills of upstate New York, where Val and his wife have a lot in the cemetery and expect to be buried. The monks were kind to Chuck, as Val had promised. They invited visitors to dinner, where one of the monks read aloud in Russian about lives of saints during the silent meal. When we returned home, I discovered a tick on Chuck's leg with a "target" of inflammation around it, but it was not a deer tick and he did not have Lyme disease.

In 2004 Val and I flew Chuck to Costa Rica to see Docelunas, Christopher's small, charming tropical resort hotel (four star) on the Pacific at Jaco, a surfers' paradise, where Val and I bodysurfed. We went to see crocodiles in the river. A friend of Christopher's took us to the nearby national park where we saw a three-toed sloth and a "Jesus Christ lizard" running on the water without breaking the surface tension.

Val and I took Chuck, who was always partial to train travel, by Amtrak in their special accommodations for the handicapped to Palo Alto, California, to visit Nicholas, his wife Karen, and little Louis at Stanford. As we flew home, he asked to go again. "Of course, if you are well enough next year." It was not to be.

In the spring of 2004 we received an invitation from Penn State to a weekend planned to honor those who had received their Ph.D.s fifty or more years prior (see vignette, "CWD's Ph.D. Honor").

As he declined and realized that death was near, one remark of

Chuck's that almost broke my heart was "I haven't done enough; I should have accomplished more."

"No, Chuck, you've done marvelously, and you did it as a family man as well as a scientist."

In a way, he was of course right. Malemud affirmed that ideas Chuck was working with were seminal. Both Malemud and I were happy to learn that four research groups around the country are carrying them forward (see Malemud's vignette "The Growth Hormone/Insulin-Like Growth Factor 1 (GH/IGF-1) Paracrine Axis Contributions by Charles W. Denko, Ph.D. M.D. to the Understanding of GH/IGF-1 in Regulating the Inflammatory Response").

I did not tell him that I have a similar regret as I age, and our Biblical threescore years and ten are mockingly short. Recently, patching a hole in my education, I finally caught up with Boswell's *Life of Johnson.* Besides the first dictionary of the English language, which Johnson completed in ten years, not his projected time limit of three, this man had written essays, literary commentaries, a six-volume criticism of Shakespeare's plays, etc., never revising a single word in anything (how I envy him that!). But he considered himself lazy — with some justification — because he liked to spend hours dining and conversing, or monologuing with friends and basking in their adulation, and spent years putting out nothing in hard copy. His reflections on life, literature, and politics, like the words of all of us, were lost in the wind. Chuck and I and no doubt other achievers have the same feeling as Johnson as we approach the big deadline: "It is a most mortifying reflexion for any man to consider, *what he had done,* compared with what *he might have done.*"[2] In the case of Chuck, he and I discussed how his life as a family man — Indian Guides, Boy Scouts with the boys, shopping and cooking on weekends, time spent with me, traveling beyond conference travel — all this reduced what he might have done as a scientist. Given that time and energy are limited, his choices were good, his life was rich, and he was blessed with abundant energy and an eighty-nine-year span.

Chuck continued to work on vignettes for my project. One feature of Parkinson's disease is deteriorating penmanship. His previously beautiful handwriting became more difficult, but I could decipher it. Also, because of the hard work that writing had become, he would put down ideas as they came to him, and I later rearranged them in chronological sequence, with, sometimes, explanatory material over my initials.

Over the weekend of October 15–16, 2005, all three sons came home for different reasons, such as class reunions. On the morning of October 18, when I came into Chuck's room, I found him cyanotic and without respiration or pulse. I administered mouth-to-mouth respiration and thumped his chest rhythmically, thereby starting both breathing and heartbeat, but he remained unconscious. The EMS came within five minutes, asked how to code him ("*Save him!*") but lost his pulse and respiration on the way to the hospital. We don't know the state of his brain.

I had planned the funeral in advance and had gathered material for his obituary (see *Plain Dealer* obituary.) On the memorial card given to visitors attending the funeral was this quotation of Ralph Waldo Emerson:

> " To laugh often and much; to win the respect of intelligent people and the affection of children; to earn the appreciation of honest critics and endure the betrayal of false friends; to appreciate beauty; to find the best in others; to leave the world a bit better whether by a healthy child, a garden patch, or a redeemed social condition; to know even one life has breathed easier because you lived. This is to have succeeded."

The boys all returned for Russian Orthodox funeral services on October 21, and Chuck was buried the following day in the Locust Grove Cemetery in his hometown of Ellwood City, on a hillside overlooking the hills of western Pennsylvania. On his side of the green granite grave marker, I placed the benzene ring for organic chemistry and a caduceus for medicine; on mine are a caduceus and a book, quill, and inkpot.

Notes

1. Val was not the only person fond of Chuck, even when he was in severe decline. People of all backgrounds responded affectionately to him. For Val's Sundays off the agency sent Joan Paynter. Over Christmas 2011 I took Joan out for lunch. This woman, a school crossing guard, surprised me with "I still miss those Sundays with Chuck." This was six years after his death.
2. James Boswell, *Life of Johnson,* Vol. 2, edited by George Birbeck Hill (Oxford Press, 1887), p. 129.

09/11/2001

We tend to remember where we were and what we were doing when historic news broke. Christopher did a vignette about the Kennedy assassination; my cousin Eunice recalled our entrance into WW II at the bombing of Pearl Harbor.

On another day of infamy, 09/11/2001, when the planes ran into the Twin Towers in New York, the Pentagon in Virginia, and crashed in Shanksville, Pennsylvania, Chuck and I were at sea, on our way to northeast Russia, just beyond the Bering Straits, having completed the Northwest Passage on the Russian icebreaker *Kapitan Klebnikov.* It was early morning, and the PA carried an announcement that the radio had received word of a catastrophe in the States. We were invited up to the radio room. Donning robes, we climbed the gangways to find out what had happened.

With only the words to go by, we never felt the complete impact that those did who watched transfixed, all day, over and over, the crumbling Twin Towers.

At the time we were almost in Russian waters. Arriving in Providenya, we learned that the U.S. was not allowing any flights in or out, and so we had extra time, about five days, in the far northeast part of Russia. We were taken to see an anthropologic dig of ancient prehistoric Inuits, 700 years earlier. We were taken to an island with two breeds of puffins breeding in enormous numbers. We were taken to an Inuit village, and visited the school, where portraits of Tolstoy, Dostoyevsky, et al., graced the walls.

Finally a flight was permitted to Nome, from which we made connections to Anchorage and home via Salt Lake City.

I was always impressed by how much more shaken the people were who had followed the entire event at not only the Twin Towers but also the Pentagon and Western Pennsylvania, on the day it happened.

Christmas 2002 Letter

November 24, 2002

Dear Friends,

Many years have passed since our last "annual letter", the year Chuck gave a paper in Buenos Aires, and the idea besieged my mind to send postcards, the first from Iguaçu Falls, with the cascade in Argentina but the view from Brazil. 2002 has produced no comparable trip, partly because we had become traveled out in 2001, having gone to Zambia for the solar eclipse on the summer solstice and then to the Canadian Arctic on a Russian icebreaker where we were detained by the fateful 9/11.

Adventures of other kinds have marked the past couple years.

With a record as late first-time grandparents, we now have three precious grandchildren: Kristina Joanna (Valentine's Day, 2000), Madeleine Grace (5/9/01), and Louis Alexandar (Russian spelling) (6/11/01). The latter, little Sasha, was adopted in Ukraine, came home with his parents, Nicholas and Karen, in December 2001, and we went to California by Amtrak to welcome him in March. His father is on the tenure track at Stanford in molecular genetics. Timothey is a psychiatrist on the staff at the University of Pittsburgh. Christopher has bought a small hotel in Costa Rica and is remodeling it.

2002 has been unhappy for the older Denko relatives. Chuck's sister Munya died in February, and brother John in November, both of cancer.

Meanwhile we continue to use each day to the full, realizing that it will never be given to us again. Although walking has become difficult for Chuck (from post-polio plus Parkinsonism), he and his colleague have gotten out three papers this year on his data linking arthritic disorders to abnormalities in growth factors. I had one book come out earlier this year, and I expect to hold another in my hand early next year. That one will be *Into A Mirror and Through A Lens.* It consists of forty poems on the mother/child relationship from conception to marriage. I am now working on a book on envy in literature and life. I intend to stop seeing patients the end of March because I can't keep up with fifty hours a year of ongoing education. We are also looking for a buyer for the apartment building because our manager and his wife are not well and, as I see it, cannot be replaced.

We spend as much time as we can (which isn't much) at our summer place on Beaver Island in the upper end of Lake Michigan. Living in Pittsburgh, Timothey and his family can take more advantage of it than the other sons.

As a Christmas event we are taking local friends to the Episcopal Medieval Feast in December. If only you all lived closer, you would be included.

I hope to be able to continue to write in the years to come. I fear the news in the letters from some of you.

As ever,

Chuck and Joanne Denko

CWD's Ph. D. Recognition

In early 2004 we received an invitation from Penn State for a weekend they were planning to honor graduates who had received their Ph.D.s fifty and more years earlier. At that time Chuck was able to travel and used a wheelchair as needed, but getting him to central Pennsylvania posed a problem.

Family members were welcome. I couldn't reach Christopher, who was probably in Europe. Timothey would attend the event with his family but by traveling directly from Pittsburgh. Nicholas was scheduled to attend a meeting in Denver during those days. At least that was closer than California, and Nicholas was able to arrange a detour to Pennsylvania for his father's recognition. I still had the problem of transporting Chuck to and from the university.

Needing a man who was strong enough to support Chuck, I asked the priest at St. Herman's House of Hospitality, which we had supported over the years, a man who had been friendly and was sympathetic to my problem. That idea failed for what seemed to me a strange reason. Father John indicated that his vows forbade his touching another man. (Aren't there priests, even Eastern Orthodox ones, who work as nurses or other medical workers?) Anyway, after a week of fruitless telephoning and other efforts, I finally got Chuck to State College by myself and into the Nittany Lion Hotel. The brothers and Timothey's family arrived as planned.

The ceremony was simple but impressive. On the wall was one of those modern recognition arrangements that look like a branching tree, with each honoree engraved on one of the metal leaves. When Chuck's name was called first, as the longest-time Ph.D. in attendance, having graduated sixty-three years prior, I rolled him up to the platform.

Other events were standard, a luncheon, exhibit of research work, etc., but the best part was a trip with Nicholas and Timothey, Patricia, Madeleine, and little Charles Michael to the Milk Pail, where the Ag School's rich milk is sold as ice cream. Over the years, whenever Chuck and I have come through that part of Pennsylvania, we have always stopped for ice cream.

Christmas Letter, 2004

December, 2004

Dear Friends,

Although Chuck's condition is not improving, we are grateful that his Parkinson's disease is relatively stable. With the help of a physical therapist, he has regained walking skills, with the help of the walker, and can navigate the downstairs, better some days than others. We have a home health aid, Val Onipko, who helps Chuck. You've heard of things happening 24/7 — well, this man works for us 12/6. Chuck's appetite continues to be impressive. I got him to Butler, Pennsylvania, Patricia's parents' home, for Thanksgiving. We go to an occasional concert, meetings of the astronomic society and the history of medicine society, Kiwanis, movies and plays, and, this upcoming Saturday, the Medieval Feast at Trinity Cathedral, for which I have reserved sixteen seats for our Christmas party. For Chuck's costume I attached gold alchemical symbols to his academic gown so this chemist could go as an alchemist. Until this spring he went a half day a week to the university, where he worked with his colleague on data he has been collecting, and the two of them got out four papers this year.

Our three sons visit whenever they can. They were all here in October. Timothey, in Pittsburgh, lives the closest and has been trying to come almost every Saturday with Patricia and the children. Nicholas works on a committee for NIH, evaluating grant proposals in his field, and goes to Washington every few months for that. For some reason the army issues his flight tickets, and they have obligingly included a daylong stopover here to visit his ailing father. Christopher has remodeled a small resort hotel in Costa Rica, and they are now moving into their first high season this month. He would like us to come down to see it.

When all three were here, I arranged a dinner at a Greek restaurant, and we made it into a family reunion. Chuck's only surviving sibling, Helen, was able to get there too. I called it my "pseudo-Thanksgiving" dinner.

I let my license run out at the end of March 2003 so that I could work on my books without patient interruption. Last year my book of mother/child poems came out. In a few weeks my book of nature poems, *Interlink,* is due out. I am still collecting vignettes about interesting experiences in the lives of anyone ancestral to our grandchildren, and I will accept any more such with great pleasure.

I enjoy buying books and toys for the grandchildren and attending the girls' ballet recitals. Otherwise, I don't buy Christmas presents, except for this heifer [Heifer, International] to be sent to a needy family in the Third World, in honor of you all.

A merry and a blessed Christmas,

Chuck and Joanne

P.S. They sent me a lovely accordion-folded gift card, so I had to photocopy it, so you all could see what this charitable institution

(Heifer) does. My photocopier doesn't like me. Heifer's gifts make much better sense than to send food to the Third World.

Boris and the Fox

We had a lovely reddish-brown dog, a golden retriever on short legs with a cocker face. He was six years old when Patricia found him for us at a shelter as a replacement for Tina, another reddish-brown dog that Timothey brought home when his friend's mother was diagnosed with cancer and she couldn't take care of him. Our new dog had been called "Buddy", a dog name I didn't care for, so we used the principle of changing to a name with the same initial consonant and with the same number of syllables and named him "Boris". Boris had no trouble adjusting. In the words of the old joke, his attitude was "Call me anything, but don't call me late for dinner!" He died at sixteen.

We also had a fox that lived nearby, probably in a den on the cliff over the lake. She sometimes ran across our property, and neighbors also spotted her. Once when we had a snowfall, on a brilliant winter day she sunbathed for several hours on the snow in the northeast corner of our land. She wrapped her tail around her nose for warmth. With my binocs I could see that her ears were rimmed with black, and her eyes were closer to green than yellow. She even had kits, two of whom came together as adolescents to the back yard. Twice the vixen came up onto the back steps, causing me to surmise that she was very hungry. Therefore I began putting out food for her after dark, dog food, knowing that she had not only to support herself but also to make milk for the babies. The dish was always empty by morning. Although I never saw her at night, Boris would sometimes bark from inside the back door.

One day Val accidentally let Boris out in back when the fox was there. Boris chased the fox over the cliffside and followed her to the beach, where the fox led him out onto the ice. Val went in pursuit to bring Boris back. After a few seconds Val saw the fox stop, turn, and face Boris, having evidently thought, "What's going on here anyway? Who's the predator and who's the prey? Why am I letting a *dog* chase *me?*" Boris immediately stopped, and for a few seconds he and the fox sized each other up, then both rotated and left in opposite directions. Val herded Boris off the ice, then caught and carried him up the cliff, lest he take off again.

Val didn't tell me about the incident for a few weeks, thinking I might blame him for not first surveying the yard.

Career

Work in Nutrition

Chuck considered himself (and was) an expert in nutrition. By this he meant something much broader than "diet", and I considered it closer to "metabolism". In fact he was grandfathered into the American Board of Nutrition as a diplomate, as a result of his work with COs in the Army Nutrition Lab in Chicago, later at Johns Hopkins School of Public Health (bibliography items 3, 4, 5, 6, 7, 8, 9).

As a nutrition office in the U.S. Army, stationed at the 98th Army General Hospital in Munich, he performed nutrition surveys on German civilians in 1946 to assess their nutritional status, which had been suspected to be poor due to wartime deprivation. By vitamin assays of the blood, he found their nutritional status to be normal.

He did nutrition research involving patients with connective tissue disorders.

He did research on inflammation and distribution of trace metals (copper and zinc) in animals on restricted diets (bibliography items 75, 76, 93).

Dr. Charles Denko's Noteworthy Patients

It could have been the luck of the draw or perhaps the admissions personnel shunted high profile and otherwise especially interesting patients to the services where Chuck was low man, but in medical school, internship, and residency he was always telling the rest of us about patients that were especially interesting either medically or as celebrities of some kind.

At Hopkins Chuck had, for example, Carlos Julio Arosemena, a colorful politician and onetime president of Ecuador, deposed in a military coup and exiled to Panama. Arosemena came for some other medical problem but was also in an early stage of Hansen's disease (leprosy). Besides the usual reasons of patient privacy, this had to be kept quiet, both not to start panic and for this man's political future.

At Illinois, Chuck was the intern assigned to Siamese twins, joined at the head and scheduled for separation. He did not get to scrub and hold retractors for hours because all the surgical residents wanted this experience, but with his aversion to the surgical specialties, he was glad the others had the opportunity.

As mentioned earlier, it was during his time at the University of Chicago that Chuck was on the service where Enrico Fermi and Mahalia Jackson were treated, and the chancellor was admitted for his annual checkup.

Thirty-five Years of Evolution of Our Understanding of Autism

Chuck's and my interdigitated story about childhood autism began at Hopkins, where five or six medical students including Chuck (but not me) sat in the office of a pioneer on the condition, Dr. Leo Kanner. One of our classmates presented the detailed history he had taken from the parents and the results of his examination of a child. Then the latency-aged son of a well-known actor was brought in for evaluation. The child showed no reaction to the doctors and students in the room, treating them exactly as if they were furniture, the classic behavior of autistic children. At that time it was universally held that not only autism but also other mental illnesses like schizophrenia were the result of bad parenting, and the mother was considered the culprit, and held accountable. I did not learn what advice Dr. Kanner gave the parents or what, if any, subsequent treatments were tried. Still, the boy grew up to be a competent and respected film star, though not as prominent as his father.

Several years later when I was a psychiatric resident in the Children's Psychiatric Hospital at the University of Michigan, my very first patient was an eight-year-old boy, Harvey, who was largely speechless, banged his head, twirled, rocked incessantly on the playground swing, all features characteristic of autistic children. His parents, at their wits' end, were also at each other's throats, but I was beginning to see what was cause and what effect: how could a marriage remain normal while dealing with such a problem?

Undoubtedly Harvey was autistic, hence a good teaching case for a new resident like myself. I was scheduled for an hour a week of one-on-one tutorial with each senior staff person, including Dr. Ray Keeler, a visiting professor from Toronto. Imagine my surprise when Dr. Keeler indicated all those features in my child patient and maintained that they represented soft neurologic signs, as yet un-understood, of this devastating condition. When I asked what I should be doing to work with the boy, Dr. Keeler replied, "Be sure the staff treats him kindly, as I am sure they will, and avoid anything stressful, like putting normal expectations on him. Beyond that, we don't know yet. And be compassionate with the parents. This is not why they painted the nursery blue."

The rest of the staff overtly and covertly made fun of Dr. Keeler, and I recall my chief saying, "Ray wouldn't know an id if he fell over one."

The next time I heard Dr. Kanner mentioned was a couple decades later, at my high school class reunion. Vance Ferguson, whom I had dated in high school, and I were catching up. He told me that he and his wife had only one child, who was autistic. They had taken him to Dr. Kanner years before, and Dr. Kanner's conclusion was not "I do not diagnose your son as autistic" but "Your son cannot be autistic because you are not the kind of parents who produce autistic children."

Back home, Vance and his wife had tried an experimental kind of therapy based on the idea that something had gone wrong in the growing-up process, and to correct this the child was expected to go back through the stages of crawling and walking. It just happened that my friend Anne, the classics major who had subsequently taught the EMR (educable mentally retarded) in St. Joe (because there was no one else to do it), had been brought into this program too and had crawled with Victor's son and others in hopes of getting them off to a better start, with no apparent improvement. Finally a friend of Vance's and his wife's, a priest in the mountains of South America, had suggested that they send the young man to him, where the priest would take care of him, and the pressures would be minimal. This seemed to be working well, and they could only hope for the future.

When I heard this story about Dr. Kanner, I was shocked by this example of a scientist performing whatever mental acrobatics it took to preserve his initial hypothesis in the face of evidence to the contrary. Seeing parents who did not warrant blame, and clinging to the belief that only bad parenting could produce an autistic child, he preferred to deny the diagnosis rather than question the hypothesis. Refusing to reexamine a hypothesis in the face of contradictory evidence, i.e., clinging to one's *idée fixe,* represents the ultimate in the paranoid position.

(This kind of reasoning was illustrated by a joke that circulated a few years later. A patient insisted that his psychiatrist was a ghost, despite all the doctor's efforts to dissuade him. This would not be the correct strategy in good therapy. Nonetheless the doctor hit on another way to prove his point to the patient: "Do ghosts bleed if you cut them?" he asked. "Of course not. Anybody knows that." So the doctor whipped out his Swiss army knife, nicked his finger, and produced a drop of blood. "See?" "Well I'll be damned. I was wrong. Ghosts *do* bleed if you cut them!" Like the psychiatrist in real life, this patient abandoned anything but his original belief in the face of new evidence.)

For decades the idea continued to be held in psychiatric circles that not only autism but also schizophrenia and other psychiatric disorders had no physical basis, but had been caused by bad mothering. When, as usually happened, the mother appeared well within the broad, hazy confines of "normal", the therapist assumed the toxic element was somehow occult, maybe not intentional or even recognized by the parents. Hence mothers enduring the grief of children with psychiatric disorders suffered the added torment of believing that they had somehow unwittingly brought it about. I have a friend who questioned with me whether her daughter's psychiatric disorder had somehow resulted from the time she had lied to the child about their dog's death, in an effort to spare her.

More years passed. After Kanner's death, at our medical school reunion, there was to be a Kanner memorial lecture on autism. The problem was that in the interval, evidence had surfaced for the condition's neurologic basis, and opinion had shifted in the direction of supporting what Keeler's voice had been crying in the wilderness decades earlier: the condition is neurological, and the cause is unknown.[1]

Note

1. I am reminded of Nicholas's report that on the day he started medical school, in the convocation, the incoming students were told, "Half of everything we will teach you will be proven wrong. Unfortunately, we don't know which half." All of us, but particularly those of us on whom the welfare of others depends, must constantly reexamine our assumptions in the light of new evidence. Nicholas's Ph.D. rests on work that he undertook when another experiment did not produce the

expected results. He then pursued those new results and was in time awarded his degree.

Dr. Denko as Diagnostician

Soon after we moved to Rocky River, a call came one evening for Chuck, from Carl Zerke, a friend he had known back in high school in Ellwood City. Now living in Florida, Carl told Chuck about the medical problems that they had had with their grandson. Several physicians they had consulted had been unable to diagnose the problem or offer help. Chuck listened intently, asked a few questions, and finally said, "Yes, I think I can help him. Bianca can bring him up to Cleveland."

On admission to the children's ward, Chuck took the complete history from Bianca, the child's grandmother, examined the boy, and began treatment. His condition was one of the rarer auto-immune diseases related to lupus: scleroderma. The boy soon showed signs of improvement and was able to return home, where Chuck coordinated treatment with the pediatrician in Florida.

The family was so appreciative and grateful for Chuck's help that Bianca did two things. She had heard from me that I was interested in carnivorous plants. In fact, when one of the drug companies used Venus flytraps as advertising, I contacted the detail man and asked for enough for one of the little boy's class-mates (I believe it was Nicholas). Knowing this, Bianca shipped me pitcher plants from their area, although I was not able to grow them.

As a gift for our boys, the Zerkes sent a baby cayman. We had trouble getting it to take food, even hamburger. When Nicholas held it close to his upturned face to examine it (remember that he was very nearsighted), the cayman bit his nose. (How many of us have survived an alligator bite?) My worries about what to do as it grew were unnecessary, as it soon died. I should have thought to take it to the nature center.

As a young adult, that former patient contacted Chuck to thank him for saving his life.

At one of my high school reunions I was happy to see Art Ablin, my old debate partner and the class salutatorian, and, as mentioned earlier, a fellow passenger on the student ship to Europe. His family had run a fishing fleet of two or three boats on Lake Michigan. Later, when his father's health failed, his mother ran a restaurant, where Chuck and I would always go when we visited. Art's mother had hoped that Art and I would marry.

At the reunion I noticed that Art made a point to greet all his classmates, not just his special friends, but when he and Chuck and I got together, he commented that nobody seemed to have any special interests. When he would ask what they were doing, they would say, "Why, nothing! I'm retired." This was in contrast to Art, who, like most physicians, worked well beyond sixty-five. He reviewed all grant proposals at U.C.S.F. Medical School (University of California at San Francisco). He also traveled. He would collect fern seeds to grow a collection back home, while his wife would be birding.

Then Art told Chuck about his painful hip, making walking problematic. As a pediatrician at UC San Francisco and later as chief of the research review board, he had had access to specialists, but no one had helped. As the dining room staff cleared away, Chuck had a waiter bring a phone book and told Art to stand with one foot on it. Magically, the pain vanished, and Chuck explained that no specialist yet had observed that Art's legs were not of equal length. With a lift on the short side, he could walk comfortably. Whenever we have met or talked on the phone since then, Art has always remembered this incident with appreciation. And I remember it with pride in my husband.

The Rumalon Story

In the early sixties, Chuck (and I) attended a European Congress of Rheumatology in Rome, at which he gave a paper on his S^{35} work in rats. A representative of a Swiss Pharmaceutical firm, Robapharm, sought him out to discuss a product of theirs, Rumalon, a watery extract of bone and cartilage derived from animals in slaughterhouses. Used for various arthritic conditions, it could be given only by injection. It had no apparent side effects. One question the Robapharm representative raised was whether improvement in patients could be attributed to a placebo effect. He asked whether Chuck would be interested in studying it in his rats. Chuck agreed to take it on and added, "Nobody has ever attributed a placebo effect to rats, and besides, I'll give controls a sham injection of the saline substrate."

His results on the metabolic activity of Rumalon in the cartilage of rats were so favorable that Robapharm not only sent us both to the Pan American Congress of Rheumatology in Santiago, Chile, in 1963, for him to present his data, but even paid for us to spend an extra week in Chile's Lake District with its smoking volcanoes. Robapharm later credited Chuck's talk with thousands of dollars of sales in South America and worldwide. (In those days "thousands" were lots of dollars.)

Subsequently, Chuck was authorized to give Rumalon to osteoarthritis (OA) patients experimentally. Some patients with OA of the hip even showed regrowth of cartilage, as evidenced by widening of the joint space by X-ray. One patient's husband was an antique car aficionado. This patient had a dramatic flair. Arriving at the next annual meeting in a wheelchair, as in former years, she got up, walked to the dance floor, and proceeded to dance with her husband, to the astonishment of their friends. She was flattered when Chuck took "her" (i.e., her films) to meetings.

Chuck found improvement and regrowth of cartilage in 20 percent of osteoarthritis patients with OA of the hip, eliminating the need for surgery, or at least delaying it. When he would show the "before and after" films to colleagues, they would often say, "You've got those up in reverse," and he would have to point out the dates burned into the films at time of exposure. No one at that time had ever had evidence of cartilage regrowth.

While Chuck had been authorized to try Rumalon experimentally in patients, getting the FDA (Food and Drug Administration) to authorize its use in this country for patients was impossible because a new regulation was in place requiring all pharmaceuticals to be synthesized (presumably for standardization).[1]

Chuck himself suffered traumatic arthritis of the hip resulting from his tipped pelvis from the lifelong disparity of length of his legs from polio, despite the surgical amelioration of his gait. He tried Rumalon on himself, found it helpful, and planned to take it the rest of his life.

Soon Chuck's contact at Robapharm had died, the son and daughter of the founder were not interested in taking over the business, and Robapharm had been sold to a French firm. By then Rumalon was available throughout the world except the USA and Canada. Much of it was produced in Argentina, as a byproduct of their cattle industry. Our laws permit patients to bring in medication from abroad for their personal use. Often these are patients with incurable cancer who understandably grasp at straws by seeking cancer-cure claims elsewhere.

Because Chuck was being helped by Rumalon, when in the mid-'90s I went to Easter Island and Chile to witness a solar eclipse, I left a day early for Santiago, Chile, found a pharmacy with a good supply, changed enough money, and bought $2,500 worth of Rumalon over the counter. The customs man in Miami waved me through. Chuck gave some Rumalon to his sister, and I gave my friend Charmaine some, but most of it he used until his death. There is just one vial left in the cupboard.

Now our over-the-counter oral products for self-medication of arthritic problems contain chondroitin sulfate (*chondro* is Greek for "cartilage"), one of the components of Rumalon, now synthesized. I take it to help keep my knee pain-free. The difficulty is that much of it is digested in the GI tract.

Note

1. Prior to that, for example, patients with hypothyroidism were given desiccated thyroid (similarly from slaughterhouses, like the cartilage and bone extract in Rumalon), which was then replaced by synthroid (levo-thyroxin). I took the Armour desiccated thyroid for years.

The Alcusal Story

During my sabbatical at the Australian National University in 1974–5, in Canberra, in the laboratory of Dr. Michael Whitehouse, I studied copper as an anti-inflammatory agent. Subcutaneous injections of copper glycinate and copper citrate were more effective anti-inflammatory agents than colchicines, indomethacin, and phenylbutazone (*J. Rheumatology* 3:54–62, 1976). Dr. Whitehouse formulated the copper complex salicylate, Alcusal. Dr. Ray Walker, a chemist, was instrumental in this work.[1]

In this country a few of my arthritis patients volunteered to try Alcusal in treating soft tissue conditions such as bursitis and tendonitis. I used it to treat athletic injuries. I gave a sample to a local athletic coach who reported Alcusal to be superior to any other agent in treating sprains and strains. Epicondylitis (tennis elbow) responded well.

In addition I have given it to my professional colleagues who have reported good results in treating insect bites and poison ivy irritation, as well as muscle pains.

I arranged with the Australian company, Alcusal Pty, to import Alcusal and exploit it in the U.S. For this purpose I submitted a protocol to our FDA, which was acceptable for efficacy trials. I received an IND 23596. I organized Alcusal of North America, chartered in Pennsylvania, planning to manufacture and market Alcusal.[2]

CWD
8/15/1998

Notes

1. One advantage was that Alcusal was topical.

2. Chuck struggled with this for years, even buying a building with the intention of converting it for the manufacture of Alcusal, but ran into repeated roadblocks from the bureaucracy, and hence this possible use of copper compounds in the treatment of soft tissue inflammatory conditions came to naught. I always had the feeling that Chuck's problem in matters like this was that, utterly honest and straightforward, he did not know or use the politicking maneuvers, the *quid pro quo* tradeoffs that normally characterize business deals, even scientific ones.

Stillborn Symposia

Dr. Denko organized two symposia, both of which came to naught.

One was on INFLAMMATION: Basic Mechanisms & Pharmacologic Control of Crystal Deposition Disorders (Gout and Pseudogout), sponsored by Fairview General Hospital Department of Medicine and Case Western Reserve University School of Medicine. He assembled an international faculty including Ali Askari, Frederic Bishko, Roland Moskowitz, George Naft, and J. David Reid, all from Case Western Reserve University in Cleveland; John Clough, Allen MacKenzie, and Arthur Sherbel from the Cleveland Clinic; Thomas Benedek from the University of Pittsburgh (Pennsylvania); Thomas Passananti and Elliott Vesell from Pennsylvania State University in Hershey; Joseph Houpt from the University of Toronto, Canada; Kay Brune, University of Basle, Switzerland; and Michael Whitehouse, Australian National University in Canberra. This never elicited enough interest and had to be canceled.

The other was intended to recognize the 150th anniversary of the first synthesis of an organic compound, urea, from ammonia and cyanic acid, by the German chemist Friedrich Wöhler. This defied the vital-force theory, which held that substances derived from living beings could not be copied using nonliving components. This project also had to be abandoned for lack of interest.

Rheumatology in Antiquity

In 1986 we attended a meeting in Jerusalem.

After the rheumatology congress in Jerusalem we were traveling south in Israel to Eilat on the Gulf of Aqaba on the Red Sea, when Chuck jumped out of his seat yelling, "Ashqelon!" He got the driver to bring the bus to a halt while he got out to take a photo of the directional sign indicating the way to that ancient city.

Why did the place name "Ashqelon" excite him so? It turned out that the Greek historian Herodotus had mentioned this as a place where Scythian soldiers had stopped on their return home after fighting farther south (I believe in Egypt). Thenceforth some citizens were found to have a rheumatologic ailment that in the time of Herodotus was attributed to the anger of the city's goddess. Less sanguine, Chuck attributed it to the fact that the Scythians had left genes with the temple prostitutes, genes that had carried the anlagen for this ailment. Hence Chuck's excitement when he saw the direction to the place where some kind of arthritis had been described by Herodotus! The other passengers looked at us with the usual stare of those who don't know the specifics of what someone has spent a lifetime studying.

Historical Vignette: A Rheumatologic Disorder in Antiquity

Arthritis in Scythian Art

For how many millennia have rheumatologic disorders afflicted mankind?

In the Hermitage Museum in St. Petersburg, Russia, is a collection of gold art objects fashioned by the Scythians about 2,500 years ago and found by Peter the Great's anthropologists in burial mounds in the area north of the Black Sea.

Included in this collection of exquisite gold objects is a bowl modeled in gold depicting a scene of a shaman (medical practitioner) examining the ankle of a patient wincing with pain. We know that the practitioner is a shaman because he wears a pointed cap associated with positions of authority. The patient is in obvious distress. [Delineating the reasons for the pain as the shaman palpates the boot-clad ankle, CWD indicated to me the swelling in some fingers of each hand, shown holding a staff or spear. This pattern is typical of rheumatoid arthritis. *JDD*]

Several of my colleagues have examined the [photo of the] bowl and agree that the ankle is swollen [how do we know, since it is in a boot? *JDD*] and the patient is in pain.

We are offering this as the first documented case of rheumatologic disorder.

CWD

Charles Malemud, Chuck's colleague, has been trying—and is still trying—to accomplish CWD's original plan for his entire paper, which he discussed with Dr. Valentina Nasonova, the retired and now deceased head of the Russian Rheumatologic Institute, who, he believed, agreed to his plan, i.e., to issue the paper that he was writing at the time jointly in his name and hers, in both English and Russian, in both Russia and the USA. Malemud's efforts to contact her for final approval and cooperation in Russia were unsuccessful, and following her death, her son, Eugeny, has taken her position. Therefore Malemud is trying to reach Eugeny to proceed with joint publication.

Chuck's Integrated Life

Charles Denko had a remarkable scientific career, based on his scientific training as a biochemist, coordinated with his medical (rheumatologic) expertise, and his teaching skills.

While working on his Ph.D. in biochemistry, Chuck's professor, mentor, and friend, A. K. Anderson, strongly advised that for the type of biochemical research relating to human health and disease that he wished to pursue, he should if at all possible have an M.D. as well as a Ph.D. Many in the basic sciences had found that collaborating with physicians on this kind of work is difficult, and therefore both viewpoints should reside in one brain. His enlisting in the army despite being 4F because of his polio leg was fortuitous. By the time of his discharge from service, the GI Bill had been passed, and this enabled him to follow Anderson's advice and have the GI Bill put him through the world's premier medical school, Johns Hopkins University (where he enjoyed the good fortune to meet me). Thus he became, after medical school, in the 1950s, one of the few with a double doctorate, earned separately, unlike now, when they are usually pursued simultaneously, with the saving of several years but less rigor. He always considered himself primarily a biochemist, and he listed his Ph.D. first, correctly, because that was the order in which it was earned.

He described how what he learned from patients he took to

the lab for further study, and what he discovered in the lab from rats' cartilage and from human blood, he used to implement his treatment of patients, not just their symptoms but the molecular changes at the root of their conditions. It was like a tango.

He proudly confided to me what a joy it was to be the first in the world to know something new by having discovered it, e.g., that the red blood cells function as little trucks carrying toxic levels of growth hormone from pituitary to arthritic joint space and dumping it into the synovial fluid. (See Malemud's "A Tale of Two Charleses".) As his thinking oscillated between the clinical symptoms wrought by disease and the biochemistry of the body, his analysis was enhanced by his interaction with students and young doctors, whose questions are often more trenchant than those of older physicians, who tend to be more rigid and conventional in their thinking. Charles was a lifelong student and began each lecture, to medical students, to colleagues, or to scientists from other parts of the world, with "Good morning, fellow students". His weekly half day scanning the newly arrived journals at the library kept him abreast of everything new that was known, thought, or tried in his field, once it had made it into print. It was another tango between teaching and learning.

Occasionally I would hear, from a former student or colleague of his, something like "The first time I heard of ________________ was in one of Chuck's lectures twenty years ago."

(His own summary of his life's work up to 1990, prepared for submission to an international contest, the Carol Nachman Prize in Rheumatology, in which he came in second, worldwide, is found in two vignettes about his life as a scientist: "Resume of Research in Osteoarthritis and Cartilage" and "Significance of My Research" and in his colleague's memoir "A Tale of Two Charleses".) How his work moved his specialty forward is detailed in Malemud's "The Growth Hormone/Insulin-Like Growth Factor-1 (GH/IGF-1) Paracrine Axis Contributions by Charles W. Denko,

Ph.D. M.D. to the Understanding of GH/IGF-1 in Regulating the Inflammatory Response".

Chuck was not good in the politics of medicine. A flaw I saw in his dealings with other medical personnel was that he never tried to push an idea to the next level. He would suggest it once and drop it if they seemed uninterested. It was this way in hospital conferences too, some of which I attended. When I brought it to his attention that he was not commenting on cases, as I knew he was well able to do, he said, "They don't want to hear from me." This was probably true. A frequent comment by a practitioner about an unusual condition is: "You never see that in practice." My silent rejoinder is, "Of course not, if you haven't learned about it." Although he was very discreet and would discuss such things only with me, I suspect that others sensed that the clinicians he respected were those who thought in terms of molecules, not just symptoms, and who treated on the basis of metabolism, not just in "cookbook" fashion. I believe that some physicians who saw up to fifty patients a day (how could it be otherwise with the shortage of physicians compared to the endless stream of ailing patients?) and had to apply a few principles or they wouldn't make it through the day, envied his leisurely analytic approach to patient care, despite his lower (academic) salary. Spending as much time as possible with his family, he was never hail-fellow-well-met with other physicians, didn't go golfing or drinking on TGIFs. He was never good at male banter anyway. In general women liked him better than men did — appreciated his gentle ways and his kindly respect for women.

One instance of his innovative thinking resulted from his having come upon the information that aspirin causes the red blood cell membrane to become slippery. This caused him to think.[1] Chuck therefore went to the head of cardiology at the hospital to suggest giving at-risk patients a small dose of aspirin each day to make their blood flow better through small arteries and capillaries, rather than forming clots. Dr. Richard Watts' reply was to the effect of "What do you know? You're not a cardiologist."[2] Fairview Hospital could have been recognized for introducing this now standard treatment, and, more important, twenty more years' worth of thousands of patients could have benefited, and lives saved. He also might have gone to other cardiologists, those more innovatively oriented, those at the university. I believe that, this not being his area of rheumatology, he could not afford to spread himself too thin by spending time pushing the aspirin idea.

He tried, also, to organize two symposia but was unable to secure the necessary interest (see vignette "Stillborn Symposia").

As a good family man, he danced another tango between work and home. He was actively involved in "boy things" such as Indian Guides and Scouts. He also shared household burdens with me and took over provendering and cooking on weekends.

To give me more free time to work on my writing projects, Chuck would take the children to visit his relatives. (See Christopher's vignette, "Food Circuit".)

Like other scientists and clinicians, he gleaned knowledge of advances in his field from specialty meetings, at which he exchanged ideas with colleagues and almost always presented papers, occasionally a poster. It soon became apparent to me that this was how Chuck's "five-year plan" for travel abroad was not just idle chatter. Not only did he and I go "abroad" every five years at first, soon more often, but some of these congresses offered opportunities for including our children and teaching them principles of travel, and broadening their perspective on the world as well. An opportunity for all of us to live in a foreign capital came as a benefit of his sabbatical at the Australian National University in Canberra. Another opportunity linking work and family was an informal American/Canadian group of rheumatologists from around the eastern end of the Great Lakes, calling itself the Interurban Rheumatologic Society. These friends met one weekend each fall in Niagara-on-the-Lake, Ontario, with families, and often included a play at the Shaw Festival. Chuck served as its final president before several members moved away and the group dissolved.

Travel, with or without slides, afforded other opportunities for Chuck to pursue his lifelong fascination with rheumatology, at its interface with the arts. On a trip around the eastern end of the Mediterranean, following Odysseus, at the summer villa of Tiberius on the Tyrrhenian Sea, we were shown the bloodthirsty emperor's commissioned sculpture of Odysseus ramming a burning pole into the only eye of the Cyclops, Polyphemus. Chuck noticed that the fingers of the sculptured figure showed the swelling of rheumatoid arthritis. The artist had copied his model this accurately, without even intending to. Chuck later learned that this sculpture came from the "true" period of exact replication in art (see reprint, "Did the Model for Polyphemus Have Acromegalic Arthritis?").

As mentioned earlier, at the Hermitage Museum in St. Petersburg, which we visited on an extension from a congress in Moscow, Chuck spotted, on a gold bowl, an engraving of a shaman examining a patient wincing in pain, with signs of rheumatoid arthritis (see vignette "Rheumatoid Arthritis in Scythian Art"). Finally, as a result of visiting Jack London country on a family vacation to Alaska and the Yukon, he became a medical detective and uncovered evidence for London's suffering and dying from lupus (see vignette, "Jack London. A Modern Analysis of His Mysterious Disease). Thus two of his three studies at the interface of rheumatology and the humanities resulted from observations he made while traveling apart from his work.

How did we finance all this? Academics' salaries are not at the high end. I never saw private patients full-time, and several times I worked in community clinics, again at low hourly rates. However, as a medical resident, Chuck had taught himself principles of investing in securities (see chapter 6, "Years of Training"), and we seized an opportunity to buy rental property with no cash outlay, only the securities as collateral. That building's income underwrote our travel and more (see chapter 8, "Sixteen Family Years on Avalon").

Most physicians and scientists work between fifty and eighty hours a week. Chuck's family time with the boys and me squeezed his workweek to the short end, about nine hours per weekday and another five over the weekend. Thus, over a lifetime, his scientific life was thousands of hours shorter than those of his single-minded colleagues in science and medicine without a balanced family life. His life as a family man encroached on his career, but not the reverse. If he had not chosen to integrate family living with his scientific career, he could have advanced farther in the biochemical bases of rheumatology. His longevity partly made up for this, giving him about a fifty-year career life despite its late start in his mid-thirties. Fortunately he had boundless energy and stamina.

His own slogan says it well: "Work hard, and love it." He echoed Teddy Roosevelt's famous line: "Far and away, the best prize that life has to offer is the chance to work hard at work worth doing."

Notes

1. Yet another example of the shortened form of Louis Pasteur's "Chance favors the prepared mind."

2. This is a perfect example of the logical fallacy known as *argument ad hominem.* This means judging a proposition not by its inherent validity but by its proponent.

Following is Charles Denko's description of his research, which he submitted to the international competition, the Carol Nachman Prize in Rheumatology, in which he came in second, worldwide.

Resume of Research in Osteoarthritis and Cartilage [through 1990]

In studying the biochemistry of cartilage, connective tissue, and osteoarthritis (OA) over the past forty years I soon recognized the fact that cartilage is metabolically active and its metabolism is amenable to quantitative evaluation. Using newly available radioisotopes, radioactive sulfate (35^{S}), I found that cartilage metabolism decreases with age (10,11). Important to my later work was the demonstration that hypophysectomy reduces 35^{S} uptake in cartilage (12). This experiment provided the tool for my study of growth hormone (GH) functions. GH increases 35^{S} incorporation in cartilage of hypophysectomized animals but decreases it in normal animals.

Subsequently I expanded the list of modalities influencing cartilage and connective tissue metabolism as measured by 35^{S} uptake to include, in humankind, inflammation and scar formation (16) and systemic sclerosis (17). In experimental animals, this process is inhibited by glucocorticoids (which also inhibit GH) (18,27), by phenylbutazone and its derivatives (36), and by deficiency of essential fatty acids (58). It is stimulated by prostaglandins (58,60), by corn oil (a dietary precursor for prostaglandins) (60), by mechanical vibration (47), by prolactin (20), and by a cartilage and bone marrow extract (CBME) (35).

Also important for my thinking about osteoarthritis (OA) was my demonstration that several forms of experimental inflammation are accompanied by liver dysfunction as demonstrated by the reduced synthesis of albumin and thiol and delayed metabolism of barbiturate. These experimental inflammations include adjuvant disease (the model for rheumatoid arthritis (RA) produced by injections of foreign protein), the model for gout and pseudogout produced by injection of urate crystals and calcium salts, and carrageenin injection (57).

Data from my studies of the biochemistry of inflammation in patients with various rheumatic diseases provide further support for my concept of OA. Changes in serum levels of acute phase proteins (transferrin, albumin, ceruloplasmin, antitrypsin, and acid glycoprotein), all considered evidence of inflammation, are similar in OA patients to the changes in patients suffering from RA, gout, pseudogout, and systemic lupus erythematosis, all disorders considered inflammatory (69). These serum protein changes are protective (68,70,85). Beta-endorphin, a polypeptide with anti-inflammatory and pain-relieving properties, is low in the serum of patients with OA, as it is in patients with diverse rheumatic disorders such as RA and gout (80). Assays in synovial fluid show that beta-endorphin and acute phase reactants are both lower in the synovial fluid of OA than in that of RA patients.

Radiographically, OA patients show characteristic joint space narrowing (indicating cartilage loss) and bony overgrowth and osteophytes. Since I had demonstrated that a cartilage-bone-marrow extract (long used clinically in Europe) stimulated cartilage metabolism in rats, I then treated volunteer patients with severe hip OA by injection of this agent. About a quarter of patients showed not only clinical improvement but bony regrowth and widened joint space on X-ray, presumed evidence of cartilage growth (62,63).

Later I investigated the growth factors influencing bone and cartilage, namely GH, insulin, and insulin-like growth factor-1 (IGF-1) in OA patients using standardized radioimmunoassay tests. Controls were normotensive, nondiabetic normals matched for age, sex, race, height, and weight. GH and insulin, both known stimulants for bone, were found to be elevated in OA, with its bony proliferation, while IGF-1, a cartilage stimulant, is severely reduced, in line with cartilage loss (98).

Normally GH causes the liver to synthesize IGF-1, but if liver function is impaired, IGF-1 production is reduced. Normally insulin is metabolized by the liver, so if liver function is impaired, insulin accumulates. GH that is not metabolized by the liver accumulates and inhibits cartilage metabolism. GH in physiologic doses is known to block insulin receptors (with only minimal effect on insulin action), thereby leading to increased insulin resistance (Bratusch-Marrain, Smith, DeFronzo: *J. Clin. End. & Metab.* 55, 1982). GH is known also to interfere with post-receptor insulin function. Therefore, as the liver functions suboptimally, insulin and GH become elevated, thereby up-regulating bony synthesis, while IGF-1 remains depressed, thereby down-regulating cartilage metabolism, the exact situation we find in OA. These processes of up-regulation and down-regulation can continue without further stimuli.

Thus my data support my new hypothesis that OA is a generalized metabolic disorder with primary lesion in the liver. OA is amenable to treatment and is reversible.

CWD, 1990

Significance of My Research

[Also submitted with his entry into the competition.]

Looking at OA as a metabolic disorder offers opportunities for both treatment and prevention.

Biochemical changes in a disease suggest that treatment should be sought to normalize the chemistry. Factors found in excess suggest looking for ways to remove or defunctionalize the offending chemical or chemicals. Conversely, when substances are deficient, treatment might consist of the substance itself, precursors or metabolites thereof, or other chemicals that function similarly. Treating a biochemical lesion in a generalized rheumatologic disorder is preferable to pursuing treatment of one joint after another. In families with strong history of OA, at-risk members might be identified at a younger age, and preventive measures instituted to normalize their biochemistry.

Further Research Directions

I would like to study the growth factor levels in secondary OA, which has such diverse origins as trauma, metabolic disorders, rheumatoid arthritis, infections, and occupational activities. Are the changes similar to those in the primary disease, and when do they appear?

I would like to improve our understanding of diffuse idiopathic skeletal hyperostosis (DISH). My preliminary data on growth factors in patients with DISH suggest that DISH is not a variant of OA and may require different treatment. With DISH occur disorders now considered as co-morbidity but which may be, I feel, expressions of a more widespread disorder that shares biochemical abnormalities with DISH. These include hypertension, cardiac disease, non-insulin dependent diabetes, and obesity.

CWD, 1990

A Tale of Two Charleses: My Reminiscences of Chuck Denko, Ph. D., M.D.

Charles J. Malemud, Ph. D.

It's almost thirty-five years now since I arrived at CWRU in 1977 from SUNY at Stony Brook. I had just completed five years of postdoctoral research working first in Aaron Janoff's laboratory on the effect of neutrophil elastase and Cathepsin G on cartilage proteoglycan degradation, and then, after our NIH funding was secured, in Leon Sokoloff's laboratory where I further studied the way in which a pituitary gland contaminant we called chondrocyte growth factor altered chondrocyte membrane transport. When I informed Leon in the spring of 1977 that Rollie Moskowitz had offered me a tenure-track assistant professorship at CWRU, he wasn't that pleased, but he said that this position seemed like a good opportunity for me to advance academically and that at least CWRU had a bona fide musculoskeletal scientist in Leroy Klein. I told Leon that once I was settled in Cleveland, I would set up a meeting with Leroy and see if we had any mutual research interests that could lead to collaboration. Although Leroy and I had many fruitful discussions, we never actually got around to collaborating.

Interestingly, there was not much discussion in the Arthritis Research Laboratory (as it eventually was called) at CWRU about potential collaborations with other rheumatologists at the other two academic medical centers in Cleveland (i.e., Metro and the

Cleveland Clinic). We all knew of the research published by Irv Kushner and colleagues at Metro, but his major research interest in the anti-inflammatory acute phase reactants seemed uninteresting to Rollie because Rollie's pet disease, osteoarthritis (OA), didn't seem to have an inflammatory component as part of either its pathogenesis or its progression. Then there was "that other guy", at this smaller hospital on the west side of Cleveland, called Fairview General Hospital. To this day, I have pondered what it is about researchers who deny the important contributions made by others in their field because the experimental evidence offered by them does not seem to fit into the dogmatic view of how things should work. This has always bothered me, and in the case of "that other guy", namely Chuck Denko, more so than with others who have fallen into this category. It seemed to me that what Rollie was really saying was "stay away"!

So for about four years I focused my budding research career on an experimental model of OA in the rabbit (which by the way does not seemingly have an inflammatory component) and my basic research studies on how human and rabbit chondrocytes keep from becoming "de-differentiated". Then I think that it was in 1982 that Chuck Denko invited me to deliver a seminar at Fairview. Looking back on this invitation it seemed to me to be merely an opportunity to hone my seminar-delivering skills at a local hospital without too much peer pressure. After all, I had already been invited to give research presentations at the New York Academy of Sciences and at the 1st Animal Models of Osteoarthritis Symposium in Wales, UK, where the audience was all of the top-tier researchers in my field. Little did I know at the time that this seminar at Fairview would clearly change my scientific life and, moreover, my thinking about how OA comes about and what changes occur in articular cartilage to cause the joints to degenerate mechanically and functionally. Well, my seminar went off without a hitch, and afterward Chuck and I had an opportunity to have a discussion in his lab. Here was this short, stocky man in a small lab (they called it the Scott Lab) with one technician doing this glorious science while trying to convince the cognoscenti how important inflammation was to OA. Moreover, Chuck's view was that OA was not merely a focal defect in synovial joint metabolism but rather a systemic disturbance encompassing, among other things, deregulated pituitary and liver metabolism. Of course, this protracted discussion left me spinning because I knew that Chuck's viewpoints were generally not accepted by the "OA mavens", including my chief. In those days, there was no such thing as PubMed where we now can readily access all of the published biomedical literature in the comfort of our office using the PC. Back then, we had to go to the library and (G-d help us) actually read the papers from the journals (what we now call hardcopy). There I found it: Chuck Denko's novel findings, which resulted in his heretical view of OA (Denko CW, Bergenstal DM: The effect of hypophysectomy and growth hormone on S35 fixation in cartilage. *Endocrinology* 57: 76–86, 1955). In this paper, Denko and Bergenstal first proposed that growth hormone (GH) would significantly influence articular cartilage proteoglycan synthesis and that experimental removal of the pituitary could alter cartilage function. Thus defects or changes in GH metabolism would alter cartilage function by influencing the production and deposition of proteoglycans, which are enormously large polyanionic molecules that bind water and in doing so are critical to the ability of cartilage to resist compression. This seminal contribution to cartilage physiology was followed up by many published studies from Chuck's lab on the role of GH, insulin-like growth factor-I (IGF-I), acute phase reactants, and serum proteins in OA. All of these papers proposed that inflammation is a step, if not the key step, in moving the indolent phase of OA to its progressive phase, which ultimately leads to synovial joint failure.

The paper by Denko and Gabriel, entitled "A new delineation

of the congeries of osteoarthritis," published in *Clinical Rheumatology* (Denko CW, Gabriel P: *Clinical Rheumatology* 2: 115–122, 1983), was the first of many papers from Chuck's tiny lab that influenced the scientific world about the need to incorporate the results of serum protein assays into the diagnosis of OA because these biochemical assays could tell us a lot about what was going on in the OA disease process. Still there was much resistance to this viewpoint. I remember serving on my first NIH grant review panel in 1983. There were no proposals that even offered to consider this novel and forward-thinking concept.

Many "unofficial" discussions ensued between Chuck and me over the next six to eight years (unfortunately we rarely saw each other except at Rheumatology Grand Rounds at CWRU). Then Chuck moved to CWRU after the Scott Lab closed. Now all of a sudden Rollie was interested in the GH/IGF-I paracrine axis, and who knew more about this than Chuck Denko? It still amazes me to this day that after all the years of Chuck's influence on our own research having been denied, he was now in demand, because all of the other hypotheses we had pursued to explain how OA began in this experimental rabbit model of OA just never panned out. Chuck's move to CWRU (I think it was in 1991)[1] made it possible for our personal and scientific relationship to flourish even more. Although by then I had become an independent investigator funded by my own NIH grants, I still maintained my collaboration with Rollie who now had made understanding defects in the GH/IGF-I paracrine axis one of the main objectives of his own research. This provided me with an opportunity to work closely with Chuck and to consolidate our thinking about OA. During this period, which lasted over thirteen years, the GH/IGF-I paracrine axis not only was fitted into the experimental OA model work but also for the first time with Chuck's guidance was pursued to explain the metabolic changes that occurred in human OA as well as in other musculoskeletal diseases. The work was summarized (and not by Chuck, but by

Rollie, can you believe it!) at the International OA Symposium held at La Sapinière outside Montreal, Canada, in 1994.

In addition to incorporating the cogent view that defects in the GH/IGF-I pathway drove OA pathogenesis and might even be, in part, responsible for the progression of the disease, Chuck and I continued to focus our attention on his idea that OA was a systemic disturbance. When I was asked to edit a monograph on "Fundamental Pathways in Osteoarthritis" for *Frontiers in Bioscience* in 1998, I suggested to Chuck that we write a summary of his research findings on the GH/IGF-I pathway, and that we should try to incorporate his results into those from my laboratory research, which focused on chondrocyte biology. This was the first time that Chuck's seminal contribution to rheumatology research that OA was a systemic disturbance (Denko CW, Malemud CJ: "Metabolic disturbances and synovial joint responses in osteoarthritis." *Frontiers in Bioscience* 4: d686–d693, 1999) was incorporated into a series of other review articles written by many of the "established" OA investigators. I think this summary of the role of GH/IGF-I in OA firmly cemented Chuck's point of view that OA was not merely a focal disease of the synovial joint but rather was a systemic, metabolic disturbance. Thus, the pain, stiffness, and swelling that are the major clinical manifestations of OA only come about when the inflammatory component of OA becomes prominent and that "toxic" levels of GH play a critical role in this pain-related component of OA.

One more tale of Chuck's splendid insights is also in order. In the course of discussing the theme for our paper for *Frontiers in Bioscience,* I asked Chuck: "How do you suppose the 'toxic' levels of GH are delivered to the synovial joint to influence the OA process?" He simply related that in his view GH must be sequestered in the red blood cell. In that regard GH in red cells was transported to the joint space where GH was dumped into the synovial fluid. *Oh, right,* I thought. *Why didn't I think of that!* Well, Chuck suggested that we test his hypothesis. He informed me that he had saved and had frozen all of the red blood cell fractions from the many blood samples he had collected over the years from his rheumatic disease patients. He then indicated that we measure the GH content of these cells. Sure enough, our radioimmunoassay of GH (with the able assistance of his technician, Betty Boja) provided unequivocal evidence that the red cell did indeed sequester GH. These data were published (Denko CW, Boja B, Malemud CJ: "Intra-erythrocyte deposition of growth hormone in rheumatic diseases." *Rheumatology International* 23: 11–14, 2003) and made a big splash in the field. In many ways this study completed the circle of evidence showing how defects in the GH/IGF-I paracrine axis could alter the progression of OA.

Later, Chuck and I successfully mined his enormous collection of clinical data (I rarely had seen such a preciseness in the clinical characterization of all of his rheumatic disease patients) on GH and IGF-I levels in several rheumatic diseases, such as rheumatoid arthritis, DISH, SLE, and fibromyalgia. This endeavor culminated in a major review of the subject published shortly before his official retirement (Denko CW, Malemud CJ: "Role of the growth hormone/insulin-like growth factor-1 paracrine axis in rheumatic diseases." *Seminars in Arthritis & Rheumatism* 35: 24–34, 2005).

During the time that we were writing many of these papers I would often travel to Chuck's home in beautiful Rocky River, Ohio. We would sit in a renovated portion of the garage, which I think he used as an office and where I believe he used to meet and greet his many visitors. We would discuss not only how the writing was proceeding but also world politics and just things in general. Chuck had a great intellect and was knowledgeable about many things, including history, art, and psychology, to name just a few of his "outside" interests.

Chuck Denko, my friend and scientific colleague, has had a significant impact not only on my career as a biomedical scientist but also on my personal view as to what a scientist should strive to be. His courage to pursue his ideas, however unpopular, made him, in my opinion, one of the most respected and important physician/scientists of his generation.

Charles J. Malemud, Ph.D.
July 8, 2011

Note

1. 1986.

The Growth Hormone/Insulin-Like Growth Factor-1 (GH/IGF-1):

Paracrine Axis Contributions by Charles W. Denko, PH.D., M.D. to the Understanding of GH/IGF-1 in Regulating the Inflammatory Response

Charles J. Malemud, Ph.D.

Introduction

Growth hormone (GH) gene expression and synthesis is a major function of pituitary gland homeostasis. GH produced in this fashion is both episodic and pulsatile, indicating that GH is strongly regulated by the pituitary. (1) The secretion of GH is significantly affected by gender, age, and sleep architecture. (2) Although the single most important function of GH is to control skeletal long bone development, (3) GH is also responsible for the synthesis and release of insulin-like growth factor-1 from the liver. (4) In this regard, reduced IGF-1 synthesis is often attributed to GH deficiency, (5) although a deficiency in GH does not cause abnormal growth *in utero* or growth arrest during maturation, (6) which is a strong indication that the GH/IGF-1 paracrine axis is not involved in skeletal development prior to the postnatal period.

Functional aberration in the hypothalamic-pituitary axis has long been associated with the inflammatory response characteristic of the rheumatic diseases. (7–11) Thus a second major function of the GH/IGF-1 pathway resides in the significant role GH/IGF-1 plays in the inflammatory response and in associated rheumatic disorders.

This short review focuses on the contributions of Charles W. Denko, Ph.D., M.D., to our understanding of how pituitary gland abnormalities contribute to the evolution of pain, inflammation, and organ dysfunction in the rheumatic diseases. In many ways, the experimental and clinical studies initiated by Dr. Denko in the late 1950s and early 1960s (12, 13) and continuing on for 5 decades (3, 14–18) resulted in a segue change to the landscape of our knowledge base that the pathophysiology of rheumatic disorders must include the connection between a hormonal imbalance in the hypothalamic-pituitary axis and the systemic disturbances that drive the progression of pain, immobility, and joint inflammation. Thus, Dr. Denko made significant contributions to furthering our appreciation for the underlying pathophysiologic disturbances that drive such diverse rheumatic disorders as osteoarthritis, rheumatoid arthritis, systemic lupus erythematosus, Sjögren's syndrome, crystal-induced arthopathy, and fibromyalgia, which continue to this day.

The Legacy of Charles W. Denko to GH/IGF-1 Research in the Era of Molecular Medicine

A continuation of studies related to the contribution of the GH/IGF-1 paracrine axis to the pathology and progression of rheumatic diseases remains a "hot topic" in the era of molecular medicine. (19–23) Additionally, novel pathways contribution to cartilage regeneration of articular cartilage during the aging process and in the arthritides have been further defined over the past five years. These include molecular pathways that link a network of pro-inflammatory cytokines to defective pituitary-hypothalamic function in several of the rheumatic disorders (24) as well as connecting defective IGF-1 production to the inefficient repair of articular cartilage in osteoarthritis. (25)

The "Somatomedin Hypothesis"

The pioneering studies of Denko and Bergenstal (13) connected the production of pituitary GH to the maintenance of articular cartilage homeostasis. The results from these studies paved the way for what eventually became known as the "somatomedin hypothesis."

An experimental study (26) as well as a series of reviews (27–30) completed the circle initiated by the findings of Denko and Bergenstal. (13) These studies showed that IGF-1 (then known as "somatomedin" or "sulfation" factor) was responsible for regulating the addition of activated sulfur (i.e., sulfate) to the chondroitin polymer moiety, resulting in the formation of chondroitin sulfate. Chondroitin sulfate was shown to be essential for stabilizing the polyanionic-rich cartilage extracellular matrix (ECM) proteoglycan, known as aggrecan, where aggrecan is responsible for the resistance of articular cartilage to compression. (31) It followed from this concept that deficient articular chondrocyte responsiveness to IGF-1 was capable of altering both the biomechanical properties of articular cartilage (32) as well as the repair of cartilage following traumatic injury (33) and in the milieu of osteoarthritis. Moreover, the restoration of chondrocyte responsiveness to IGF-1 has long been considered a significant paradigm for improving the repair of articular cartilage in various forms of arthritis. (34)

GH As a Potential Critical Mediator of Pain

In addition to the critical role of GH in the GH/IGF-1 paracrine axis, Denko had originally proposed that toxic levels of GH could be responsible for the pain associated with arthritic synovial joints. This view, which was summarized in 1999, (3) held that only after GH reached supra-physiological levels would the pain of arthritis be evident as a clinical symptom of the disease process.

Follow-up studies showed that circulating GH was sequestered in red blood cells. (35) Denko hypothesized that this phenomenon was responsible for the significantly higher levels of GH in arthritic synovial fluid compared to normal synovial fluid. (16) Thus, modulating the level of GH in the peripheral circulation could become a useful pharmacologic strategy to limit the pain associated with various inflammatory disorders, including irritable bowel disease, (36) fibromyalgia (37, 38) and neuropathic disturbances associated with defective nociceptive pain mechanisms and altered vasoactive peptide function. (39, 40)

Conclusions

The pioneering experimental and clinically relevant studies performed by Charles W. Denko and his colleagues have had monumental "staying-power," reflecting the current high level of interest in modifying the levels of GH, IGF-1, and endogenous neuropeptides to regulate the inflammatory response associated with various types of arthritis and other disorders of inflammation. Evidence of this can be found in the wealth of peer-reviewed scientific literature from the past decade and a half as well as the current development of pharmacologic agents to modify the levels of these molecules. A considerable amount of new data indicates that modification of the GH/IGF-1 paracrine axis will eventually result in the suppression of arthritis inflammation and the retardation of its progression.

References

1. Robinson, ICAF. (2000) Control of growth hormone (GH) release by GH secretagogues. In: *Mechanisms and Biological Significance of Pulsatile Hormone Secretion.* pp. 206–220.

2. Ojeda, SR, SM McCann. (2000) "The anterior pituitary and hypothalamus." In: *Textbook of Endocrine Physiology,* 4th Ed., pp. 128–162.

3. Denko, CW, CJ Malemud. (1999) *Frontiers in Bioscience* 4: d686–d693.

4. Sussenbach, JS, et al. (1991) "Structural and regulatory aspects of the human genes encoding IGF-1 and -II." In: *Molecular Biology and Physiology of Insulin and Insulin-like Growth Factors,* pp. 1–14.

5. Jones, JI, et al. (1995) *Progress in Growth Factor Research* 6: 319–327.

6. Cohen P, RG Rosenfeld. (2000) "Growth regulation." In: *Textbook of Endocrine Physiology,* 4th Ed., pp. 286–302.

7. Aspden, RM, et al. (2001). *Lancet* 357: 1118–1120.

8. Chikanza, I, L Fernandes. (2000) *Expert Opinion on Investigational Drugs* 9: 1499–1510.

9. den Berg, WB. (1999) *Zeitsschrift fur Rheumatologie* 58: 136–141.

10. Blumenfeld I, E Livne. (1999) *Experimental Gerontology* 34: 821–829.

11. McAlindon, TE, et al. (1993) *Annals of the Rheumatic Diseases* 52: 229–231.

12. Denko, CW, DM Bergenstal. (1955) *Endocrinology* 57: 76–86.

13. Denko, CW, DM Bergenstal.(1961) *Endocrinology* 69: 769–777.

14. Denko, CW, P Gabriel. (1985) *Journal of Rheumatology* 12: 971–975.

15. Denko, CW, et al. (1990) *Journal of Rheumatology* 17: 1217–1221.

16. Denko, CW, et al. (1996) *Osteoarthritis and Cartilage* 4: 245–249.

17. Denko, CW, B Boja. (2001) *Journal of Rheumatology* 28: 1666–1669.

18. Denko, CW, CJ Malemud. (2005) *Seminars in Arthritis and Rheumatism* 35: 24–34.

19. Davis, UM, et al. (1997) *Arthritis & Rheumatism* 40: 332–340.

20. Roman, O, et al. (2003) *Chronobiology International* 20: 823–836.

21. D'Elia, HF, et al. (2005) *Arthritis Research & Therapy* 5: R202–R209

22. Gaissmaier, C, et al. (2008) *Injury* 39 Suppl 1: S88–S96.

23. Biermasz, NR, et al. (2009) *Journal of Clinical Endocrinology & Metabolism* 94: 2374–2379.

24. O'Connor, JC, et al. (2008) *Cellular Immunology* 252: 91–110.

25. Van der Kraan, PM, et al. (2002) *Osteoarthritis and Cartilage* 10: 631–637.

26. Skottner, A, et al. (1987) *Journal of Endocrinology* 112: 123–132.

27. Daughaday, WH. (2000) *Pediatric Nephrology* 14: 537–540.

28. Le Roith, D, et al. (2001) *Trends in Endocrinology and Metabolism* 12: 48–52.

29. Le Roith, D, et al. (2001) *Endocrine Reviews* 22: 53–74.
30. Isaksson, O, et al. (2001) *Growth Hormone IGF Research* 11 Suppl A: S49–S52.
31. Heinegärd, D. (2009) *International Journal of Experimental Pathology* 90: 575–586.
32. Kuettner, KE, et al. (1991) *Journal of Rheumatology* 27: 46–48.
33. Fortier, LA, et al. (2011) *Clinical Orthopaedics and Related Research* 469: 2706–2715.
34. van de Loo, FA, et al. (2008) *Current Rheumatology Reviews* 4: 266–276.
35. Denko, CW, et al. (2003) *Rheumatology International* 23: 11–14.
36. Akbar, A, et al. (2009) *Alimentary Pharmacology & Therapeutics* 30: 423–435.
37. Neeck, G, W Risedel. (1999) *Annals of the New York Academy of Sciences* 22: 325–338; discussion 339.
38. Malemud, CJ. (2009) *Clinical & Experimental Rheumatology* 27 Suppl 56: S86–S91.
39. Xu, XJ, et al. (1991) *Neuropeptides* 18: 129–135.
40. Hobson, AR, Q Aziz. (2009) *Current Opinion in Pharmacology* 7: 593–597.

Charles J. Malemud, Ph.D.
Professor of Medicine & Anatomy
Department of Medicine, Division of Rheumatic Diseases
Case Western Reserve University School of Medicine
Cleveland, Ohio 44106

Distinctive Features

CWD's Firsts

Chuck never fit standard patterns. Sometimes this was because he had been born into an Eastern European background at a time when such people were not well accepted by the Protestant Anglo-Saxon majority, or if they were "making it", it was because of special talent or at the cost of added effort to "prove themselves".

At Penn State he got them to accept Russian and French for his Ph.D. requirement for "two foreign languages" (which for all the rest of the candidates were French and German). He argued that good chemistry papers were already coming out of Russia at that time, and more from Russia than from France.

Later, in the army despite being 4F, he did not qualify for the three recognized religions, Catholic, Protestant, and Jewish, but got them to mark his dog tags "RO" for Russian Orthodox. (I would have suggested "EO" for "Eastern Orthodox", which could have included Greek and others.)

As long as I knew him, he argued that "Tchaikovsky" was a mistransliteration through German, and that the Cyrillic letters for the initial consonant sound should be transliterated only Ch, hence Chaikovsky. He wrote several letters to the musicologists writing program notes for the Cleveland Orchestra. One followed Chuck's suggestion, or possibly arrived at this transliteration independently, but another, with a German name, retained the "Tch".

CWD's Rejections

Although Chuck and I were both accepted by Johns Hopkins Medical School, we were both rejected by Harvard. Chuck noted their arrogance in what the admissions officer told him: "We don't take applicants from cow colleges." [Penn State]

Twice in later years he was offered a position at the Harvard Medical School, but he declined. The first time it was because the pay was so paltry that I would have had to support him, which he didn't consider appropriate. I don't remember his reason the other time, but it was not because of the earlier snub.

When Chuck was one of the few (possibly the only) 4Fs in the army, he was offered an assignment to work as a chemist on the Manhattan Project (the atomic bomb). He declined because although his M.S. was in inorganic chemistry, his main interest was physiologic chemistry, the area of expertise that he advanced throughout his career in the army and in his life's work in the biochemistry of connective tissue. On this occasion, too, the rejection was his.

CWD's Contacts with Notables

Chuck worked toward his Ph.D. at Penn State during the Depression when enrollment was low and Penn State was small and congenial, more like a college. Besides the chemistry he was learning, he also had the opportunity to attend lectures by notables the university brought in, and even, in some cases, receptions given for them. One such lecturer was Amelia Earhart, the aviatrix who was the first woman to fly across the Atlantic and later went down in the Pacific on the last leg of a round-the-world flight. She inspired an entire generation of women, and was a role model for many of my generation's mothers. Another visitor was the Russian composer and musician Rachmaninov. On the occasion of his visit, the Russian professor, who was also the Russian Orthodox priest, invited his students to a special reception to have an opportunity to meet and speak with this Russian native speaker, who spoke little or no English.

While visiting friends in New York, Chuck met Tolstoy's youngest daughter, Alexandra. In the terminology of her father's writing days, as his secretary, she was his "typewriter". "Sasha", her father's pet name for her, had bought property, which included a motel, along the Hudson River in upstate New York, and invited members of the Russian community up for weekends. She invited Chuck also, but he was just then transferred out and unable to accept.

He met Walter Hamden, an actor, and Robert Frost, the poet of New England, both in the Penn State lecture series.

Later, at Johns Hopkins University, we had a number of esteemed professors. The head of internal medicine, A. McGee Harvey, at thirty-three was the youngest ever to hold that post. Alfred Blalock (pediatric surgeon) and Helen Taussig (pediatrician) were famous for their new cardiac surgery on infants born with congenital cardiac anomalies. In the words of our party skit, they "turned blue babies into pink babies by hocus-pocus". Chuck's younger brother, Peter, with a cardiac anomaly, was born too soon to be saved by such a procedure.

I had no such special patients, but I happened to be a favorite with our famous obstetrics professor, Dr. Alan Guttmacher. This was because of an incident in his class, when he outlined the handling of a particular obstetrical problem. The next class period, having forgotten that he had gone over this, he asked us what to do in a case like this. He pointed at me and called on "Dr. Decker". As I parroted back his lecture, he was muttering about how one so young could show such mature clinical judgment.

My classmates, who knew very well how one so young had imbibed such clinical judgment, were choking back their mirth behind their hands, but Guttmacher somehow didn't notice. Later, Dr. G offered me a residency, which would have been a real plum, but the life of an obstetrician, bad enough for a married man, was not in accord with my plans for marriage and a family. Years later, when I was having obstetrical problems, Dr. Guttmacher sent me to the only gynecologist in the world, Dr. David B. Davis, who did a kind of plastic surgery on my pelvis that made possible our family.

I had another obstetrical recognition, however, albeit from a humbler source. As an intern at the University of Illinois Research and Education Hospital in Chicago, I, like everyone else, rotated through obstetrics. One of our professors was working with a new way to administer anesthesia, extradurally, which avoided possible damage to the spinal cord but required inserting a needle into the spine at just the right depth. One day several obstetricians from South America were visiting and wanted to observe this procedure. I stood by while our professor tried several times and missed. The patient became increasingly restless, whimpered, and finally said, "I want my doctor!"

"I'm your doctor," said the professor.

"I want my little girl doctor," she whined.

"I'm right behind your head," I reassured her while the professor glared at me, but then got his needle in right.

When another woman finally delivered her eighth child (and we, routinely and without permission from this so-called "grandmultipara", tied off her tubes because further pregnancies posed increased risk), she ran out of ideas, and so she named the baby for me. The youngest patient I delivered was thirteen, and I managed to get the baby out without a tear.

During our Cleveland years, an old classmate of Chuck's, Andy Tkach, who was personal Whitehouse physician to Nixon, offered Chuck a job as his assistant. Of course Chuck didn't consider it, intending to continue with his research on connective tissue disease. Besides, Tkach's wife advised against it. "It's a great job for the person, but it's a terrible life for the family," she said. "Andy's gone much of the time, both in and out of Washington, and we're left alone."

When Chuck had a meeting or other reason to be in Washington, he would sometimes have lunch with Tkach in the White House dining room. Once, the postmaster general was there too, and complained about his arthritis, and so Chuck advised him to consult a particular rheumatologist he respected in Washington. For many years rheumatology was a specialty on the fringes, and patients were often not referred appropriately when they could have been helped. When Chuck lunched there, the butler usually gave him a cigar with the White House logo on its band, which he gave his delighted father.

Chuck corresponded with John Glenn (senator, former astronaut) about the fact that what was considered good for the country ("growth") was bad for those on fixed incomes ("inflation"). Glenn had some of Chuck's argument read into the Congressional Record. Chuck was also in contact with longtime senator Howard Metzenbaum.

Finally, Victor McKusick, a medical student two or three years ahead of us, spent his professional life on the hereditary diseases, and Chuck wrote a chapter for his book. At our son Nicholas's graduation from medical school, Victor gave the commencement address. He drew our attention to the fact that within his lifetime we had gone from the erroneous belief that *H. sapiens* has forty-eight chromosomes (the correct number is forty-six) to a mapping of the human genome.

Chuck's Polio Disability

Having suffered polio at age one, which resulted in shortening and weakness of his left leg, in childhood Chuck received surgery severing a binding ligament. Subsequent physical therapy strengthened the muscles, resulting in a greatly improved gait although with a limp. Therefore Chuck was able to live a remarkably full and rich life, even hiking long distances in the mountains. But when he was unable to do certain things, he encouraged the boys and me to do the few things he could not. In the early years of our marriage these occasionally pertained to riding horseback. He explained that horses were trained to accept a rider only from the left, the side on which he could not support his weight to mount. Therefore he never rode on four-legged beasts.

When we camped at Grand Canyon on our way to a rheumatology meeting in San Francisco shortly after we were married, Chuck encouraged me to take the daylong trip down Bright Angel Trail on a mule. (That was one of the adventures my Aunt Blanche, coming home like Marco Polo with her traveler's tales, had told me about when I was a child.) In those days you could arrive at park headquarters and sign up, whereas now I understand there is a months-long reservation period. I was lucky enough the day we arrived to be the last of thirty to sign on for the three trains of ten each, for the next day. Chuck's paper wasn't quite ready, and so while I had my adventure, he sat in the campground and put the finishing touches on it for the meeting.[1] As Chuck and I drove through the West on that trip, I pointed out many small bits of hexagonal columnar basalt, like those I had seen years earlier with my mother at the Giant's Causeway in North Ireland. There was a much larger example at the Devil's Postpile National Monument in California. (Years later when we camped to Los Angeles to board ship for Australia, we went via the Grand Canyon for the boys' experience, and I was sorry that they were too young for the mule trip.)

Similarly, when Lake Mead was planned, and the result would be to flood the beautiful Rainbow Bridge, Chuck agreed to stay behind while two women friends and I packed in with a guide on an overnight saddle trip. Besides seeing the spectacular bridge itself, we slept on cots under a desert sky just strewn with thousands of stars. A drug company had called for vacation pictures with just one human figure, to flood physicians with their postcard advertising campaign for their new product for gastric irritation. Their caption would read, "Nothing will help your ulcer patient like a vacation, unless it's [I forgot the name of the med]." I sold one-time use of the slide I took of our guide on a horse with its ears pricked forward, and the canyon country drifting off to infinity. In those days the $250 they paid me was enough to pay for our entire trip.

When Nicholas and Timothey had both finished college, we took them to East Africa, primarily Tanzania, to see the savannah animals, the Ngorongoro Crater, and the Rift Valley where the Leakeys made their finds. Then we proceeded on to Rwanda and Zaire to visit the gorillas. Chuck saw all the East African savannah animals but was unable to climb the slippery bamboo slopes to the mountain gorillas. (It was very difficult for me.) I regretted his having to miss this adventure, but, as always, he wanted the rest of us not to skip anything on his account. (Another guide drove him to the place where gorillas often crossed the road, but, unfortunately, not that day.) Our climb took us four and a half hours, and the guides, small men weighing 140 pounds and wearing dress shoes, with chests of cold drinks on their heads, would boost me at the worst places. (After the final climb of the trip I gave my hiking boots to one guide, to his delight.) We were instructed to act submissive for our hour in the presence of the gorilla family, close enough to see their individual hairs. It was heartwarming to see the silverback, the patriarch, actually babysitting, letting his offspring by various females climb and play on him and suck their toes. Many human fathers could learn from the silverback. In this way gorillas bought protection by tourists' visits, since part of our fees went to the conservation system.

Chuck had heard somewhere of a replica of an ancient Roman statue of a warrior in the Pushkin Museum in Moscow. This statue came from the "true" period of art about two millennia ago, noted for detailed representation of the subject. In this case the warrior showed signs of rheumatoid arthritis, as the subject must have had, since it was copied so accurately. Therefore when we went through Moscow on our way to Lake Baikal, I scheduled an extra day for Chuck to see and photograph this. It was on the second floor, up a high marble stairway with a handrail so wide that I could barely span it. Chuck was still walking with a cane, and I followed, although I doubt I could have caught him, as he toiled laboriously up that colossal climb. It demonstrated his enormous drive and determination to do what needed to be done to achieve his ends.

After taking the train to Irkutsk, we had another extra day, planned for us to meet Aleksey Golovko, the physicist whose solar laboratory we had visited on the previous trip, who had agreed to take us to the geology museum we had visited on the prior trip for us to give our specimens from my home, Berrien County, fulgurites and fossil crinoids.

On the boat trip itself Chuck missed shore excursions without a pier, where we had to disembark and embark over a plank. He and another handicapped scientist remained on the boat and chatted. I was sorry that he missed the stromatolite. None of us saw the world's only freshwater seals in the wild because of a storm, but we saw them in an aquarium ashore where they were being studied.

In Antarctica Chuck was able to go ashore by zodiac on all sixteen landings, visit the penguin colonies and the research stations (American, British, Polish, and Chinese Great Wall Stations), and do everything but climb the volcano on Deception Island and go swimming in its effluent.

In August 2001, his choice was a Northwest Passage trip on the Russian icebreaker *Kapitan Klebnikov,* starting from Resolute. The captain and the ship's doctor came to try to dissuade him from the trip, but he persuaded them he could manage it. When the rest of us were landed by helicopter, he was given helicopter rides to see foxes, geese, and, his favorite, muskoxen, because they formed a protective ring around their young. He missed nothing on this, his final eco-trip, at eighty-five.

In Chuck's last four years his polio disability and his Parkinson's colluded to make walking more difficult, until he went to a walker, and later a wheelchair.

For many years I had planned the difficult trips first because we had no way to know how long he (or I) would be able to travel.

Note

1. For another meeting he made a poster and asked what I thought of it. "It looks like a first grader's project," I said. But it attracted much attention. It was a matter of content over form.

Chuck's Emotional Side

Chuck always maintained that Russians are emotional and loving, and he contrasted their usage of "Mother Russia" with the German "Fatherland". However, long before we as a society began making the point that males should get in touch with their soft, loving, emotional side, he himself was a man able and unafraid to cry.

On my very first trip from Baltimore to Ellwood City to meet his family, I saw the first instance of this. Just minutes before our arrival, his nephew Bobby's little cocker spaniel, Chipper, had been killed by a car. On learning this, Chuck's face contorted and tears ran down.

For many years, life went our way except for many obstetrical problems, but by the time Christopher's behavior was beyond the pale, I recall the time when, after struggling unavailingly for half an hour to talk sense to Christopher on the telephone, Chuck sat on the bed and sobbed.

There were other occasions for weeping, the causes of which I have forgotten, but I remember a recent incident when he was well into his final decline with Parkinson's disease. Our friend Gerry Thorrat had read that Cleveland's Jewish newspaper was collecting material relating to the Holocaust. With his consent, she contacted their editor, who called and interviewed Chuck on the telephone. The part of his Occupation experiences that was germane to her interest was his assignment to find, wherever possible, remaining relatives of Jewish orphans, blond children who had been taken by the Nazis from their families in Poland and Czechoslovakia and Ukraine and given to German families to rear as Aryan. This was especially difficult because in most cases the parents were themselves victims of the Holocaust. The intention was to find a relative, any relative, a third cousin twice removed, for example, with whom to place the child so as to give him some feeling of family continuity. As Chuck described this work over the telephone, he cried — sixty years after the event (see *Cleveland Jewish News* account).

This sensitivity translated into gentleness. The physical expression of his gentleness was his baby-soft hands. Throughout our marriage, for the duration of his health, he washed my hair and was proud of keeping the sunny blond look that first attracted him to me. (In this way, but not for this purpose, he saved me time and us the money of half a century of trips to the beauty parlor, paying, in effect, for several long trips. Over my lifetime I have met only one other woman whose husband took on the shampooing job. To me, this is an example of showing love by doing, not just by talk, which is proverbially cheap.)

The major flaw I found in Chuck, creating problems over many years, was his failure to call up strength when I thought it was needed, in the disciplining of children. (As Dorothy Parker once said, "That woman speaks eighteen languages, and can't say No in any of them.") I learned very quickly not to say, "When your father gets home, we'll see what to do about this" because when I tried that, addressing the bad behavior never came to anything. And so I just did whatever I thought the situation warranted. At the same time I became increasingly angry that I could not just enjoy the good part of parenting, as Chuck was doing, and share the bad part, discipline, which I felt would have been only fair. This was a cause of ongoing dissension between us. It resulted in the children having nothing but good memories of him, many bad ones of me. One might argue that if the boys felt I was too hard on them, it would have been reasonable for them to expect Chuck to come to their defense rather than just watching silently, but they never complained. They knew they deserved my handling.

There were many good sides to Chuck's gentleness. His humor was clever but never sarcastic or cruel. Twice he was voted the most humorous man in the class, in high school and college. He was a welcome guest, always willing to help. Once, while the rest of us were laughing and joking in the living room, I heard him in the kitchen offering, "I can peel carrots" and our hostess replying, "I'll be happy if you just sit there and talk to me."

Until the end of his life he remembered the hurt of always being chosen last for sandlot baseball teams because of not being able to run fast, although already improved to the point of being able to walk with a limp, and even run with difficulty. (As an excellent compensatory mechanism, when he was in high school, he announced sporting events over the local radio station and wrote for the *Ellwood City Ledger.*) When he went into decline, we converted the garage into a bed/sitting room with bath. A physical therapist came to exercise him to maintain his strength. For the first time in over fifty years of marriage, I heard him mention this old wound about sandlot baseball teams, to the kind therapist, who happened to be black. Later Chuck told me he thought this man would understand because of having a disadvantage of his own to overcome. Until this late date, I had never heard about his childhood pain. It must have been much worse before the corrective surgery.

The Cruelty of Parkinson's Disease

Since we are all mortal, we must all have a terminal event. The lucky ones have a swift, painless, and merciful demise and are not aware of it, e.g., in their sleep. Others are slated by Atropos, the mythical Fate, who cuts the thread of our life, to undergo a long, downhill course, with a sometimes painful, often disabling, terminal disorder. Such was Chuck's fate with Parkinson's disease.

In some cases, before an elderly person's decline is apparent even to the physician in the tiny sliver of time he has to observe the patient, a family member in close and continuous contact can recognize impairment. Although Chuck's death did not occur until October of 2005, my first awareness that something (not yet diagnosed) was wrong came in the late '90s. At a meeting of chemists at Geneva College, various alumni gave their reminiscences. I had suggested that he was no longer thinking fast enough to do this extemporaneously, and that he would present himself to better advantage if he read his remarks. He did not acknowledge this problem, tried to speak "off the cuff", and did not do it fluently. It was his last such attempt.

During the same period Chuck was having more difficulty walking, which eventually we realized resulted from the effects of both recurrent polio and Parkinson's disease. He went from cane to walker. A fall put him into the hospital and subsequently into a nursing home where he had intensive physical therapy for walking with his walker. But the nursing home was not permanent.

Soon thereafter Dr. Milton Good, the neurologist (who happened to have trained at Bronson Methodist Hospital in Kalamazoo, where my mother had her nurse's training and I was born), diagnosed Chuck's condition, although he showed little in the way of the classic signs of Parkinsonian tremor and cogwheel rigidity in the arms.

My next evidence of Chuck's cognitive decline from Parkinson's disease came on our circumnavigation of New Zealand over the "faux millennium", 1999–2000. He had not counted out his medication correctly, and I had to have the ship's doctor get us the New Zealand equivalent. But he was able to do everything — see the yellow-eyed penguins, the nesting wandering albatrosses, and the tuataras in captivity. Since our ship was ordered out to sea lest the computers crash at midnight, cutting out a visit to a glowworm cave, and since Chuck and I had been promised this, having missed it when we had a day in Auckland on our way to the sabbatical, I got the tour guide to send us later to Waitomo from Auckland by taxi to see glowworms (see my poem "Austral Galaxy at Waitomo" in *Interlink*).

During these years Chuck continued working, although it was becoming increasingly difficult. After I worried for many years about his lateness after his late-afternoon rounds, the feared call came from Lakewood Hospital. Chuck had rolled his Volvo by hitting a parked car, due to loss of depth perception. The police found him hanging, unhurt, from his seatbelt, and I found him chatting with the nurses in the emergency room. (This was not his first accident. About six months earlier he had totaled another car, but somehow I had assumed it was a one-of-a-kind accident and did not terminate his driving, although Christopher said I should have. And Christopher was right.) On the second occasion, Chuck never protested my taking his keys. For a time he worked mornings, taking a taxi to the university, and I would pick him up at noon, an hour's roundtrip in light traffic. When this program became too difficult for him, Charles Malemud, Chuck's colleague (and former student) came to our house to work with him and organize his data for publication. Malemud is still working on publication of Chuck's final paper, on the evidence for rheumatoid arthritis in the engraving on the Scythian gold bowl in the Hermitage Museum in St. Petersburg (see vignette "Arthritis in Scythian Art").

His appointment at Case Western Reserve kept being renewed, and he had been promised a full professorship, but they kept dawdling until he had exceeded the age limit, to his and my disappointment (see vignette "A Tale of Two Charleses").

Years earlier when stairs became too difficult for him, we had a stairway elevator installed. In anticipation of future need, we had the garage converted into a bedroom/sitting room/bath so he could avoid the stairs altogether. Ken Spiro, our builder, even tracked down special commercial flooring, in use at the university, that Chuck had found the ideal texture, neither slippery nor clinging.

The problem we faced was Chuck's transportation to CWRU to work as long as possible. He wanted me to drive him to the lab to work with Charles Malemud and return to get him one morning a week. Each roundtrip would be at least an hour and a quarter, often more, depending on traffic. I thought that the time had come to use taxis, but, realizing that for a taxi driver to find someone in a hospital complex would be difficult, we compromised by having a taxi take him to the east side and me get him at our agreed-upon time and place. Later Malemud came to our house to work one morning a week. (Chuck had helped Charles during a time of personal crisis, as well as having been his mentor and friend for years.)

During the summer of 2001 we took his last two trips, one to the southern part of Africa, where Christopher helped him embark and disembark (see vignette "Travel Around the Edges") and to the Northwest Passage by icebreaker (see chapter 10, "His Final Years"). He missed nothing but had personal helicopter flights because of the very rough tundra.

He was taken twice to the hospital, once after a fall and once with a bladder infection. Although the hospital was necessary, they did not get him out of bed as ordered, and his mobility suffered. He was sent to a nursing home and had very beneficial physical therapy before returning home. I noticed from the bulletin board that one activity they offered was "word games" and I made sure they took him to it. But his deterioration was illustrated when he complained, "I was the best in the class, but still they wouldn't let me go home."

Val and I got him to California via Amtrak, to visit Nicholas and family, and flew home. He said, "I want to go again," and I agreed, "If you're well enough next year." But that was not to be.

Several months later Val and I also flew him down to see Christopher's resort hotel, Docelunas. How much he was aware of the significance of this I don't know, because he asked, "How did you hear about this place?"

As Chuck tried to feed himself French toast with syrup, he admitted, "This'll determine whether I get another trip."

"No, your travel doesn't hinge on fine motor coordination. We don't care if you spill a little syrup."

His medication produced hallucinations. (Dr. Good, his neurologist, said that some medication for epilepsy does this also, and his daughter, with epilepsy, had to learn to ignore the hallucinations — they were preferable to seizures.) Chuck's consisted of a "party in the snow next door" and a "dog at Severance Hall". He also had to learn to ignore them.

One day he asked at home, "Who is running this establishment?"

I replied, "This establishment is your home, and I am running it."

It is a terrible thing to see the once fine mind of someone you love come to this.

Travel Around the Edges

I like the principle of making one operation serve more than one, possibly several, purposes, e.g., doing several errands on one trip to the business part of town. In travel this becomes: When in the vicinity of something of natural or historic or cultural interest, detour to see it.

This included visiting friends. I had warned them not to invite us unless they meant it because we might show up. On our way to China we made time for a stopover in Seattle to see Lem and Mel Petersen, whom I had known from St. Joe when I was growing up and later when we were both in Chicago. When crossing Iowa, we arranged to stop to see my college debate partner Luella and her husband Herk Kameraad, by then a minister. They loved having someone from outside their church to talk to, about the problems of running a church in a small town. Often as we passed through New York City, we would stop to see our medical school friend Izabella Aldon Salman; in Teaneck, New Jersey, and Bernice Goldberg, whom I had met on the Komodo dragon trip.

Mainly, however, my "travel around the edges" consisted of allowing extra time before or after a congress or other main event, to see something else of interest in that part of the world, such as Gregor Mendel's (the father of genetics) monastery and garden in Brno on our way to Prague.

One example came in connection with the ocean voyage we took on the "Little Red Ship", first of the small cruise ships, which we boarded in Tenerife in the Canaries. We were to fly in to Tenerife via Madrid, but I arranged for us to start two days early. Arriving in Madrid, we stayed overnight and went to the Prado Museum, famous for its Spanish art. We were still a day early in Tenerife, which I had planned for a day trip to Gomera, another of the islands, noted for its "whistling language", which was demonstrated by the waiters where we lunched. It consisted of placing words on a whistle, so that a message could carry from one mountaintop to another. Not only had we had our two extra days for these excursions, but many of our fellow passengers arrived in Tenerife a day late due to a hurricane in the Atlantic. Arriving a day early is not a bad idea for such contingencies.

Another example of "travel around the edges" occurred on Chuck's next-to-last major trip. It was scheduled for another eclipse, this one in Zambia, and Victoria Falls, a trip on the Rovos Rail, the Edwardian "blue train" with mahogany paneling and brass fittings through Zimbabwe, which their dictator Robert Mugabe had already trashed, and a few days at a private preserve just outside Krueger National park (where I was delighted to see not only the "Big Five", but also a pangolin, a fascinating mammal with scales that I had seen only stuffed at the Cleveland Museum of Natural History). (See my poem "Pangolin and Me" in *Interlink*.) This trip was planned to include Christopher, the eclipse chaser, to help Chuck, and Nicholas's wife, Karen, for her first time in Africa. Again I allowed two extra days to join the group in Johannesburg. The first we spent in Atlanta and took a taxi out to see Stone Mountain, a memorial to the Confederacy by Gutzon Borglum, famed for Mount Rushmore. Arriving a day before the group in Johannesburg, we took a taxi to Soweto (Southwest Township), where black apartheid took its first defeat just twenty-five years prior. Our guide proudly drove us down the only street in the world with the homes of two Nobel laureates, Nelson Mandela and Archbishop Desmond Tutu. He showed us an enormous hospital where medical students and young doctors from Western countries often serve. There was a large rally that day, and Christopher attended, one of a handful of white youths in a completely peaceful, well-behaved festival.

Geneva's Science Wing

Geneva always recognized Chuck and his accomplishments, unlike Hope, which sent me only the standard alumni communications. In 1969 Geneva gave him its Distinguished Service Award. We attended various science alumni meetings, and both of us gave talks at Geneva. Knowing that I had always yearned for Academe, Chuck recommended me to Geneva, where I eventually became a visiting professor and gave an occasional lecture or seminar in areas I had studied.

With Geneva and chemistry dear to his heart, we gave the college money, the earnings of which were to go for chemistry scholarships or, if there were no applicants, scholarships in other sciences.

They also asked for a contribution for a new wing for their science building, and we agreed to give them a large sum in amounts decreasing over a period of several years. There was a ribbon-cutting ceremony, and Timothey, Patricia, and Madeleine, and Nicholas, Karen, and Louis were there. I had wanted the donation to be anonymous and was embarrassed by all the hoopla, did not want the name Denko on the wing, and did not like the fact that this was written up in several newspapers and on the news in western Pennsylvania. Patricia's parents and Chuck's sister Helen called us about it.

Over the years we received occasional thank-you notes from scholarship recipients, usually two at the same time, so I assumed they were assigned by a staff person at Geneva. I was shocked by one such note, after Chuck's death, when we were about halfway through the designated giving pattern for the science wing. While the note from the young woman that year was a perfectly good thank-you note, the young man's note was replete with misspellings, nor did he mention chemistry or anything academic. This is his note:

> *[undated]*
>
> Dear Sirs.
>
> I would like to thank all those that have suported me these 4 years at Geneva. God has truly blessed me while I have been here. I have grown not only mentaly but also spirtually. I know that it was Gods will for me to be here. However I could not pay the whole bill. You were the hands of God. It was only by your gracious heart that was able to experience Gods Blessing at this time and this place. So I offer my most sincere and heart-feilt thanks for the roal you have plaied in my life thou we have never meet. May God bless you in abundance for what you have done for me.
>
> *Your Brother in Christ,*
[signature]
In His Steps

I returned the original to the new president of the college, but kept a copy.

In my letter I indicated that I expected the scholarship money to go to persons who were scholars, whereas this person should not ever have been accepted into the college until he showed evidence of having had remedial English. When I received no reply, I requested that the scholarship money be applied to the science wing fund; their response indicated that the terms of the gift precluded this. They ignored my expectation that scholarship grants should require a letter written under supervision (so someone else, such as a wife, couldn't write the letter). For several years I received no communication addressing my concerns. Therefore I stopped the contributions to the science wing fund.

Two years later I received a letter from Geneva's "Director of Donor Services" giving me the names of the current scholarship recipients. I replied, thanking her for the letter and requesting photocopies of the application letters of these recipients, but I received no reply.

I expected that my stopping the annual check to the science wing fund would get their attention, but only three years later did they call requesting a conference. When this was accomplished in March 2011 it was in my accountant's conference room, and I made no promises concerning future gifts. Dr. Smith, Geneva's president, offered to send suggested amendments to our bequest.[1]

I am outraged that Chuck's hard-earned money should have been supporting someone for four years who was not even learning the language, and the language I refer to is English. I have no way of knowing whether he learned any chemistry.

Note

1. When I received Dr. Smith's suggested tightened rules, I made them even more stringent, requiring the applicant to give evidence of being already a scholar, speaking and writing grammatical English, and in no need of any remedial work that (s)he should have learned earlier. Such a graduate will be a CHARLES W. DENKO SCHOLAR, and this should appear on the diploma. I have not received evidence that this has been done.

Obituaries and Tributes

Journal of Rheumatology
2006; 33/9

In Memoriam

Charles W. Denko, Ph.D., M.D.
1916–2005

In 1986, after a professional lifetime of research in the biochemistry of connective tissue diseases, Charles (Chuck) Denko increased his time to full at the Cartilage Research Laboratory of the Case Western Reserve University (CWRU) School of Medicine to begin fruitful interdisciplinary studies on the role of growth hormone (GH) and insulin-like growth factor-1 (IGF-1) in rheumatic disorders and in sleep architecture disturbances, which were still under way at the time of his death on October 18, 2005.

Chuck Denko was born August 12, 1916, in Cleveland, Ohio, USA, the eldest child of Wasil and Evdokiya Denko. The Denkos moved to Ellwood City, Pennsylvania, in 1917, where Chuck spent his childhood and formative years. At one year of age, Chuck contracted polio, which left one leg shorter than the other, with muscle atrophy. Despite this disability, which improved with surgery, Chuck was an excellent student who entered the class of 1938 at Geneva College because of its outstanding reputation in chemistry. After graduation, Chuck entered Pennsylvania State University, receiving the M.S. in Organic Chemistry and the Ph.D. in Physiologic Chemistry in 1943. After working for a short time in chemistry research, Chuck participated in World War II at the Army Nutrition Laboratory in Chicago. When the war in Europe ended in May 1945, Chuck was sent to serve in the Sanitary Corps during the European Occupation, where he inspected the "displaced persons" camps, and destroyed empty penicillin bottles to keep them out of the hands of black marketeers. He was also instrumental in returning to relatives Jewish children taken from their families before and during the war to be raised as Aryan. After the war, Chuck entered Johns Hopkins University School of Medicine, where he received the M.D. degree in 1951. From 1951 to 1952, he interned at the University of Illinois in Chicago and completed his residency in Internal Medicine at the University of Chicago in 1956. He then completed research fellowships at the University of Michigan (1956–58) and Ohio State University (1958–68) before joining CWRU in 1968, where he rose to become Clinical Associate Professor of Medicine.

Chuck Denko was Director of the Scott Research Laboratory at Fairview Hospital in Cleveland, Ohio, from 1968 to 1986. He also spent a half-day a week teaching, and practiced rheumatology two half-days a week at CWRU. He was a member of the American College of Rheumatology and the Inflammation Society, and the author of over one hundred scientific papers and book chapters. Many of Chuck's earliest experimental studies in rheumatology focused on the role of hormonal influences on cartilage glycosaminoglycan synthesis, especially the role of prolactin, endorphin, and enkephalin in modulating chondrocyte metabolism and in inflammation both *in vitro* and *in vivo*. He also conducted pioneering bench research studies on monosodium urate crystal-induced inflammation in rodents. A systematic analysis of the clinical management of patients with osteoarthritis (OA) under his care led Chuck to conclude that OA was more than just a result of a mechanical wear and tear of cartilage; rather, OA was a systemic disturbance, where OA pain as well as synovial joint pathology and cartilage degeneration were modulated by hormonal influences. He was the first United States rheumatologist to test the efficacy of Rumalon (a cartilage and bone marrow powder) in the clinical management of OA, monitoring cartilage structural restoration by an analysis of the patient's radiographs.

When Chuck joined the Cartilage Research Laboratory at CWRU in 1986, he began a systematic study of the role of the GH/IGF-1 paracrine axis in rheumatic diseases and in sleep apnea, in collaboration with Rollie Moskowitz and Kingman Strohl, respectively. The rheumatic disease studies resulted in a series of research papers that included a novel quantitative assessment of serum and synovial fluid GH/IGF-1 levels in patients with symptomatic and asymptomatic OA and diffuse idiopathic skeletal hyperostosis (DISH). Several of these papers were published in *The Journal [of Rheumatology]* from 1990 to 1994. Subsequent studies indicated a role for GH/IGF-1 in the hypermobility syndrome as well. In the final decade of his research career, I had the privilege of working with Chuck to finalize the data collection and interpretation of his many studies of the GH/IGF-1 pathway in rheumatoid arthritis (RA), systemic lupus erythematosus (SLE), DISH, and fibromyalgia that culminated in a review analyzing the results of our own studies on the GH/IGF-1 pathway in these conditions, as well as experimental and clinical studies in this area published by other investigators. This review was recently published. (1) In the two years prior to his death, Chuck published several additional papers with me that explored the relative influences of GH, IGF-1, and somatostatin in OA, RA, and SLE. Chuck's last scientific paper, on the influence of body mass index and blood glucose on insulin, GH, and IGF-1 levels in patients with symptomatic DISH, was also recently published. (2)

In addition to Chuck Denko's scientific and clinical accomplishments in rheumatology, he was an eminent scholar of rheumatology in history and in antiquity. Among his other contributions, Chuck reported on the likely diagnosis of SLE in the writer Jack London, (3) and on the strong possibility that the model for the statue of Polyphemus at the villa of Tiberius had acromegalic arthritis. (4) He also studied a depiction of arthritis among Scythian gold artifacts. Chuck traveled on all seven continents, observing animal behavior. His archives are housed at Geneva College, where he received his baccalaureate degree.

Chuck Denko would begin each lecture with the phrase "Good morning, fellow students," for he considered his audience lifetime students like himself. Chuck's insightful comments about the vagaries of clinical management of rheumatic diseases were gleaned from his many years of experience in treating these chronic conditions. Chuck Denko was a well-respected scientist and contributor to rheumatology research and clinical management. He will be missed by all who knew him, learned from him, and profited from their interactions with him.

References

1. Denko CW, Malemud CJ. "Role of the growth hormone/insulin-like growth factor-1 paracrine axis in rheumatic diseases." *Semin Arthritis Rheum* 2005;35:24–34.
2. Denko CW, Malemud CJ. "Body mass index and blood glucose: correlations with serum insulin, growth hormone, and insulin-like growth factor-1 levels in patients with diffuse idiopathic skeletal hyperostosis (DISH)." *Rheumatol Int* 2006;26:292–7.
3. Denko CW. Jack London. "A modern analysis of his mysterious disease." *J Rheumatol* 1993;20:1760–3.
4. Denko CW. "Did the model for Polyphemus have acromegalic arthritis?" *J Rheumatol* 1995;22:2191–2.

Charles J. Malemud, Ph.D.
Professor of Medicine and Anatomy,
Division of Rheumatic Diseases,
Case Western Reserve University School of Medicine
and University Hospitals of Cleveland

Cleveland Plain Dealer
October 21, 2005; Metro/Obituaries B5

CHARLES DENKO, PHYSICIAN, LECTURER, STUDIED DISEASES RELATED TO ARTHRITIS

Wally Guenther, Plain Dealer *Reporter*

ROCKY RIVER – Dr. Charles Denko, 89, a biochemist/physician at Case Western Reserve University where he researched connective tissue diseases related to arthritis and rheumatism, died Tuesday at Fairview Hospital.

Denko's major research discoveries centered on the biochemical abnormalities in various forms of arthritis that were previously believed to be caused by wear and tear of the joints, said his wife, Dr. Joanne Denko, a psychiatrist.

His findings through the years were published in more than 100 scientific articles. He also presented his findings and lectured at medical schools and rheumatology conferences around the world.

The Rocky River resident had the title of emeritus associate professor at Case. Although he gave up his teaching duties several years ago, he continued his research at Case until July, when he became ill, his wife said.

When he was named director of the Scott Research Laboratory at Fairview General Hospital in 1967, he also began his association with Case's medical school. The laboratory closed in 1986.

His portrait was hung in the Army Medical Museum and Library in Washington, D.C., in the 1950s as one of 400 people at that time who made significant contributions to medicine.

Denko overcame polio at the age of 1. The symptoms returned in later years, forcing him to use a cane, a walker, and finally a wheelchair, his wife said.

He was born in Cleveland but raised in Ellwood City, Pa. He received a chemistry degree from Geneva College, Pa., and a master's degree in organic chemistry and doctorate in physiologic chemistry from Penn State University.

During World War II, Denko was deferred because of his polio, but he talked the military into accepting him and worked in the Army Nutrition Laboratory in Chicago.

He was sent to Europe after the war to study the nutritional status of the Germans, including supervising displaced-persons camps. He helped many Jewish orphans to be relocated with their relatives.

Denko was assigned to destroy used penicillin bottles to prevent black marketeers from reusing the bottles, his wife said. He left the army in 1947 with the rank of major.[1]

After the war, Denko received his medical degree from Johns Hopkins University.

He taught at Ohio State University, the University of Michigan, West Virginia University, and the University of Chicago before joining Case.

In 1993, the medical world accepted Denko's investigation published in the "Journal of Rheumatology" that author Jack London died in 1916 of lupus, not suicide as first believed.

Denko and his wife had been married for 55 years.

Also surviving are sons, Christopher of Washington, D.C., Nicholas of Menlo Park, Calif., and Timothey of Pittsburgh; four grandchildren; and one sister.

Services will be at 3:30 p.m. today at SS. Peter and Paul Russian Orthodox Church, 12711 Madison Ave., Lakewood.

Arrangements are by the Zeis-McGreevey Funeral Home, 16105 Detroit Ave., Lakewood.

Note

1. He mustered out as captain, was offered rank of major if he stayed.

Beaver Beacon
December 2005

Charles Denko

Dr. Charles Denko, a biochemist and physician at Case Western Reserve in Cleveland and 15-year owner of the southernmost Donegal Bay cottage, passed away on October 18th.

Dr. Denko's major research discoveries centered on the biochemical abnormalities in various forms of arthritis that were previously thought to be caused by wear and tear of the joints. Through the years his findings were published in over 100 scientific articles. In the 1950s his portrait was hung in the Army Medical Museum and Library in Bethesda, Maryland, as one of 400 people who made a significant contribution to medicine.

He was born in Cleveland but raised in Pennsylvania. He suffered polio as a youth, which left him with a short leg and severe hobble. One day a stranger driving past stopped and came over to him, and told him that the Shriners would be able to help him at their hospital in St. Louis. He went there and underwent leg-lengthening surgery, which required several months of recuperation.

He won a full scholarship to college, and earned a Ph.D. in 1943 for his synthesis of gold compounds for treating arthritis. He was declared 4F, but wangled his way into the army as a medical researcher; he studied metabolism in conscientious objectors. He was later sent to Europe and assigned the task of repatriating the children, mostly Jewish, whom the Nazis had seized as "Nordic types" on their eastward march. On one occasion he stopped in Landshut and asked to see the cell where Hitler had been imprisoned as a young man. The warden took him to another cell also, and introduced him to a prisoner who would be executed on the following day for "crimes against humanity", a man Dr. Denko knew had devised a test for diphtheria, for which he knowingly sacrificed the lives of many people, but which would nevertheless help millions.[1]

Dr. Denko was also involved in destroying the vials the new penicillin came in because they were being stolen by black-marketeers and used for selling fraudulent (and damaging) concoctions — the same crime the character portrayed by Orson Welles committed in *The Third Man.*

He mustered out in 1947, and went through med school on the G. I. Bill. His research and teaching appointments brought him to the University of Illinois, the University of Chicago, the University of Michigan, and Ohio State before Case Western. His recent work on biochemical abnormalities established that osteoarthritis is a metabolic disorder.

A man who saw most of the world in his later life, he had many interests in many subjects. For example, he wrote the definitive paper on Jack London, establishing that his death in 1916 was not a suicide but from lupus.

He is survived by his wife, the poet Joanne Denko, three sons (Christopher, Nicholas, and Timothey), four grandchildren, and a sister.

Note

1. The Schick test had not sacrificed lives. The irony was that Schick, an ethical and respected scientist who had devised the beneficial test for diphtheria before Hitler's time, became corrupted under Hitler. Schick used twins for worthless research and then sacrificed both.

T-Bones: *A newsletter from the Division of Rheumatology*

The Department of Medicine, Case School of Medicine
November 2005

In Memoriam

Charles W. Denko, MD, PhD, Emeritus Associate Professor of Medicine in the Division of Rheumatic Diseases, died on October 18, 2005. He was 89 years old.

Dr. Denko was named Director of the Scott Research Laboratory at Fairview Hospital in 1967 and began his association with the Case Western Reserve University School of Medicine at that time.

After the Scott Laboratory closed in 1986, "Chuck" joined the Division of Rheumatic Diseases, where – in collaboration with Rollie Moskowitz, MD, and Betty Boja – a study of the growth hormone (GH)/insulin-like growth factor-1 (IGF-1) paracrine axis in rheumatic diseases began in earnest. Several seminal publications resulted from these studies, which were published in the *Journal of Rheumatology* and other rheumatic disease specialty journals, from 1990-1996.

In 1998, Dr. Denko began a fruitful collaboration with Charles Malemud that resulted in the postulation of osteoarthritis as a systemic disturbance characterized by a dysfunction in GH/IGF-1 published in *Frontiers in Bioscience* in 1999. These studies culminated in a review of GH/IGF-1 disturbances in the rheumatic diseases published in *Seminars in Arthritis and Rheumatism* in August 2005.

Prior to his passing, Dr. Denko was still working on the relationship between body mass index and hyperglycemia in rheumatic diseases and on a description of rheumatoid arthritis in ancient Scythia (Southern Russia).[1]

Dr. Denko is survived by his wife of 55 years, Joanne Denko, MD, a psychiatrist and eminent scholar; sons Christopher, Dr. Nicholas and Dr. Timothey Denko; a sister and five grandchildren.

Respectfully submitted by Charles J. Malemud, Ph.D.

Note

1. It was that engraving on the gold bowl.

Rocky River Kiwanis Club *November 2005:* Gong & Gavel

In Memoriam Dr. Charles Denko

Dr. Denko has been a member of Rocky River Kiwanis since 2003. We applaud Dr. Joanne and "Chuck" for staying active and attending our meetings regularly in the face of his health problems. Our sympathy and best wishes to Dr. Joanne and all their extended family.

Ellwood City Ledger

Thursday, February 23, 1995

Letter to the Editor

Class of 1934 member salutes one classmate

Recently the Lincoln High School Class of 1934 held its 60-year class reunion.

We were Depression students and did not have all the advantages that today's children take for granted. However, we did have one big advantage and that was our leisure time with not so much pressure.

This is not just a nostalgia trip but to tell you about probably our class' most famous graduate — Charles Denko, who was our class president.

He came from poor immigrant parents and, like most of us, had little money to further his education. He was fortunate in receiving a scholarship to Geneva College where he graduated with highest honors.

After graduation from Geneva College, he continued his education at Penn State University where he received a Ph.D. degree in organic and physiological chemistry. This was in 1943.[1]

In 1945, he entered the U.S. Army and served as a nutrition officer, biochemist and microbiologist in the Sanitary Corps in the United States and the European Theater.

Returning to civilian life he earned his medical degree at Johns Hopkins University in Baltimore, Md.

He and his wife, Joanne, a psychiatrist and writer, have traveled the world visiting every continent. He has had many honors heaped on him and has had many research papers published championing ideas that have gained acceptance years later.

He is included in a permanent national medical library display of history's 10,000 most influential scientists.[2] At the present time, he is still working at Case Western Reserve in the arthritis clinic, a position he holds without pay.

It would take many pages to tell of all the things he has done and all the places he has visited since his growing-up years in Ellwood City, but as Chuck's classmate, I would like to salute him and say I am proud of him as well as the Class of 1934.

I believe this tribute is long overdue to one of our most talented and productive citizens.

Esther Gotjen
Ellwood City
Class of 1934 Graduate, Lincoln High School

Notes

1. The organic chemistry degree was an M.S.
2. This is a collection of only 400 medical scientists to that time.

Charles W. (Chuck) Denko, Ph.D., M.D. — Teacher

Even with my eyes closed, I could tell Chuck Denko was beginning a seminar because he would always preface his remarks with the statement, "Good morning fellow-students." That was Chuck's tagline, always. In the role of teacher, he was there to disseminate knowledge and to learn, for he too was a student, always ready to accept input from his colleagues.

Chuck brought to all of his teaching encounters, his vast clinical acumen and his thorough knowledge of the subject matter. He was a learned person who was able to convey his ideas to an audience in a friendly and enlightened manner. Of course, Chuck offered insights as well which I thought was always his "strong suit" as a teacher. Early during my stay in Cleveland, Chuck invited me to lecture at Fairview Hospital. At that time, I learned from him the trials and tribulations of being a "change-agent" in scientific research. So as a teacher, Chuck not only mastered a teaching style, but also the ability to provide his audience with the scientific support for his controversial ideas on rheumatic diseases, pathology and physiology, as well as the potential that his concepts could be brought to fruition at the "bedside." Chuck was a scientific trailblazer and I am proud to have collaborated with him, to have learned from him, and to see that his fundamental understanding of the contribution of the hypothalamic/pituitary/adrenal axis to rheumatic disorders is finally receiving the international acclaim it so rightfully deserves.

Charles J. Malemud, Ph.D.
March 30, 2005

Letter of Condolence from Father Don Thomas, M.S.

85 New Park Avenue, Hartford, CT 06106-2184

October 24, 2005

Dear Joanne and Family,

This letter is sent to you with no intention of renewing your sorrow over the death of your beloved husband, Charles, but I did want to send along my sincere expression of sympathy to all of you on the occasion of Charles' death. Billy and Johanna called me last week to inform me of the news, and they also asked me to celebrate a Mass for the repose of His soul, which I did last week upon hearing the news. May God grant him eternal rest and peace, and may God reward Charles for all the good he accomplished in the course of his life here on earth. You would know more about that than any of us, but even to us in his last years it was eminently clear that he was gifted in many areas and shared those gifts with many.

I am certain that in your lives and in the circle of his many friends he will be missed very much. I want to assure you of continued remembrances in prayer, and may God also strengthen all of you in your time of loss and sorrow.

Keep well, Joanne, and keep occupied with your many interests as well. The memory is a fantastic faculty which will enable you to relive many marvelous times you have had together as a couple and as a family. May God be with you daily, and thank you also, Joanne, for all the good you have done and continue to do in your life. Bye for now....

Love and prayers always,
Father Don Thomas, M.S.

Note

Father Thomas is Kristina Thomas' granduncle. At family events, such as Kristina's birthday parties, her granduncle on the Thomas' side and her grandfather on her Denkos' side would enjoy each other's company.

Levai Tribute to Dr. Charles Denko, Ph.D.

I first met Chuck many years ago on the occasion of his marriage to Joanne. Whenever I hear *Some Enchanted Evening,* I recall this happy event.

Chuck has made an indelible impact on my life. Later, unable to walk steadily, he slowly mounted the thirteen steps up to the top of our summer home. "What a magnificent view of the lake!" he exclaimed. I watched him descend the same way — a step at a time on his backside. He has helped me understand the power of an indomitable will.

Now, as I approach ninety years, I think of Chuck as I climb the thirteen steps. The hardest steps are not always climbed with our feet.

Thanks, Chuck.
Blaise Levai, B.D.

Note

Blaise Levai is the minister husband of my college roommate, Marian Korteling, who became a physician, went to India as a missionary with her husband, returned when India rejected Christian missionaries, became a child psychiatrist, and continues to work as a locum tenens for psychiatrists on vacation.

Nephew's Letter of Appreciation

March 21, 2004

Dear Uncle Chuck:

I have heard that you are not doing well. I am sorry to hear that news and want you to know that I have been thinking about you lately.

Over the last few months, a small wooden flute[1] has been seen in my house on the floor of my children's playroom. They play it off and on, and each has his own interests in the sounds that it makes. That flute was a present to me from you and Joanne many years ago when I was about the age of my oldest son Alex. Alex now likes to hear its sounds as he blows into its wooden mouthpiece and covers its tuning keyholes. My two-year-old, Jackson, tries to take it from Alex and play his own song. No matter who is playing it or where I see it on the floor or couch, its sight reminds me of you.

You have been an inspiration to me since I was very small. I have always admired your dedication to knowledge and learning and the fascinating wisdom that I have heard from you whether as a warning to my four-year-old self to not swallow gum or later stories of the horsemen of Scythia that I recently recalled when I read Gibbon describing the energy of the Scythian tribes from the East sweeping into Europe.

Your gifts to me have been small and large, tangible and intangible, and like the flute on the floor of the playroom, they will be with me always, an example to emulate and a memory to cherish. The world is a better place because of you and I wish you well today and always.

Your loving nephew,
John Scott Denko

Note

1. It is a Native (South American) flute.

Dad's Most Admirable Qualities

As my father's Parkinson's disease progressed, he continued always to push himself physically as hard as possible, knowing that as functioning ebbed, it could never be recaptured. Examples of this abound, with Dad's insistence on walking from the car to our new home, despite the ease and availability of his wheelchair, with me carrying a chair for him to sit on periodically, as we made our way from point A to point B, catching up on life's events when he would sit to rest.

One event in this vein remains in my consciousness to this day, and can stand as an allegory for many of Dad's most prized qualities. Before my family moved to our "dream house", we lived in a smaller house that was ill equipped to house my parents when they would visit us in Pittsburgh. For one such visit we reserved a room at an elegant small hotel that was on the registry of historic landmarks. This detail is germane as such a building was able to function despite the absence of an elevator.

At the late hour of the evening, and with snow and ice on the ground, Dad and I decided to use the wheelchair to navigate from the car to the check-in of this lovely hotel. When we arrived, the clerk, a man probably not yet in his twenties, quickly detected Dad's mobility issues (the wheelchair likely being a major clue). He politely informed us that this hotel lacked an elevator and perhaps we'd be more comfortable down the street where such accommodations were more easily available. The clerk appeared to be quite concerned about the possibility of a fall, and I think he did not relish the possibility of a lawsuit. I felt myself becoming a bit angry, with a feeling of rejection and being told we were not all that welcome. Dad, on the other hand, remained without visible signs of any unpleasant emotion. He calmly and politely informed the clerk that he understood the man's concern for his well-being, appreciated the hotel's fear of a customer being injured, but also that "I did not get where I am by avoiding difficult situations". Dad told the man he thought he'd be able to navigate the stairs,[1] and he thought the hotel was very nice, and that he'd like to spend the night. The clerk did not know how to proceed, and, after a few more feeble attempts at dissuasion, capitulated to Dad's wishes.

I had competing emotions of pride in Dad, some shame at the situation, trepidation for the task to come, and some feelings of impatience, which I shunted away. We wheeled to the bottom of the stairs. I helped Dad arise, and he turned to sit on the bottom step. He then, one stair at a time, used his legs and arms to push and lift himself up one step at a time. The pace was slow but steady, and we arrived at the top, and his room, in one piece.

What I found to be the most remarkable aspect of this event was how Dad treated the clerk. By this time Dad had already given his alma mater a million dollars,[2] had been at the peak of his profession, and had any number of reasons to behave in a haughty manner. He did no such thing. He did not become defensive or angry (which I felt brewing inside me), and he treated this person precisely the way he would have treated his son or his wife.

TCD

Notes

1. I was with Chuck, and the difficulty did not end with the stairs. I helped him get into the very high, canopied bed.
2. Later, and not quite accurate. See vignette "Geneva's Science Wing".

Newspaper Articles

New York Times
December 5, 1943; Review of the Week Editorials

Gold for Arthritis

New experiments may decrease dangers of using the metal

Compounds of gold have been used for the past fifteen years in the treatment of arthritis. Many physicians object to them because they are highly toxic. One per cent of those treated with gold die.

Two new possibilities for the gold treatment may arise out of researches conducted at Pennsylvania State College by Drs. A. K. Anderson and Charles W. Denko. One is the development of new, nontoxic gold compounds called auroxanthates, which, when injected into rats, build up resistance to toxic compounds injected later; the second is concerned with the discovery that before the rats die from the effects of the toxic compounds there is a significant increase in non-protein nitrogen of the blood.

Drs. Anderson and Denko do not profess to know whether or not their nontoxic compounds have curative properties. But they have shown that when the compounds are injected into rats, resistance[1] is developed to subsequently injected toxic compounds. Rats that have received small doses develop a tolerance to larger amounts. Not until clinicians repeat the experiments on human patients will it be known if arthritis can be controlled in human patients. It is possible that a non-toxic injection may build up a tolerance, which would permit the use of the therapeutic toxic compound.

The revelation that non-protein nitrogen in the blood increases before death in rats, after toxic reaction, may be important to physicians. If the blood of arthritic patients were analyzed frequently an increase in non-protein nitrogen would be a warning that the gold treatment must be stopped. In rats an increase in non-protein nitrogen always resulted in damage to the kidneys.[2] Sometimes the increase was detected even in rats that showed no kidney damage. Drs. Anderson and Denko conclude that the damage may sometimes be invisible.

Notes

1. As often occurs, this article shows incorrect usage of the term "resistance" when "tolerance" is meant, in the sentence "But they have shown that when the compounds are injected into rats, resistance is developed to subsequently injected toxic compounds." This error is corrected in the subsequent sentence.
2. I believe the science writer has this reversed. It is kidney damage that causes elevated non-protein nitrogen.

Note to My Grandchildren:

I was particularly determined to include this article so that you could appreciate how remarkable your grandfather was even early in his career. Rarely does any newspaper carry the work of graduate students, and in this case they sent a reporter from New York City to central Pennsylvania to interview Chuck and his professor. Back in 1943 *The New York Times* was excellent journalistically, and it still has first-rate science coverage. I am quoting the article despite the fact that *The New York Times* is charging me $1,130 for permission.

Cleveland Jewish News

June 23, 2000

He Reunited Families in Aftermath of War

Ask Dr. Charles Denko what he does and he will tell you he applies chemistry to people who have arthritis. The 84-year-old rheumatologist has been doing research on the subject at Case Western Reserve University for over 50 years.[1] But before that, the Rocky River resident applied human chemistry and understanding to an even more crippling situation.

During 1945 and '46, Denko, who is Russian Orthodox, supervised public health in the displaced persons camps in Austria for the U.S. Army. Armed with a Ph.D. degree in biochemistry (he was yet to get his M.D.), he oversaw among other things, sanitation in the camps and the care and feeding of the mainly Jewish refugees.

His most memorable undertaking was the repatriation of children, Denko explained in a phone interview. As the Nazis swept through places like Poland, Byelorussia and Czechoslovakia in the early years of the war, they "took children who looked Nordic (i.e., had blond hair and blue eyes) and sent them to Germany to be adopted."[2]

In the dislocation of war and the forced roundups, German soldiers "found these kids wandering around, and their army set up a retrieval mechanism" for them. As for getting away with these blatant abductions, Denko asks rhetorically, "Who bothers a victorious (German) army?"[3]

Once the youngsters, most of whom were Jewish, were taken back to Germany, officers and other powerful people "probably got the first pick," he says.

But these families were hardly engaged in a humanitarian mission. Instead, like the "disappeared" in Argentina decades later, these children were probably taken in by childless couples who planned to raise them as good Germans. With no intention, of course, of ever giving them back to their rightful families.

"The children, generally between the ages of 8 and 12, were well dressed and clean, unlike the people I saw in the concentration camps," says Denko. Their existence was discovered at war's end because "the Germans kept good records" and the International Red Cross (IRC) was able to "latch on to these records."

Using those records as a road map, the IRC located several hundred of these children and, removing them from their German homes, brought them to the DP camps.

An effort was made, Denko says, to group children from the same country or region together, with "the older ones trying to take care of the younger ones." One youngster he remembers most vividly was, like the others, blond and blue-eyed, but a little older (12 or so) and a little taller than the rest. He would get his group of charges together and "try to pacify them," Denko recalls. "'We will be all right,' he told them. Gathering the younger ones under his arms, he tried to get them not to cry and not be afraid. They seemed to get strength from him."

Recounting this story publicly for the first time, Denko breaks down in tears. It is a while before his is able to continue.

When he does, he explains that because he spoke "a little" German, Russian, French and Polish and "understood the problems" of these youngsters, he was in charge of supervising their repatriation.

First, however, he had his superiors to convince. His colonel, for example, was concerned that some of the children might be sick and felt only the healthy ones should be repatriated. But the yet-to-be-doctor knew of a stronger medicine; the healing qualities of returning to one's own family.

When the children were apprised of the planned repatriation, "virtually nobody asked to go back to Germany," Denko says. Furthermore, he adds, the children had not forgotten their (respective) native languages.

The next hurdle was locating the missing families. No small task in chaotic, war-decimated Europe. Denko says that in most cases they were able to identify and find the youngsters' real families. Not necessarily their parents or immediate relatives, given the fact that 6 million Jews had perished, but an aunt, a cousin, "anyone within the child's extended family that we could find." Denko estimates he was responsible for the return of at least 30 of these children.

The Red Cross was able to bring about one-third to one-fourth of the families to Austria for a reunion. But when I ask Denko to describe one of those reunions, he bursts into tears again. "It was difficult," he finally admits, between sobs.

In an unrelated incident, while Denko was inspecting sanitation at one of the DP camps, he came across a Jewish man accused by several of his fellow Jews of being an informer for the Nazis. As a result, the man was being taken to Palestine to be hanged. When, upon questioning the officer in charge, Denko found that the accusation had not been proven, he insisted on turning the accused over to the Army's Counter-Intelligence Division (CID).

Weeks later, while Denko was walking down a street in Salzburg, the same man ran up to him and began covering Denko's hand with kisses. The CID had investigated his case, the man told the startled Denko, determined he was not an informer, and he was set free. So, in addition to reuniting children with their families, he had also saved a life!

After returning to the States, Denko entered medical school and got on with his life. He never again had contact with any of the people he helped.

Reflecting on those long-ago years, Denko says his experience with the children, in particular, "made me aware of the fact that to be with family, to be with people like yourself..." was the best medicine for human beings.

Talking of family, Denko also tells me that many of his relatives were living in Brest, Belarus, when the Germans came. The relatives told him how they had suffered during the war and had to hide out in the woods. "Maybe you'll put that in the story, too," he adds.

Not surprisingly, Denko says he gets "upset" with revisionists, people who claim the Holocaust never happened. "I try to associate with people like myself," says this good man. "Unfortunately, there are not enough of us."

Notes

1. Obviously Cynthia Dettelback did not follow the several venues of Chuck's career.

2. This German program of taking Aryan-looking Jewish orphans to be brought up as German was called "Lebensborn". Many such orphans would probably not have survived the war without it. It is mentioned in William Styron's novel and the film *Sophie's Choice*, in which Sophie (played by Meryl Streep) tries unsuccessfully to get the commandant to send her little boy to this program to save his life.

3. The "victorious German army" that abducted Jewish children was moving eastward in the early part of WWII.

The Plain Dealer

Sunday, July 19, 1992

Studying a 1916 Death

WRITER SAYS LUPUS KILLED LONDON

By Grant Segall, *Plain Dealer* Reporter

Rocky River

Charles Denko limps through his wet yard in Rocky River, plants his walking stick on the bluff, points to Lake Erie's horizon and talks about the green flash.

"We've seen it several times," he says. "The rays of the sun as they go down filter everything out except green." It happens on the clearest evenings and lasts for a moment, he says.

Denko, an associate professor at Case Western Reserve University School of Medicine, has spent his 75 years scanning horizons for flashes. He has been to every continent. He has published many research papers in his field, rheumatology, championing ideas that gained acceptance years later. He is included in a permanent National Medical Library display of history's 10,000[1] most influential scientists. He and his wife, Joanne, a psychiatrist and writer, have crammed their Rocky River home with heaps of books, magazines, and bric-a-brac that mirror the owners' busy minds.

Now he is promoting a new theory about the poor health and early death of Jack London (1876–1916), the best-selling author of "Call of the Wild," "White Fang" and other adventure stories.

London had a few things in common with Denko. He was a prolific writer, a tireless traveler, a controversial thinker, and, if Denko's theory is right, a victim of a lifelong illness.

Denko's illness is polio. He fought it off as a child in Elwood City, Pa., but its symptoms are returning in old age, forcing the use of a walking stick.

London's love of wolves inspired him to name a novel "The Sea Wolf" and his dream home, Wolf House. Denko believes London's illness was lupus, a rheumatic illness named for the wolf-like fury with which it drives the body to attack itself.

London was diagnosed over the years with many seemingly unrelated ailments, from scurvy to gout. But he lived as hard as he could. An illegitimate child whose family chased prosperity from one town to another, London became a river pirate, sailor, hobo, jailbird, gold miner, war correspondent, novelist, rancher and socialist crusader. He drank hard for years and ate raw fish and raw meat.

A servant entered London's study in Glen Ellen, Calif., one morning and found the 40-year-old author unconscious, doubled over, breathing harshly and blue in the face. A mostly empty vial of morphine lay on the floor nearby. Several doctors rushed to treat him, but he died a few hours later.

One of the doctors later called the death a suicide. He said that, depending on how full the bottle had been, London could have taken up to 12.5 grains of morphine, an often-fatal dose.

The other doctors blamed London's longtime kidney disease, for which the morphine had been prescribed. They signed a death certificate pinning the death on "uremia following renal colic."

Denko thinks all the doctors missed the mark. He says suicide would fit the stereotype of a temperamental artist better than the facts about London.

"He had no reason to commit suicide," Denko says. "He had fame, money, a beautiful wife devoted to him...."

Besides, London had often used morphine before, probably building up enough tolerance to withstand 12.5 grains. Denko also says the writer would have drained the vial completely if he'd wanted to die. Also, the doctors pumped London's stomach immediately and gave him an antidote to morphine, with no success.

Denko says the death certificate was probably right as far as it went: uremia was the immediate cause of death. But, to a man of Denko's curiosity, that was like blaming a cough on a sore throat. It does not delve deeply enough.

He caught London's trail on a Yukon trip in the mid-1970s. He attended a reading at which a speaker mentioned that London had been treated for scurvy in the Yukon and recovered quickly. Denko raised his hand, asked some pointed questions, and said scurvy rarely heals fast, leads to quick recoveries or relapses. Besides, the Yukon has plenty of native foods that prevent scurvy, such as cranberries and wild roses.

A decade later, a business trip took Denko to California. He used the chance to inspect some of London's medical records, interview his daughter and meet his biographer, Russ Kingman, who runs the Jack London Bookstore in Glen Ellen. Denko concluded that all of London's ailments could be chalked up to lupus.

Lupus is "the great imitator," Denko says. It darts around the body unpredictably, mimicking different illnesses in different patients. It may cause the bleeding gums normally associated with scurvy, the swollen joints of gout and the kidney pain of uremia.

Most people who see London's photographs notice the handsome face, blue eyes and tousled hair. Denko points out the spindly fingers and curving thumbs – common signs of lupus, he says.

Top doctors treated London over the years, but none seem to have suspected lupus. The disease was not well known on the West Coast, Denko says. "It would have taken somebody very sharp to figure it out."

Denko presented his theory at a medical conference a few years ago and says he got a favorable response. He finally wrote a paper about it last year. "I work very slowly," he explains with a laugh.

Kingman, the biographer, published the paper in the bulletin of the Jack London Society. "It's fabulous," he says in a phone interview from Glen Ellen. London would have admired Denko's thorough research, Kingman says. "He didn't believe in inspiration. He said, 'Dig.'"

According to Denko, the paper is slated to appear in an upcoming anthology of London research. He hopes his theory will sway other researchers to reinterpret London's life and work, which contains many passages about illnesses. "People who spend their lives studying his writing will have a better way to interpret it," he says.

Denko ran the research department of Fairview General Hospital until the department folded in 1986. Since then, he has continued his research at CWRU without pay.

He pauses in puzzlement when asked what makes him keep digging. "I think we ought to clear up misunderstanding," he says.

Note

1. I don't know how this 10,000 crept in. It would be difficult or impossible to list 10,000 scientists of all kinds in history at that time. His portrait was one of just 400 medical scientists.

Plain Dealer Article
Sunday, February 28, 1988

Caring and Curing

In 1988 feature writer Grant Segall asked to interview us for an article for the *(Cleveland) Plain Dealer.* On the appointed day, first a photographer showed up, for which we had not prepared especially. Not a great newspaper reader, I didn't realize that it was either de rigueur or a sine qua non to accompany every such article with one or two photos. Therefore one has us at the kitchen table and the other in the living room stacked high with articles and books, and the dog, Tina, lying at our feet.

Deb Baldanza, a new member in my main writer's workshop, had recently written a piece, which appeared in the *Akron Beacon Journal,* about her years-long struggle to find help for what turned out to be lupus. Grant must have seen that article, because the introductory anecdote he didn't get from us. He asked us for the names of people he could contact to confirm (or deny) what we told him, and he later told me he had never encountered a story in which no one offered any discrepancy with what he got from the subject(s). Compared with the usual newspaper article, riddled with (usually) small errors and inconsistencies, this one has only one exaggeration. We never were active in service organizations; Kiwanis was certainly not a "gaggle". Otherwise Grant held himself to a high standard of accuracy.

One point he made to me later, but did not include, was that he had never encountered anyone with the urgent sense of mortality that I expressed. This was because I was still working on my early books under my pen name and looking for a publisher. (I still feel the same way because I have two more books to see in print. I realize that every day I draw another day out of my ever-dwindling bank account, and I never know the balance.)

Following is the *Plain Dealer* feature story of 1988.

Caring and Curing

A rare pair goes beyond call of duty to benefit others

If Drs. Joanne and Charles Denko of Rocky River were more conventional people, Deb Gaefke Baldanza doubts that she and her little boy would be alive.

Joanne, a psychiatrist, would not have taken it upon herself to call Baldanza, whom she knows only from a few meetings of a writers' workshop, and ask, "Has somebody diagnosed what's wrong with your skin?"

As Baldanza recalls, "If any other person had called me with that question, I would have said 'Back off; it's none of your business.'" But Joanne had struck her as both unusually caring and careful.

First Joanne asked about the new blotches on Baldanza's skin, then about her health in general. It turned out that the Lakewood woman, then 26, had suffered many seemingly unrelated problems since childhood, from a possible heart attack to miscarriages in all but one of several pregnancies.

Joanne came to a typically blunt conclusion: "I think you have lupus, and I think you should get the best help you can, and that happens to be my husband."

If rheumatologist Chuck Denko had a conventional doctor's restraint, he might not have won Baldanza's confidence. She was tired of other doctors chalking up her problems to nerves, so she blurted to Chuck, "If you can't tell me what's wrong with me, I'm going to kill myself!"

"That is the stupidest thing I've ever heard!" Chuck shot back.

Baldanza started to cry. He reached out, patted her hand, and said something medical schools don't teach: "Sometimes it's time to give up. I promise I'll tell you when that is."

But the truth is, Chuck never gives up hope. "I've never seen a case that I thought I couldn't improve," he says today.

A blood test showed no sign of lupus, a potentially fatal tissue disease. But Chuck, a leading researcher, knew of strains that elude the test and noticed a high protein level that often accompanies lupus. So he treated Baldanza as if she had the disease.

She got better in a few months and managed to carry a second child to term. Today she says, "There is no question in my mind that I and my boy wouldn't be here without Chuck and Joanne."

Joanne, a stickler for words, says the couple has no interest in being "normal" in the sense of "normative," or average. "My husband is always saying that if the average person is so wonderful, do you want to go to an average architect to create your house?"

Joanne, 60, still blond and slim, sees patients privately and publishes psychiatric books and articles, prizewinning poetry, and widely circulated journalism, some of it under a pen name.

Chuck, 71, bearded, with hair to his shoulders, speaks five languages, lectures around the world, and has a portrait hanging in a National Medical Library exhibit of history's 10,000[1] most influential medical scientists. He ran Fairview General Hospital's research department until it closed in 1986, and keeps up one of the job's old duties without pay — teaching and researching at Case Western Reserve University, where he is an associate professor of medicine.

The Denkos play as hard as they work. They reached their seventh continent, Antarctica, last year.

But the couple's zeal draws flak as well as fanfare. They believe in what Joanne calls "sagesse oblige," a play on "noblesse oblige." It means an obligation for sages to use their brains to help others.

The trouble is, others may not appreciate the help.

Mensa, a society of people who score in the top 2% of the population on intelligence tests, denied Joanne a customary second term last fall as its Cleveland area secretary, the highest local post. The election winner, Peter Spearing, said Joanne lost for trying to prod the members toward social service instead of social pleasure. For one thing, she canceled a talk they had scheduled in her absence on mechanical aids for sex.

Some members called her a censor, but Joanne believes a leader is supposed to lead, not pander. "I thought there were many other reasonable things for an organization oriented around intelligence to do," she says.

Yet she has applied her own intelligence to sex. She was the first researcher to report on what she dubbed klismaphilia — the erotic use of enemas. She has even been quoted in *Penthouse*.

She often pens many indignant letters to editors or individuals, such as a visiting lecturer who had mocked a question of hers. But friends say she's actually shy, and she agrees.

"Sometimes it's very hard to speak out, but I wouldn't like myself if I didn't," she says in her small, precise voice.

Chuck is more earthy, often teasing Baldanza by calling the son she bore during treatment "my baby." But he, too, has talked himself out of an office. When the Denkos lived in Columbus, Chuck was dropped from the board of a Russian Orthodox church[2] after defending a rebuffed volunteer.

In rheumatology, he has often championed ideas years before they caught on, such as a now-accepted link between inflammation and chemicals called prostaglandins.

He also takes the unpopular view that arthritis is not an inevitable price of age — neither he nor Joanne have a bit of it — but a specific malfunction that will be cured someday. "Thousands of little old ladies ailing in nursing homes (will) get up and take walks and enjoy their remaining years," says Chuck.

Ironically, Chuck is even more admired abroad than at home, according to a CWRU colleague, Associate Professor Charles Malemud.

It's not enough that the Denkos belong to a gaggle of service groups. They're always serving someone one-on-one, too: bringing large-type books to an acquaintance with poor sight, counseling an orphaned friend of their son's, tramping through Huntington Metropark on a frigid day to reunite a cat with its owner.

The Denkos were decades ahead of their times in the 1940s in becoming a duo of doctors. Jacqueline[3] Joanne Decker, an only child, graduated from a three-room schoolhouse in rural southwestern Michigan at 16[4] and from Hope College in Michigan with highest honors at 20. Next came a Johns Hopkins University medical degree and a University of Michigan master's in psychology[5] — a degree not even required of psychiatrists.

Chuck was born in Cleveland and survived an early brush with polio. He grew up in Ellwood City, Pennsylvania, a state that had no public medical school[6], so he could afford only to get a Ph.D. in organic chemistry[7] at Penn State.

A favorite professor came down with arthritis and urged him to look for a cure. "I'm still doing it," Chuck says, laughing ruefully. "It takes a long time."

Chuck researched vitamins for military rations during World War II, then went to Johns Hopkins Medical School on the GI bill. Students were seated in alphabetical order there, so Denko sat near Decker. The couple married in 1950, graduated and lived in several Midwestern cities before settling in a lakefront home in Rocky River twenty years ago.

Joanne had several miscarriages, then gave birth to three sons. She worked part time while they were young, and she and Chuck groomed them with typical care: posting charts of chores, enrolling them in after-school classes, and camping with them around the world.

The parents hold their sons to the same standard of "sagesse oblige" as themselves. "The word 'achievement' is considered a dirty word these days," Joanne says. "But without it, we might as well be orangutans. Cheetahs are more beautiful than human beings. A clam on the barrier reef metabolizes just as well."

The middle son, Nicholas, 23, a cancer researcher at the University of Pennsylvania, is applying to patent a device that separates proteins. But the parents are disappointed that he has put off going to medical school,[8] despite a lavish scholarship offer. They say that taking care of patients has helped their research over the years, and vice versa.

Joanne, who writes daily from 5:00 to 7:00 a.m., coauthored a book about the psychological symptoms of hypoparathyroidism,[9] an extremely rare disease she spotted in a patient after other doctors missed it. Chuck, who saw patients until he left Fairview, had government permission to use experimental drugs on them and used to get what colleague Malemud calls fantastic results.

The couple's curiosity leads them to everything from the Cleveland Astronomical Society to Mrs. Hudson's Lodgers, a club of Sherlock Holmes' fans. Joanne made her ballet debut at 50 in an amateur group and collects homonyms — words spelled differently but pronounced alike.

In a fitting tribute to the Denkos' partnership, they have been invited to write chapters on their respective fields for a forthcoming survey of diseases to be published by University of Cambridge, England.[10]

The Denkos hope not to fade into that history until they have had more effect on it. Joanne could be speaking for Chuck when she says, "I would like to imagine myself quoted in 100 years. We are all shaped by our culture. Very few of us shape our culture, but I would like to think I do so."

I believe very strongly that our most underexploited natural resource is intelligence.

— Dr. Joanne Denko

Notes

1. Actually, as in my vignette, Chuck's portrait was to be one of 400 at Army Medical, not 10,000. There hadn't been 10,000 medical scientists from Paracelsus to the mid-20th century.

   I was surprised by the line attributed to Chuck when Deb Baldanza suggested suicide. Chuck never gave up on anyone, but in this case he was buying time with her by promising to tell her when to give up.

   Segall's suggestion that I was "blunt" in suggesting lupus as Deb's diagnosis reminds me of something we learned in medical school: The last physician to see a patient has the best chance to make the diagnosis because the course offers an accumulation of clues. Compare my diagnosis of idiopathic hypoparathyroidism after others had missed it.

2. No, this was the Gahanna Community Church.

3. They spelled my real first name "Jacquelyn".

4. Actually the country school where I received a marvelous, almost tutorial education, with three rooms with three grades in each, went from B (beginners where we learned to read the first week) through eighth. I graduated from high school at sixteen.

5. The M. S. is in psychiatry.

6. This is true, but he didn't intend to go to medical school at that time. His first love was chemistry.

7. Actually, physiologic chemistry.

8. But Nicholas was right. He started his double doctorate a little later but had additional cancer research experience in the meantime.

9. Grant left out the critical word here: *idiopathic* hypoparathyroidism. Often at thyroid surgery these four tiny glands lying on the thyroid get damaged. So a patient with a history of such surgery and certain symptoms can be so diagnosed. It is when the parathyroids go into diminished function on their own that the condition can be missed because it is so rare.

10. They used Chuck's but didn't take mine, which was an article on mental illness in preliterate peoples.

Reprints of CWD's Popular Writing

The Children's Hour

Between the dark and the daylight,
When Johnny turns on the power,
Comes a daze in pa's occupations
That is known as the Children's Hour.

—With apologies to Longfellow's ghost

Between school and suppertime comes the period of entertainment on the radio devoted to children. At least the sponsors call it entertainment. The pleasant baritone of the announcer admonishes Johnny that he must eat Wheaties for breakfast; drink Ovaltine, California Syrup of Figs, or Cocomalt three times a day; brush his teeth with Phillips' Milk of Magnesia toothpaste; and chew Wrigley's gum to be like his adored Skippy, Little Orphan Annie, or Buck Rogers.

To start the evening right Johnny listens to Dick Tracy "trace crime to its lair and bring justice to triumph." And Dick doesn't mean maybe when he starts out from radio call to radio call to save his girl by dazzling gunplay or to capture counterfeiters, bank robbers, and firebugs. From starting gong to concluding gong, Ming Lee, Whitey, Red Foster, and the rest of the gang haven't a ghost of a chance against bold Dick Tracy.

Of course Orphan Annie, "the little chatterbox," isn't quite as good as Jack Armstrong. Shucks, Orphan Annie is just a girl! But Jack is great at baseball, football, and basketball; he can run, hurdle, climb mountains, and pilot planes. He can solve any mystery; he rounds up Public Enemy Number One as fast as each new one appears.

A shrill childish voice is next heard moaning, "I lost my man." Then another six-year-old torch singer gets the blues and advises

Johnny, "Don't let your heart go gaga." Between songs Uncle Sammy tells little Joseph Herman, aged nine, of South Brownsville, Pa., and little Mary Ann Jones, aged seven, of Portage, Pa., to look in the piano, the icebox, grandmother's hatbox, the pigs' feed box, under the stove, or under the back porch for delightful surprises.

Four times a week—on Monday, Tuesday, Wednesday, and Thursday—Buck Rogers takes our rapt listener with breathtaking strides into the twenty-fifth century. Here Johnny rocket ships among Jupiter, Saturn, Mars, and Venus. With the buzzing of rocket pistols, gas analyzers, disintegrators, flying belts, sleep ray projectors, and repulsion motors Buck makes life miserable for the "depth people" and "the midgets of Venus."

From the twenty-fifth century the earth swiftly turns back 100,000 years to Og, Son of Fire. Here "in the dim and distant past when people lived in caves," Og and his friends give battle to roaring saber-tooth tigers, trumpeting mammoths, hissing lizards, howling wolves, and shouting "red beards."

Johnny never has his fill of terrifying sound effects, for there is also Chief Lone Wolf to welcome all the braves and princesses gathered around the campfire. They whoop it up and cheerfully deal out death to enemy redskins for Wrigley's delicious Spearmint, Doublemint, Juicy Fruit, and P-K gum. After this thrilling program the streets and yards of the neighborhood resound to the shouts of "Wa-ha-sa-wah-kee" and war cries of the Lone Wolf Tribe.

Next Tarzan rules supreme. Woe betide the trees and shrubbery, the unfortunate dogs and cats of the vicinity! Every tree and clump of bushes conceals its horde of Tarzans, yelling to their mates or ready to pounce upon any unsuspecting, luckless dog or cat that ventures too near the hideout.

In spite of the best—or worst—that the sponsor can do to upset Johnny's digestion, ruin his sleep, and cut short his years of growth by wily Chinamen, falling airplanes, earthquakes, and shipwrecks, Johnny always comes back for more. Every afternoon from five to quarter after six Johnny is before the radio — sitting tensely on the edge of his chair or sprawled on the floor or kneeling with his head bowed to the loudspeaker — listening while Dick Tracy trails cunning Ming Lee, or Jack Armstrong helps to capture "The Spider." Only an occasional "Gee!" or "Oh boy!" escapes his lips as the fortunes of his heroes rise and fall in "thrilling episode after thrilling episode" presented by the Itsie Bitsie Witsie Cereal Company each Monday, Tuesday, Wednesday, and Thursday at this same time.

— Charles Denko
The Chimes, 1936
(Geneva Publication)

Did the Model for Polyphemus Have Acromegalic Arthritis?

Journal of Rheumatology
Volume 22, Number 11, 1995 – pages 2191–2192

To the Editor:

On a recent trip to the Eastern Mediterranean, I retraced the homeward journey of Odysseus after the Trojan War, as described by Homer. (1) In Naples, we were taken to the Archeologic Museum in nearby Sperlonga, site of the summer villa of Tiberius, Roman emperor from AD 14 to 37. In the museum is a collection of sculptures found in the garden of the villa. According to the curator, the sculptures were produced by an unknown Greek artist on commission by Tiberius. His cruelty and blood lust led to his selection of the incidents portrayed, including the blinding by Odysseus of Polyphemus, a one-eyed giant, sometimes called Cyclops, offspring of Poseidon and a mortal. Homer describes him as "the giant with the loud (deep) voice" who had a "thick neck," a "monster with a ferocious (savage) soul."

In the tableau of figure 1, Odysseus and his companions prepare to plunge a pointed pole (in *The Odyssey,* a heat-tempered tree trunk) into the only eye of Polyphemus. He is, of course, portrayed as a giant, twice the height of Odysseus. His anatomic features that are judged compatible with acromegalic arthropathy appear in both hands. (2) In figure 2, the right hand shows swollen terminal interphalangeal joints, as well as swollen proximal interphalangeal joints and swollen metacarpal phalangeal joints. The skin creases over the joints are prominent, suggesting excessive soft tissue, also seen in the fingers of the left hand (figure 1), which appear fleshy with knobby tufts. Some of the joint swelling in the right hand may be due to thickened, redundant skin. The rib cage is prominent with marked nodosity of the costochondral junctions.

Additional features of acromegaly[1] were sought. The facial deformity and beard make assessment of frontal bossing and prognathism difficult. Cheekbones appear prominent. The penis appears normal; testicles are at the small end of normal. The toes of the left foot are enlarged, especially the first toe. The left ankle is enlarged.

Since Homer wrote his historic work 1,000 years before this statue was created, he did not describe this model of Polyphemus. Homer did not describe an acromegalic person with one eye. The sculptor found his model and sculpted him as he was.

Several questions arise with this statue, which dates from the "true" period when Greek sculptors represented figures as they appeared, realistically in truth. How did the sculptor portray an adult cyclops? Could he have had such a living adult cyclopean subject? If there were such a case, the congenital abnormality that caused the single eye would have been very close to the pituitary, the source of acromegaly. It is interesting to speculate but unlikely to have occurred because there is no case in recorded medical history of a cyclopean birth surviving, with or without medical care. Besides, the Greek custom of exposing abnormal births would have hastened the death of such an infant.

Gigantism is another matter, and the figure twice the height of Odysseus could well have been sculpted from a living model to represent Polyphemus. Yet the sculptor had no way of knowing about acromegalic arthritis, but he depicted the arthropathy in the knuckles of the right hand and the sausage fingers in the left, both accurate for acromegalic arthritis. It is unlikely that the youthful model would be suffering from severe symmetrical osteoarthritis, tophaceous gout, or psoriatic arthritis, all commonly asymmetrical. There is nothing in *The Odyssey* to tell the sculptor to make his subject arthritic.

The most plausible explanation is that the sculptor used a giant model whom he reproduced faithfully, including his arthropathic hands, except for the single eye, which he portrayed from imagination.

How can we explain the existence of a 2,000-year-old sculpture of this kind? I believe it is the earliest evidence of the existence of acromegalic arthropathy (arthritis). It is unlikely that a giant with arthropathy existed only in the sculptor's imagination.

In summary, the case for the existence of acromegalic arthritis 2,000 years ago appears acceptable.

References

1. Lattimore R: *The Odyssey of Homer*, Book IX. New York: Harper Perennial, 1967:137–51.
2. McGuire JL: Acromegaly. In: Kelley WN, Harris ED, Ruddy S, Sledge CB, eds. *Textbook of Rheumatology,* 3rd ed. Philadelphia: W.B. Saunders, 1989:1658–60.

From "Rheumatoid Arthritis in Scythian Art", *The Journal of Rheumatology* 1993; 20:10, 1760–1763.

Charles W. Denko, M.D., Ph.D.[2]
School of Medicine, Case Western Reserve University, Cleveland, OH 44106

Notes

1. CWD did not need to point out to rheumatologists that acromegaly is a kind of gigantism, with enlargement of the head, hands, and feet.
2. This shows how editors would reverse CWD's degrees. The Ph.D. came first and was done independently of the M.D.

Jack London. A Modern Analysis of His Mysterious Disease

Charles W. Denko

Modern medicine can illuminate the tragically short life of Jack London, a fiction writer whose popularity in the first half of this century rivaled that of Mark Twain. When this novelist and short story writer died, the *San Francisco Examiner* published on December 14, 1916 an article by William Brady on "The mysterious disease that killed Jack London, the most original and forceful novelist of our day, who just died suddenly and prematurely at the age of forty, the victim of uremic poisoning."

More prosaic and clinical was the death certificate signed by Dr. William S. Porter who had treated London's kidney disease for several years: "Uremia following renal colic. Not attributed to dangerous or insanitary conditions of employment. Duration, one day. Contributory, chronic interstitial nephritis. Duration, three years." The strange combination of illnesses from his early twenties until death at forty in this adventuresome man given to strenuous physical activity raises questions seeking an explanation better than the one given in his day. I have gathered information that ties together several discrete bouts of illness in London's short life that meet modern criteria for a diagnosis of systemic lupus erythematosus.

In the early years of the 20th century, when London's symptoms sent him to a variety of medical practitioners, probably only a handful of physicians worldwide would have been likely to consider this diagnosis. In the years since, knowledge of lupus has expanded and guidelines have been published. My suspicions were aroused during a family vacation in the Yukon where I heard about London's bout with scurvy, which did not fit the picture of scurvy as I remembered from my house training in Chicago.

Early illness. On a brief sojourn prospecting in the Klondike Gold Rush in 1897–98, twenty-two-year-old Jack London, living as he did on the common camp menu of bread, beans, and bacon, reported that he developed scurvy from lack of vegetables and fruit. His self-diagnosis of scurvy was based on clinical features of the "Klondike Plague," namely, bleeding and swollen gums and painful joints.

None of London's companions, living in the same cabin, and presumably eating the same diet, was reported to have any signs or symptoms of scurvy. This militates against the diagnosis. A cabin mate, Dr. B.F. Harvey, urged London to leave since he believed that there was no cure for scurvy. This was despite the fact that native Canadians for centuries brewed tea from pine needles to extract vitamin C to prevent and treat scurvy.

With two companions, London set out from the claim on Henderson Creek, facing 1500 miles of river travel. In Dawson, Yukon Territory, they sold the lumber from the raft and used the money for food and medicine. London spent most of his days in Dawson in Father Judge's hospital. Father Judge advised London to leave Dawson as soon as possible since his "scurvy" was so advanced. The trip downriver on the riverboat was uneventful and restful after leaving Dawson.

On Saturday, June 18, 1898 they arrived in Anvik, Alaska, at 10:00 p.m. London writes:

> Given fresh potatoes and can of tomatoes for my scurvy which has now almost crippled me from my waist down. Right leg drawing up, can no longer straighten it, even in walking must put my whole weight on toes. These few raw potatoes and tomatoes are worth more to me at the present state of the game than an El Dorado claim.

London's symptoms improved, which he attributed to the treatment. Curing severe "scurvy" with a minimal dose of vitamin

C provided by a few raw potatoes and can of tomatoes is contrary to my experience and that of other clinicians in treating scurvy. Usually a cure would require hundreds of milligrams of pure vitamin C, (1) many times the amount London could have received during the hours he spent in Anvik.

I feel London's bout of severe scurvy could be better explained as an attack of acute lupus involving the mouth and joints, two areas commonly attacked by episodic lupus.

Chronic illness. After returning to Oakland, London had a variety of medical symptoms. He required medical attention for mouth and tooth care through 1899. At this time it is unlikely that his mouth and dental problems were another manifestation of scurvy since he was eating a normal California diet, adequate in vitamin C.

In his twenties London married his second wife, Charmian, who kept a diary documenting the progression of London's illness in detail until the end of his life. At one point he was unable to pass the medical examination for insurance. Charmian noted that London, at age twenty-eight, suffered severe headaches that recurred over the years. "Nearly blind with headache," she wrote in one entry. London used this type of headache in his stories. In *The Sea Wolf,* the character Wolf Larsen suffered severely from a headache described so graphically that it suggests that it might have been autobiographical for London.

In 1908, when London was thirty-two, Charmian described a bad case of facial neuralgia. Such atypical facial pain is one of the common central nervous system manifestations of lupus. In Charmian's references to London's medical course are notations that he had suffered repeated pulmonary problems, grippe, bronchitis, colds, and chest pain. Although he had a scar on his lung, no active tuberculosis was found. In 1914, on the military transport *Ossabow* to cover the Mexican Revolution, he was diagnosed to have pleurisy, a criterion for lupus.

Skin symptoms of all kinds are common in lupus, particularly following sun exposure. London had recurrent rashes over sun-exposed areas. He had been diagnosed as having urticaria at thirty-one. After four hours in the sun he developed severe sun poisoning, huge swollen blotches that defied an explanation by his physician. His throat was swollen so badly that he was unable to swallow water. He may have suffered from angioedema.

In the South Pacific at age thirty-two, he experienced generalized itching and swollen and painful hands followed by peeling of the skin. His toenails grew exceedingly thick as they do not infrequently with both psoriasis and lupus. Pellagra and psoriasis were considered in the diagnosis of his skin problems but were not substantiated by the physician in Sydney, Australia, where he went for treatment.

Rheumatic symptoms were repeatedly described, beginning in 1898 when he was a young man in the Yukon and continuing until his death in 1916. In 1904, Charmian described in her notes that London at twenty-eight had such severe pain in his knees and ankles that he had to be at bed rest for sixty-five hours. This followed the minor trauma of jumping down about three feet onto a round stick. He was aboard the *Siberia* en route to cover the Russo-Japanese War.

In 1908 in the South Pacific during London's months-long bout of dermatologic disorders, which I interpret as a flare of lupus, he also suffered symptoms in other parts of the body. Prominent among these were swollen painful hands followed by peeling of the skin. Other symptoms included fever, rash with urticaria, malaise, headache, facial neuralgia, even a bout of delirium. He dealt with his anxiety and pain by smoking incessantly. He took opiates for his diarrhea and quinine for his fever.

Pictorial evidence for arthritis, swelling of joints, is provided in Russ Kingman's book *A Pictorial Life of Jack London.* (2) In one picture taken during his last year of life London is shown working on a manuscript with both hands clearly visible. The left hand shows hyperextension of the thumb, spindling of the index finger, and swelling of the middle finger. The right hand presents a swollen knuckle at the base of the fourth finger. The final picture for which he posed, taken in 1916, shows the right hand with a swollen knuckle. This time it was at the base of the second finger.

During a visit to Glen Ellen, California, several years ago, I asked Becky London, London's daughter by his first marriage, about her father's health. She had shown me her family pictures of her father. "Did he have much trouble with arthritis?" I asked.

She replied, "It's funny you should ask. The last two years of his life he had a lot of trouble walking because of pain and swelling in his feet."

London had repeated bouts of fever diagnosed as malaria. In a letter to Eliza Shepard, his sister and ranch manager, in 1908, he alluded to the curative powers of fever for his rash and joint pains. "Fever cures about everything else a man has." Because of their belief that it was malaria, London must have received antimalarial drugs, such as quinine, a modern treatment for lupus, to which other symptoms of lupus responded. Fever itself may not have been the agent that caused remission of London's aches and pains; quinine could have relieved not only his malaria, if he had it, but also his lupus-related fever and joint pains, without anyone knowing the relationship.

In 1913, at age thirty-seven, London was found to have kidney disease. Charmian reports he underwent an appendectomy at Merritt Hospital in Oakland, California, where his physician told him the appendectomy went well, but that the tubules of his kidneys were in terrible shape. The hospital record documents granular casts on urinalysis.

Modern diagnostic concepts of systemic lupus erythematosus. The symptomatology of lupus is highly varied. It is an idiopathic disease characterized by acute and chronic inflammation involving many organs, often relapsing, even leading to chronic pathology. The existing criteria proposed for classification of lupus derive from a continuously evolving concept of the disease. The American College of Rheumatology's proposed classification is based on eleven criteria. To identify patients with lupus for clinical studies, a person shall be said to have systemic lupus erythematosus if any four or more of the eleven criteria are present, serially or simultaneously, during any interval of observation. (3) I believe London's illness fulfilled these criteria.

One criterion is photosensitivity, defined as a rash as a result of unusual reaction to sunlight, by patient history or physician observation. At age thirty-one, according to Charmian's history, "Jack had a terrible sunburn with huge swollen blotches that defied an explanation by Dr. Charles B. Cooper." While cruising in the South Pacific and while en route to Sydney, she wrote, "Jack has a rash all over. Intense itching."

A second criterion is oral or nasopharyngeal ulceration, usually painless, observed by a physician. Jack had numerous visits to the dentist beginning at age eighteen and continuing through his lifetime. The severity and chronicity of Jack's dental problems despite prompt medical care suggests that his mouth problems were not the ordinary dental conditions. Perhaps he had developed an associated Sjögren's syndrome, which could aggravate his oral and dental problems.

Criterion 3 is "nonerosive arthritis involving two or more peripheral joints, characterized by tenderness, swelling, or effusion." Pictures of London's hands in Kingman's book provide evidence of joint swelling as mentioned previously.

Criterion 4 is renal disorder, documented by his hospital records from Merritt Hospital in Oakland, Ca., showing granular casts in his urine. Sjögren's syndrome may also have contributed to his renal problems since interstitial nephritis is recognized as a renal complication. His personal physician, Dr. W. S. Porter, stated on the death certificate that he had treated London for three years for kidney impairment.

Alternate theories of the death of Jack London. Charmian's notations on Jack London's health include comments on factors of his death. One possibility rumored by the author George Sterling attributed London's death to suicide by overdosing with morphine. He had no evidence for this. Dr. A. M. Thomson, first of the doctors who attended London in his final bout of illness, denied the suicide theory. He and two other physicians were present when a fourth physician, Dr. W. S. Porter, signed the death certificate stating uremia to be the cause of death. London used morphine by prescription to obtain relief from abdominal pain diagnosed as renal colic. At his death a vial of pills was found; it contained four remaining pills. Persons intent on suicide customarily empty the bottle. Treatment for morphine poisoning was given by his physicians without success, including stomach pumping and antidote for morphine poisoning.

Why would Jack London want to kill himself? He was a success as a writer, financially secure, married to a devoted wife, and there was no other woman. Drinking had been a problem in Jack London's earlier life, but his last two years were dry. Charmian's diary reveals very few times that he did any heavy drinking. London was a heavy smoker. His diet, heavy in protein, was mentioned by Charmian in her diary as being unwise for one already poisoned by uremia.

The most likely explanation for London's death remains an abdominal complication of lupus. He was working, writing, as was his custom. Obviously death was not regarded as imminent by his physician, his wife, his family at the ranch, or himself. I believe that an abdominal complication that has been reported to cause sudden death in lupus is responsible. Complications include perforated colon, infection, hepatic failure, renal failure, or gastrointestinal hemorrhage. (4) Early observers used the term "lupus erythematosus" to describe this constellation of symptoms because the severe lesions on the faces of untreated victims suggested the ravages of a wolf bite. Jack London's fame was, in part, due to writing about wolves. Even his beautiful, ill-fated dream house was given a "wolf" association, dubbed Wolf House by George Sterling. It suffered a violent, fiery end, destroyed by fire attributed to spontaneous combustion. It is ironic that Jack London himself succumbed to an acute flare of lupus, the wolf disease. [1]

Acknowledgment

I am indebted to Russ Kingman of Glen Ellen, California, London's hometown. Kingman, the family's official biographer of London, placed at my disposal several documents, the medical history of Jack London written by Charmian London, a photocopy of the hospital record of London's 1913 admission to Merritt Hospital, Oakland, California, and Kingman's *A Pictorial Life of Jack London.* Added information came from Becky London, also from Glen Ellen, London's younger daughter, and from Mrs. Sue Hodson, Associate Curator, The Huntington Library, San Marino, Calif. These sources are available to scholarly investigators.

References

1. Rivlin RS: "Disorders of vitamin metabolism deficiencies, metabolic abnormalities and excesses. Vitamin C (ascorbic acid) structure and biochemical function." In: Wyngaarden JB, Smith LH JR, eds. *Cecil Textbook of Medicine,* Vol. 2. Philadelphia: Saunders, 1988, 1234–6.
2. Kingman R: "Last days on the ranch." In: *A Pictorial Life of Jack London.* New York: Crown, 1979:270–4.
3. "Revised criteria for the classification of systemic lupus erythematosus." In: Schumacher HR Jr, Klippel JH, Robinson DR, eds. *Primer on Rheumatic Diseases,* 9th ed. Atlanta: Arthritis Foundation, 1988:319.
4. Zizic TM, Shulman LE, Stevens MB: "Colonic perforations in systemic lupus erythematosus." *Medicine 1973*;54:411–26.

Charles W. Denko, Ph. D., M. D.

Note

1. Chuck did not mention that "lupus" is Latin for "wolf". He found this ironic.

Hard Data

Charles W. Denko, Ph.D., M.D.
Curriculum Vitae

Education

1951 – M.D. John Hopkins University, Baltimore, Maryland

1943 – Ph.D. Pennsylvania State University, University Park, Pennsylvania (Physiological Chemistry) Thesis: *Synthesis of Organo-Gold Compounds and a Study of their Biochemical Effects in Rats.*

1939 – M.S. Pennsylvania State University (Organic Chemistry)

1938 – B.S. Geneva College, Beaver Falls, Pennsylvania (Chemistry)

1934–1922 Public Schools of Ellwood City, Pennsylvania

Professional Experience

1970 Associate – Assistant Clinical Professor of Medicine, Case Western Reserve University, Cleveland, Ohio

1986–1968 Director of Research, Fairview General Hospital, Cleveland, Ohio

1982–1973 Consultant in Rheumatology, Veterans Administration Hospital, Cleveland, Ohio

1975–1974 (6 month sabbatical) Visiting Fellow, Department

of Experimental Pathology, Australian National University, Canberra, Australia

1967–1966 Research Associate, Institute of Nutrition, Ohio State University, Columbus, Ohio

1965–1959 Assistant Professor of Medicine (Rheumatology), Ohio State University College of Medicine, Columbus, Ohio

1959–1957 Assistant Professor of Internal Medicine, University of Michigan, Ann Arbor, Michigan

1959–1956 Consultant in Rheumatology, Veterans Administration Hospital, Ann Arbor, Michigan

1957–1956 Instructor in Internal Medicine, University of Michigan, Ann Arbor, Michigan

1956–1955 Research Associate (Instructor) Medicine, Argonne Cancer Research Hospital, University of Chicago, Chicago, Illinois

1955–1953 Postdoctoral fellow in Medicine, (Arthritis Foundation), University of Chicago Clinics, Chicago, Illinois

1953–1952 Senior Assistant Resident, Medicine, University of Chicago Clinics, Chicago, Illinois

1952–1951 Rotating Intern, University of Illinois Research and Educational Hospitals, Chicago, Illinois

1947–1945 Nutrition Officer, Biochemist, Microbiologist, U.S. Army (captain) Sanitary Corps, U.S. and E.T.O.

1945–1944 Research Chemist (SMA Research Laboratories) Wyeth Institute of Applied Biochemistry, Chagrin Falls, Ohio

1943–Instructor in Biochemistry, West Virginia University, Morgantown, West Virginia

1943–1940 Graduate Assistant in Biochemistry, Pennsylvania State University, University Park, Pennsylvania

Professional Memberships (Past and Present)

American Association for the Advancement of Science

American Chemical Society

American Institute of Chemists

American Medical Association

American Rheumatism Association – Section of the Arthritis Foundation

American Society of Clinical Pharmacology and Therapeutics

Cleveland Academy of Medicine

Cleveland Rheumatism Society – President 1971–1972

Cyrus C. Sturgis Michigan Internists' Club

Ohio Rheumatism Association

New York Academy of Science

Professional Certificates

A. Medical Licenses

Pennsylvania, 1984, No. MD-031155-E; by endorsement

Ohio, August 26, 1959, No. 23435; by endorsement

Michigan, October 7, 1957, No. 222574; by examination

(Includes Basic Science Examination as prerequisite)

Illinois, August 22, 1952, No. 31489; by examination

Maryland, July 19, 1951; by examination

B. Specialty Certificates

American Board of Nutrition

a. Specialist in human nutrition, April 14, 1952, No. 81

b. Specialist in clinical nutrition, May 15, 1969, No. 273

Nuclear Regulatory Commission, License No. 34-12719-01

C. Rheumatologist

American Rheumatism Association, 1975

Professional Honors

A. Academic

Graduation – Highest Honors, Geneva College, 1938

Post-doctoral Fellow of the Arthritis Foundation, University of Chicago, 1953–1955

Fellow of the American Institute of Chemists, February 8, 1956

Senior Investigator of the Arthritis Foundation, 1960–1965

Portrait in series-significant contributors to Medical Science at National Medical Library, Bethesda, Maryland, 1956

Fellow of American College of Clinical Pharmacology and Chemotherapy, March 26, 1965, Certificate No. 311

Honorary Member, Australian Rheumatism Association, May 20, 1975

B. Biographies

Who's Who in Chemistry, first edition

Leaders in American Science, 5th and 6th editions

American Men of Science, 8th–14th editions

Who's Who in the Midwest, 9th–20th editions

Who's Who in Science

Ohio Lives

Dictionary of International Biography

Who's Who in Ohio

Who's Who in America (1986 ed.)

Who's Who in Science and Technology (1986 Ed.)

Who Was Who in America, Volume 22, 2010 - 2011
Who's Who in the Midwest, 1986 - 1987, 20th Edition
(pub. 1985)

Professional Civic Appointments – Past

Committee for Evaluation of Research in Orphan Drugs, National Institute of Health

Medical Advisory Committee, Lupus Foundation of America, NEO Chapter

Hospital Appointments – Past

A. Assistant Physician, University Hospitals

Personal

Business Address: Home Address:

Charles W. Denko, Ph.D., M.D.
21160 Avalon Drive

Rocky River, Ohio 44116
Rheumatology/Medicine
University Hospitals
2074 Abington Road
Cleveland, Ohio 44106

Publications – Highlights

Studies on human volunteers eating controlled diets showed that B-complex vitamins are produced in the human digestive tract in large quantities. A tryptophan intake of 240 mg daily will enable a normal human adult to remain in nitrogen balance.

Connective tissue metabolism in the rat has been evaluated by numerous modalities using incorporation of radioactive sulfate as the tracer. Decreased metabolism follows hypophysectomy, deficiency of essential fatty acids in the diet, hormonal administration such as the corticosteroids, drugs such as phenylbutazone. Stimulation of connective tissue metabolism can be accomplished by mechanical vibration, and cartilage-bone marrow extract. Prostaglandin A^2 produced stimulation in some tissues and reduction in cartilage and bone.

The role of prostaglandins as essential mediators of inflammation was pointed out in experimental inflammation due to crystal deposition (urate, calcium pyrophosphate, hydroxyapatite, cholesterol) and in adjuvant induced inflammation. An anti-prostaglandin action of colchicine in blocking formed prostaglandins was described.

Clinical studies elucidated the multi-system features of the sicca syndrome or Sjögren's Syndrome. A characteristic myopathy was described in these patients. Changes in acute phase serum proteins were delineated in patients with rheumatic disorders. These changes are postulated to be protective. Experimental studies support this hypothesis. The protective action of ceruloplasmin and other copper salts was demonstrated. Lowered tissue levels of transferrin and albumin were protective in experimental inflammation. Increased acidglycoprotein reduced inflammation.

A cartilage-bone marrow extract was found to reverse the radiologic changes in osteoarthritis of the hip and to improve clinical symptoms. A new theory of pathogenesis of osteoarthritis was proposed, namely, the liver was deficient in converting adequate growth hormone to a cartilage stimulant, somatomedin.

The neurotransmitter, beta-endorphin, was found to be reduced in the serum of patients with rheumatic disorders. Synovial fluid studies demonstrated that synovial membrane produced beta-endorphin in some rheumatoid patients. Beta-endorphin was demonstrated to have anti-inflammatory activity exerted by nullifying the pro-inflammogenic action of prostaglandins.

Current Activities

In the past year I have been full-time in research in the Rheumatology Division where I study regulatory neuropeptides and teach. My special interest in rheumatic disorders is osteoarthritis (OA), commonly regarded as a failure in repair of cartilage. Growth hormone (GH) and GH-dependent growth factors, insulin and insulin-like growth factor (IGF-1) or somatomedin are being measured by radioimmunoassay. On comparison to normal persons, the serum of OA patients contains too little IGF-1, the cartilage stimulant, and too much insulin, the bone stimulant.

With the cooperation of colleagues, Dr. R.W. Moskowitz and Ms. Betty Boja, these data have been presented at the Pan American Congress of Rheumatology in Buenos Aires, Argentina. Our data have been accepted for presentation at the American Rheumatism Association Meeting in June in Washington and at the European Congress in Athens, Greece, in July.

In an animal model of OA the sand rat or gerbil, OA develops spontaneously. Attempts are underway to modify the course of this animal disease by administering modifiers or regulators of the neuroendocrine system.

Invited Lectureships; Faculty for Postgraduate Course, and Specialty Societies Meetings

A. Conference on Chelation Therapy in Connective Tissue Disorders, Wayne State University, Detroit, Michigan, May 1968.

B. International Congress of Rheumatology, XII. Secretary for Sections on Biochemical Pharmacology, Piestany (Slovakia), Czechoslovakia, October 1969.

C. Postgraduate Course Sponsored by American Society for Clinical Pharmacology and Therapeutics and the Cleveland Clinic at the Cleveland Clinic, Cleveland, Ohio, January 1972.

D. Inaugural Meeting, Connective Tissue Society of Australia and New Zealand, at Melbourne University, Melbourne, Victoria, Australia, March 1975.

E. Annual Meeting, Australian Rheumatism Association at Sydney, New South Wales, Australia, May 1975.

F. Monash University, Clayton, Victoria, Australia, Department of Biochemistry, March 1975.

G. Visiting Professor of Medicine, Southern Illinois University School of Medicine, Springfield, Illinois, October 1975.

H. Inflammation Research Association Symposium, New York, October 1976.

I. Research Department Seminar, A.H. Robins Company, Richmond, Virginia, March 1977.

J. Johns Hopkins Medical Surgical Association 25th Class Reunion, Baltimore, Maryland, June 1977.

K. Florida Academy of Family Practice, Miami, Florida, September 1977.

L. University of Panama Medical School, Panama, Republic of Panama, July 1978.

M. Robapharm, Incorporated. Seminar for Technical Staff, Basle, Switzerland, November 1978.

N. Visiting Professor of Pharmacology, School of Medicine, Erasmus University, Rotterdam the Netherlands, August 1979.

O. International Symposium on the Role of Trace Metals in Inflammation at University of Arkansas, Little Rock, Arkansas, August 1981.

P. Texas Tech University School of Medicine, Amarillo, Texas, August 1981.

Q. Chinese Academy of Medical Sciences, Institute of Materia Medica, Beijing, People's Republic of China, September 1982.

R. Shanghai First Medical College, Shanghai, People's Republic of China, September 1982.

S. European Rheumatology Congress, Moscow, U.S.S.R., June 1983.

T. American Association for Clinical Chemists, Cleveland, Ohio, September 1983.

U. Chicago Medical School, North Chicago, Illinois, November 1983.

V. Geneva College Medical Alumni Meeting, Beaver Falls, Pennsylvania, November 1983.

W. Medical Education Meeting, American Heart Association, Northeast Ohio Affiliate, Cleveland, Ohio, December 1983.

X. Russell Rizzo Memorial Symposium on Joint Disease, St. John and St. John West Shore Hospitals, Cleveland, Ohio, September 1985.

Y. Pan American Congress of Rheumatology, Buenos Aires, Argentina, November 1986.

Z. Paper on Serum Insulin, Somatomedin and Growth Hormone, American Rheumatism Association Meeting, Washington, D.C., June 1986 and European Congress of Rheumatology, Athens, Greece, July 1986.

AA. Symposium: "Update – Rheumatoid Arthritis." London, England UK, February 1988.

CWD
1988

Date of Death: October 18, 2005.

Charles W. Denko Bibliography

1. Denko, C.W., and Anderson, A.K.: "Studies on the Toxicity of Compounds in Rats." *Journal of Laboratory and Clinical Medicine* 29: 1168–1176, 1944.

2. Denko, C.W., and Anderson, A.K.: "The Synthesis of Some Organic Compounds of Gold." *Journal of the American Chemical Society* 67: 2241, 1945.

3. Denko, C.W., Grundy, W.E., Porter, J.W., Berryman, G.H., Friedmann, T.E., and Youmans, J.B.: "The Excretion of B-Complex Vitamins in the Urine and Feces of Seven Normal Adults." *Archives of Biochemistry* 10: 33–40, 1946.

4. Denko, C.W., Grundy, W.E., Wheeler, N.C., Henderson, C.R., and Berryman, G.H., with Friedmann, T.E., and Youmans, J.B.: "The Excretion of B-Complex Vitamins by Normal Adults on a Restricted Intake." *Archives of Biochemistry* 11: 109–117, 1946.

5. Cogswell, R.C., Berryman, G.H., Henderson, C.R., Denko, C.W., and Spinella, J.R., with Friedmann, T.E., Ivy, A.C.,[1] and Youmans, J.B.: "Absence of Rapid Deterioration in Moderately Active Young Men on a Restricted Intake of B-Complex Vitamins and Animal Protein." *American Journal of Physiology* 147: 39–48, 1946.

6. Berryman, G.H., Henderson, C.R., Wheeler, N.C., Cogswell Jr., R.C., Spinella, J.R., Grundy, W.E., Johnson, H.C., Wood, M.D., and Denko, C.W., Friedmann, T.E., Harris, S.C., Ivy, A.C. [1] and Youmans, J.B.: "Effects in Young Men Consuming Restricted Quantities of B-Complex Vitamins and Protein, and Changes Associated with Supplementation." *American Journal of Physiology* 148: 618–647, 1947.

7. Denko, C.W., Grundy, W.E., and Porter, J.W.: "Blood Levels in Normal Adults on a Restricted Dietary Intake of B-Complex Vitamins and Tryptophan." *Archives of Biochemistry* 13: 481–484, 1947.

8. Denko, C.W., and Grundy, W.E.: "Minimum Tryptophan Requirement and Urinary Excretion of Tryptophan by Normal Adults." *Journal of Laboratory and Clinical Medicine* 34: 839–843, 1949.

9. Denko, C.W.: "Pteroylglutamic Acid Clearance in Normal Adults." *Journal of Applied Physiology* 3: L 559–562, 1951.

10. Denko, C.W., and Layton, L.L.: "Differential Sulfate Fixation in the Spleen Tissue of Normal and Leukemic Mice." *Cancer* 5: 403–404, 1952.

11. Layton, L.L., and Denko, C.W., assisted by Scapa, S., and Frankel, D.R.: "Influence of Age Upon Chondroitin Sulfate Synthesis by the Tissues of Normal dba Mice." *Cancer* 5: 405, 1952.

12. Denko, C.W., and Bergenstal, D.M.: "The Effect of Hypophysectomy and Growth Hormone on S35 Fixation in Cartilage." *Endocrinology* 57: 76–86, 1955.

13. Denko, C.W., Ruml, D., and Bergenstal, D.M.: "Clinical Experience with Phenylbutazone in 205 Patients." *American Practitioner and Digest of Treatment* 6: 1865–1869, 1955.

14. Denko, C.W., and Schroeder, L.R.: "Ecchymotic Skin Lesions in Patients Receiving Prednisone." *Journal of the American Medical Association* 164: 41–43, 1957.

15. Denko, C.W., Goldberg, M.A., Milka, E.S., and Roth, L.J.: "Effect of Hydrocortisone on C14OOH – P-Aminosalicylic Acid Distribution in Cartilage of the Rat." *Proceedings of the Society for Experimental Biology and Medicine* 95: 483–484, 1957.

16. Denko, C.W., and Priest, R.E.: "Distribution of Radiosulfur, S35 I. In the Human Adult, II. In the Young and the Adult Rat." *Journal of Laboratory and Clinical Medicine* 50: 107–112, 1957.

17. Denko, C.W., and Stoughton, R.B.: "Fixation of S35 in the Skin of Patients with Progressive Systemic Sclerosis." *Arthritis and Rheumatism* 1: 77–81, 1958.

18. Denko, C.W.: "The Effect of Hydrocortisone and Cortisone on Fixation of S35 in the Stomach." *Journal of Laboratory and Clinical Medicine* 51: 174–177, 1958.

19. Denko, C.W., and Priest, R.D.: "Utilization of Maternal Sulfate by the Embryo and Suckling Rat." *Archives of Biochemistry and Biophysics* 79: 252–256, 1959.

20. Denko, C.W.: "The Effect of Prolactin on S35 Fixation in the Costal Cartilage of the Hypophysectomized Rat." *Endocrinology* 65: 147–151, 1959.

21. Pentz, E.I., Moss, E.T., and Denko, C.W.: "Factors Influencing Taurine Excretion in Human Subjects." *Journal of Clinical Endocrinology and Metabolism* 19: 1126–1133, 1959.

22. Denko, C.W., and Bergenstal, D.M.: "The Sicca Syndrome (Sjögren's Syndrome). A Study of Sixteen Cases." *American Medical Association Archives of Internal Medicine* 105: 849–858, 1960.

23. Denko, C.W., and McCoy, F.W.: "Current Use of Gold Therapy in Rheumatoid Arthritis." *The Ohio State Medical Journal* 56: 1492–1499, 1960.

24. Denko, C.W.: "Serum Salicylate Levels in Arthritis Patients Receiving Acetylsalicylic Acid, Buffered Acetylsalicylic Acid and Salicylate with P-Aminobenzoic Acid." *Archives of Inter-American Rheumatology* 4: 5–17, 1961.

25. Yee, N.Y., McCann, D.S., Keech, M.K., Denko, C.W., and Boyle, A.J.: "2, 5 Dihydroxyphenylpyruvic Acid in Human Urine." *Archives of Dermatology* 84: 293–301, 1961.

26. Denko, C.W., and Zumpft, C.W.: "Chronic Arthritis in the Adult Associated with Splenomegalia and Leukopenia." Pp. 244–246, Volume II *Atti del X Congresso della Lega Internazionale contro il Reumatismo,* p. 1546, *Minerva Medica,* Torino, 1961.

27. Denko, C.W., and Bergenstal, D.M.: "Effects of Growth Hormone and Corticosteroids on S35 Fixation in Cartilage." *Endocrinology* 69: 769–777, 1961.

28. Denko, C.W., and McCoy, F.W.: "The Conservative Management of Rheumatoid Arthritis." *Ohio State Medical Journal* 58: 49–52, 1962.

29. Denko, C.W., and McCoy, F.W.: "Current Concepts in Management of Rheumatoid Arthritis." *Ohio Clinical Medicine* 59: 877–888, 1962.

30. Layton, L.L., Yamanaka, E., and Denko, C.W.: "Demonstration of Human Reagins to Foods, Cat Dander, and Insect, and Ragweed and Grass Pollens." *The Journal of Allergy* 33: 271–275, 1962.

31. Denko, C.W., and Zumpft, C.W.: "Chronic Arthritis with Splenomegaly and Leukopenia." *Arthritis and Rheumatism* 5: 478–491, 1962.

32. Denko, C.W.: "Treatment of Patient with Gout." *The Ohio State Medical Journal* 59: 1098–1101, 1963.

33. Denko, C.W., and von Haam, E.: "Reiter's Syndrome: Clinicopathological Study of a Fatal Case." *Journal of the American Medical Association* 186: 632–636, 1963.

34. Denko, C.W., and Davis, L.P.: "A Correlative Clinicopathological Study of Systemic Lupus Erythematosus in Forty-three Patients." *Archives of Inter-American Rheumatology* 7: 25–43, 1964.

35. Denko, C.W.: "Efectos de un extracto de medula osea y cartilago sobre la figacion de S35 en el cartilago." *Revista Medica de Chile* 92: 265–267, 1964.

36. Denko, C.W.: "The Effect of Phenylbutazone and Its Derivatives Oxyphenbutazone and Sulfinpyrazone on S35 Incorporation in Cartilage and Stomach." *The Journal of Laboratory and Clinical Medicine* 63: 953–958, 1964.

37. Denko, C.W.: "The Effect of a Bone Marrow and Cartilage Extract on Osteoarthritis." *Rhumatologie* 16: 365–366, 1964.

38. Denko, C.W.: "Antibodies in the Sicca Syndrome (Sjögren's Syndrome)." *Arthritis and Rheumatism* 8: 970–975, 1965.

39. Denko, C.W.: "Current Concepts of Osteoarthritis." *Medical Times* 93: 1148–1152, 1965.

40. Denko, C.W., DeFelice, E.A., and Shaffer, J.: "Namoxyrate in Rheumatic Disorders." *Current Therapeutic Research* 7: 749–758, 1965.

41. Denko, C.W.: "Cutaneous Manifestations of Connective Tissue Disorders." Chapter 12, *Newer Views of Skin Disease* (ed.) Yaffee, Little, Brown, and Company, 1966.

42. Dickey, R.P., Stevens, V.C., Vorys, N., Denko, C.W., and Ullery, J.C.: "Rate of Chondroitin Sulfate Synthesis in the Cervix during Pregnancy." *American Journal of Obstetrics and Gynecology* 95: 4–45, 1966.

43. Stevens, V.C., Dickey, R.P., Vorys, N., Denko, C.W., and Ullery, J.C.: "Synthesis of Chondroitin Sulfate by the Human Cervix during the Menstrual Cycle." *American Journal of Obstetrics and Gynecology* 95: 959–962, 1966.

44. Denko, C.W., Goodman, R.M., Miller, R., and Donovan, T.: "Distribution of Dimethyl Sulfoxide – S35 in the Rat." *Annals of the New York Academy of Science* 141: 77–84, 1967.

45. Denko, C.W.: "Hypnotics and the Geriatric Patient." *Clinical Medicine* 75: 27–34, 1968.

46. Denko, C.W.: "The Effect of the Physical Modalities, Heat and Vibration on S35 Uptake by Cartilage and other tissues." Pp. 147–153 in the *Proceedings of the Fourth Pan-American Congress of Rheumatology,* Mexico, Exerpta Medica Foundation, 1969.

47. Denko, C.W.: "Mechanical Vibrations and S35 Incorporation." *Environmental Research* 2: 143–148, 1969.

48. Denko, C.W., and Old, J.W.: "Myopathy in the Sicca Syndrome (Sjögren's Syndrome)." *American Journal of Clinical Pathology* 51: 631–637, 1969.

49. Denko, C.W.: "Hypnotics and the Geriatric Patient." *Geriatric Digest* 7: 28–33, 1970.

50. Denko, C.W., Purser, D.B., and Johnson, R.M.: "Amino Acid Composition of Serum Albumin in Normal Individuals and in Patients with Rheumatoid Arthritis." *Clinical Chemistry* 16: 54, 1970.

51. Denko, C.W., and Whitehouse, M.W.: "Effects of Colchicine in Rats with Urate Crystal-Induced Inflammation." *Pharmacology* 3: 229–242, 1970.

52. Denko, C.W., Moskowitz, R.W., and Heinrich, G.: "Interrelated Pharmacologic Effects of Prostaglandins and Bradykinin." *Pharmacology* 8: 353–360, 1972.

53. Denko, C.W.: A Phlogistic Function of Prostaglandin E. in Urate Crystal Inflammation. *Journal of Rheumatology* 1: 222–230, 1974.

54. Denko, C.W.: "Effect of Prostaglandins in Urate Crystal Inflammation." *Pharmacology* 12: 331–339, 1974.

55. Denko, C.W.: "Anti-Prostaglandin Action of Colchicine." *Pharmacology* 13: 219–227, 1975.

56. Denko, C.W.: "A Phlogistic Function of PGE1 in Calcium Pyrophosphate Dihydrate Crystal-Induced Inflammation." *Journal of Rheumatology* 2: 251–257, 1975.

57. Denko, C.W., and Whitehouse, M.W.: "Experimental Inflammation Induced by Naturally Occurring Microcrystalline Calcium Salts." *Journal of Rheumatology* 3: 54-62, 1976.

58. Denko, C.W.: "35S and 3H-proline Incorporated in Rats Deficient in Essential Fatty Acids." *Journal of Rheumatology* 3: 210-211, 1976.

59. Denko, C.W.: "Modification of Adjuvant Arthritis in Rats Deficient in Essential Fatty Acids." *Agents and Actions* 6: 636–641, 1976.

60. Denko, C.W., and Petricevic, M.: "Prostaglandin A2 and 35S Uptake in Connective Tissue." *Prostaglandins* 14: 701-707, 1977.

61. Petricevic, M., Wanek, K., and Denko, C.W.: "A New Mechanical Method for Measuring Rat Paw Edema." *Pharmacology* 16: 153–158, 1978.

62. Denko, C.W.: "Treatment of Osteoarthritis with Rumalon R." Letter to the Editor. *Arthritis and Rheumatism* 21: 494–496, 1978.

63. Denko, C.W.: "Restorative Chemotherapy in Degenerative Hip Disease." *Agents and Actions* 8 (3): 268–279, 1978.

64. Denko, C.W., and Petricevic, M.: "Sympathetic or Reflex Footpad Swelling Due to Crystal Induced Inflammation in the Opposite Foot." *Inflammation* 3: 81–86, 1978.

65. Denko, C.W.: "Chernogubov's Syndrome: A Translation of the First Modern Case Report of the Ehlers-Danlos Syndrome." *Journal of Rheumatology* 5: 347–352, 1978.

66. Petricevic, M., Denko, C.W., and Messineo, L.: "Temporal Changes in Histone Acetylation." *Mechanisms of Aging and Development* 8: 241–248, 1978.

67. Denko, C.W., and Petricevic, M.: "Hydroxyapatite Crystal-Induced Inflammation and Prostaglandin E1." *Journal of Rheumatology* 6: 117–123, 1979.

68. Denko, C.W.: "Protective Role of Ceruloplasmin in Inflammation." *Agents and Actions* 9: 333–336, 1979.

69. Denko, C.W., and Gabriel, P.: "Serum Proteins – Transferrin, Ceruloplasmin, Albumin, 1-Acid Glycoprotein, 1-Antitrypsin – in Rheumatic Disorders". *Journal of Rheumatology* 6: 664–672, 1979.

70. Denko, C.W.:" Phlogistic Properties of the Serum Proteins, Albumin and Transferrin." *Inflammation* 4: 165–168, 1980.

71. Denko, C.W., and Petricevic, M.: "Modification of Cholesterol Crystal-Induced Inflammation." *Agents and Actions* 10: 353–357, 1980.

72. Denko, C.W., and Gabriel, P.: "Age and Sex Related Levels of Albumin, Ceruloplasmin, α1-Antitrypsin, α1-Acid Glycoprotein and Transferrin in Serum." *Annals of Clinical and Laboratory Science* 11: 63–68, 1981.

73. Denko, C.W., Gabriel, P., and Petricevic, M.: "Urinary Excretion of Material with -β-Endorphin Immunoreactivity." *Clinical Chemistry* 27: 207–208, 1981.

74. Petricevic, M., Denko, C.W., and Messineo, L.: "Temporal Changes of [3H] Uridine and [14C] Thymidine Incorporation and Total Organ DNA and RNA in Rat Thymus." *Thymus* 2: 355–359, 1981.

75. Denko, C.W., Petricevic, M., and Whitehouse, M.W.: "Inflammation in Relation to Dietary Intake of Zinc and Copper." *International Journal of Tissue Reactions* 3: 75–76, 1981.

76. Denko, C.W., Petricevic, M., and Whitehouse, M.W.: "35S Incorporation in Rats in Relation to Deprivation of Copper and Zinc in the Diet." *International Journal of Tissue Reactions* 3: 121–125, 1981.

77. Orlowski, James P., Lonsdale, Derrick, and Denko, C.W.: "Beta-Endorphin Levels in Infant Apnea Syndrome: A Preliminary Communication." *Cleveland Clinic Quarterly* 49: 87–92, 1982.

78. Denko, C.W.: The Arthropathies, Clinical Condition, Chapter 1, Part i, Part ii, "The Role of Copper, Zinc, and Calcium in Their Etiology," in *Anti-Inflammatory Compounds,* W.R.N. Williamson (Ed.), Marcel Dekker, Inc., New York, NY, 1982 (for series "Drugs and the Pharmaceutical Sciences" by J. Swarbrick).

79. Denko, C.W., Aponte, J., Gabriel, P., and Petricevic, M.: "Serum Beta-Endorphins in Rheumatic Disorders." *Journal of Rheumatology* 9: 827–833, 1982.

80. Petricevic, M., Denko, C.W., Messineo, L.: "Age-Related Changes in Total DNA and RNA and Incorporation of Uridine and Thymidine in Rat Brain." *International Journal of Biochemistry* 15: 1103–1107, 1982.

81. Denko, C.W., and Gabriel, P.: "A New Delineation of the Congeries of Osteoarthritis." *Clinical Rheumatology* 2: 35–42, 1983.

82. Messineo, L., Denko, C.W., and Petricevic, M.: "Age-Related Changes in Total DNA and RNA and Incorporation of Uridine and Thymidine in Rat Liver, Kidney and Spleen." *International Journal of Biochemistry* 15: 1103–1107, 1983.

83. Denko, C.W., and Wanek, K.: "Anti-Inflammatory Action of Alpha-1-Acid-Glycoprotein in *Urate Crystal Inflammation." Agents and Actions* 15: 539–540, 1984.

84. Denko, C.W.: "Regeneration and Inflammation: Handbook of Inflammation," vol. 5, chapter 10. *Regeneration, Repair, and Their Control by Pharmacological Agents*, I.L. Bonta, M.A. Bray and M.J. Parhnam, eds., Elsevier Science Publishers, Amsterdam, 1985.

85. Denko, C.W.: "Cryoglobulin-Induced Inflammation." *Agents and Actions* 17: 92–96, 1985.

86. Denko, C.W., and Gabriel, P.: "Effects of Peptide Hormones in Urate Crystal Inflammation." *Journal of Rheumatology* 12: 971–977, 1985.

87. Denko, C.W., Aponte, J., Gabriel, P., and Petricevic, M.: "Beta-Endorphin, Immunological and Biochemical Changes in Synovial Fluid in Rheumatic Disorders." *Clinical Rheumatology* 5: 25–32, 1986.

88. Denko, C.W.: Chapter 1: "Rheumatic Disorders," pp. 1–22, in *Anti-Inflammatory Compounds,* W.R. Nigel Williamson (ed.), Marcel Dekker, New York, 1987.

89. Denko, C.W.: Chapter 50: "Mechanisms of Action of Neuropeptides: A Group of Naturally Occurring (Endogenous) Anti-Inflammatory Analgesic Compounds," pp. 449–450, in *Side Effects of Anti-Inflammatory Drugs, Part II, Studies in Major Organ Systems*, Rainsford, K.D., and Velo, G.P. (eds.) MTP Press Ltd, Boston, 1987.

90. Denko, C.W.: Chapter 2: "Osteoarthritis: A Metabolic Disorder," pp. 29–35, in *Developments in Antirheumatic Therapy,* Rainsford, K.D., and Velo, G.P. (eds.), *Inflammation and Drug Therapy* Series, vol. III, Kluwer Academic Publishers, Boston, 1989.

91. Denko, C.W.: Chapter 1: "Copper and Zinc in Inflammation," pp. 1–5, in *Copper and Zinc in Inflammation,* Milanino, R., Rainsford, K.D., and Velo, G.P. (eds.) *Inflammation and Drug Therapy* Series, vol. IV, Kluwer Academic Publishers, Boston, 1989.

92. Denko, C.W.: "Reply to letter from J. Dequekes, M. Coppen, P. Geusens." *Journal of Rheumatology* 18: 937, 1991.

93. Denko, C.W.: Chapter 9: "A Role for Neuropeptides in Inflammation," pp. 177–181, in *Biochemistry of Inflammation,* J. T. Whicher, S. W. Evans (eds.), *Immunology Medicine* Series, vol. 18, Kluwer Academic Publishers, Boston, 1992.

94. Denko, C.W.: Chapter 8: "Osteoarthritis," in *The Cambridge World History of Human Disease,* K.F. Kiple (ed.), Cambridge University Press, Cambridge, UK, 1993.

95. Yunus, M.B., Denko, C.W., and Masi, A.T.: "Serum Beta-Endorphin in Primary Fibromyalgia Syndrome: A Controlled Study." *J Rheumatol.* 1986 Feb; 13(1): 186–7. PMID: 2939238 [PubMed – indexed for MEDLINE]

96. Johnson, T.R., Blossey, B.K., Denko, C.W., and Ilan, J.: "Expression of insulin-like growth factor-1 in cultured rat hepatocytes: effects of insulin and growth hormone." *Mol Endocrinol.* 1989 Mar; 3(3): 580–7. PMID: 2664476 [PubMed – indexed for MEDLINE]

97. Moskowitz, R.W., Ziv, I., Denko, C.W., Boja, B., Jones, P.K., and Adler, J.H.: "Spondylosis in sand rats: a model of intervertebral disc degeneration and hyperostosis." *J Orthop Res.* 1990 May; 8(3): 401–11. PMID: 2182801 [PubMed – indexed for MEDLINE]

98. Denko, C.W., Boja, B., and Moskowitz, R.W.: "Growth promoting peptides in osteoarthritis: insulin, insulin-like growth factor-1, growth hormone". *J Rheumatol.* 1990 Sep; 17(9): 1217–21. PMID: 2290165 [PubMed – indexed for MEDLINE]

99. Moskowitz, R.W., Boja, B., and Denko, C.W.: "The role of growth factors in degenerative joint disorders". *J Rheumatol Suppl.* 1991 Feb; 27: 147-8. PMID: 2027117 [PubMed – indexed for MEDLINE]

100. Strohl, K.P., Boehm, K.D., Denko, C.W., Novak, R.D., and Decker, M.J.: "Biochemical morbidity in sleep apnea." *Ear, Nose and Throat J.* 1993 Jan; 72(1): 34, 39–41. Review. PMID: 8444124 [PubMed – indexed for MEDLINE]

101. Denko, C.W., and Boja, B.: Growth factors in asymptomatic osteoarthritis – insulin, insulin-like growth factor-1, growth hormone. *Inflammopharmacology.* 1993; 2: 71–76, (correspondence included).

102. Denko, C.W.: "Jack London. A modern analysis of his mysterious disease." *J Rheumatol.* 1993 Oct; 20(10): 1760–3. No abstract available. PMID: 8295191 [PubMed – indexed for MEDLINE]

103. Denko, C.W., Boja, B., and Moskowitz, R.W.: "Growth promoting peptides in osteoarthritis and diffuse idiopathic skeletal hyperostosis – insulin, insulin-like growth factor-1, growth hormone." *J Rheumatol* 1994 Sep; 21(9): 1725–30. PMID: 7799357 [PubMed – indexed for MEDLINE]

104. Strohl, K.P., Novak, R.D., Singer, W., Cahan, C., Boehm, K.D., Denko, C.W., and Hoffstem, V.S.: "Insulin levels, blood pressure and sleep apnea." *Sleep.* 1994 Oct; 17(7): 614–8. PMID: 7846459 [PubMed – indexed for MEDLINE]

105. Denko, C.W.: "Did the model for Polyphemus have acromegalic arthritis?" *J Rheumatol.* 1995 Nov; 22(11): 2191–2. No abstract available. PMID: 8596176 [PubMed – indexed for MEDLINE]

106. Denko, C.W., Boja, B., Moskowitz, R.W.: "Growth factors, insulin-like growth factor-1 and growth hormone, in synovial fluid and serum of patients with rheumatic disorders." *Osteoarthritis Cartilage.* 1996 Dec; 4(4): 245–9. PMID: 11048621 [PubMed – indexed for MEDLINE]

107. Denko, C.W., and Malemud, C.J.: "Metabolic disturbances and

synovial joint responses in osteoarthritis." *Front Biosci.* 1999 Oct 15; 4: D686-93. Review. PMID: 10525474 [PubMed – indexed for MEDLINE]

108. Denko, C.W., and Boja, B.: "Growth hormone, insulin, and insulin-like growth factor-1 in hypermobility syndrome." *J Rheumatol.* 2001 Jul; 28(7): 1666–9. PMID: 11469476 [PubMed – indexed for MEDLINE]

109. Denko, C.W., Boja, B., and Malemud, C.J.: "Growth hormone and insulin-like growth factor-1 in symptomatic and asymptomatic patients with diffuse idiopathic skeletal hyperostosis (DISH)." *Front Biosci.* 2002 Apr 1; 7: a37-43. PMID: 11897552 [PubMed – indexed for MEDLINE]

110. Denko, C.W., Boja, B., and Malemud, C.J.: "Intra-erythrocyte deposition of growth hormone in rheumatic diseases." *Rheumatol Int.* 2003 Jan; 23(1): 11-4. Epub 2002 Sep 11. PMID: 12548436 [PubMed – indexed for MEDLINE]

111. Denko, C.W., and Malemud, C.J.: "The serum growth hormone to somatostatin ratio is skewed upward in rheumatoid arthritis patients." *Front Biosci.* 2004 May 1; 9: 1660–4. PMID: 14977577 [PubMed – indexed for MEDLINE]

112. Denko, C.W., and Malemud, C.J.: "Age-related changes in serum growth hormone, insulin-like growth factor-1 and somatostatin in systemic lupus erythematosus." *BMC Musculoskelet Disord.* 2004 Oct 20; 5(1): 37. PMID: 15496230 [PubMed – indexed for MEDLINE]

113. Denko, C.W., and Malemud, C.J.: "Body mass index and blood glucose: correlations with serum insulin, growth hormone, and insulin-like growth factor-1 levels in patients with diffuse idiopathic skeletal hyperostosis (DISH)." *Rheumatol Int.* 2006 Feb; 26(4): 292–7. Epub 2005 Feb 10. PMID: 15703952 [PubMed – indexed for MEDLINE]

114. Denko, C.W., and Malemud, C.J.: "Serum growth hormone and insulin but not insulin-like growth factor-1 levels are elevated in patients with fibromyalgia syndrome." *Rheumatol Int.* 2005 Mar;

25(2): 146–51. Epub 2004 Jul 24. PMID: 15759159 [PubMed – indexed for MEDLINE]

115. Denko, C.W., and Malemud, C.J.: "Role of the growth hormone/ insulin-like growth factor-1 paracrine axis in rheumatic diseases." *Semin Arthritis Rheum.* 2005 Aug; 35(1): 24–34. Review. PMID: 16084221 [PubMed – indexed for MEDLINE]

116. Denko, C.W.: Chapter "Diseases Associated with Abnormalities of Structural Proteins"; segment "The Ehlers-Danlos Syndrome." In *The Heritable Diseases of Connective Tissue,* McKusick, Victor A.

Note

1. A.C. Ivy, a respected scientist who advised Chuck's group, in his later years became involved in promoting krebiozen, a cancer treatment made from horse serum in Mexico. Despairing patients with nowhere else to turn would try this. It generated a lawsuit, and krebiozen was found to contain only creatine. Chuck believed Ivy was innocent of fraudulent intent.

Permissions

Portraits of Charles W. Denko on the dust jacket and on page 140 used with permission of Bachrach Photographers, Holliston, Mass.

In chapter "Obituaries and Tributes":

Obituary, October 21, 2005: © 2005, *The Plain Dealer.* Used with permission of *The Plain Dealer.*

Article, "Studying a 1916 Death," July 19, 1992: © 1992, *The Plain Dealer.* Used with permission of *The Plain Dealer.*

Article, "Caring and Curing," February 28, 1988: © 1988, *The Plain Dealer.* Used with permission of *The Plain Dealer.*

Obituary of Dec. 2005 used with permission of the *Beaver Beacon.*

Memoriam in *T-Bones:* A newsletter from the Division of Rheumatology, Nov. 2005, used with permission of Case Western Reserve University School of Medicine.

"A Modern Analysis of His Mysterious Disease " used with permission of the *Journal of Rheumatology,* 1993; 20(11): 1760–63.

"Did the Model for Polyphemus Have Acromegalic Arthritis?" used with permission of the *Journal of Rheumatology,* 1995; 22(11): 2191–92.

Malemud, C. J.: "In Memoriam: Charles W. Denko, PhD, MD 1916–2005" used with permission of the *Journal of Rheumatology,* 2006; 33(9): 1866–1867.

Memoriam in *Gong & Gavel,* November 2005, used with permission of the Rocky River Kiwanis Club.

Article, "Gold for Arthritis," Dec. 5, 1943: © 1943 by *The New York Times.* Used with permission of *The New York Times.*

Article, "He reunited families in aftermath of war," June 23, 2000, written by Cynthia Dettelbach, editor: © 2000 by the *Cleveland Jewish News.* Used with permission of the *Cleveland Jewish News (www.cjn.org).*

Letter to the editor by Esther Gotjen, February 23, 1995, used with permission of the *Ellwood City Ledger*